How to Reverse and Prevent
Heart Disease and Cancer

Practical Tools based on
Breakthrough Research

Naras Bhat, MD, FACP

How to Reverse and Prevent
Heart Disease and Cancer

Published and marketed by Dr. Kumar Pati at **New Editions Publishing**
1675 Rollins Road, Suite B3, Burlingame, California 94010
Phone (415) 697-4400, Fax (415) 697-7937

Book Design by Dilip Gohil Designs, Pleasant Hill, California
Illustrations by Jay Mazhar, Hercules, California

Printed in the United States of America

Library of Congress Catalog Card Number: 95-069189

ISBN: 0-9624780-0-9

TABLE OF CONTENTS

For my wife, Kusum, and my children, Anita, Jyoti, and Joy –
who shared the vision and mission of this book

For my father – who reversed and healed his disease
using the principles given in this book.

For my mother – who inspired me
to learn about my ancient heritage.

For my patients – who decide to reset their heart.

Acknowledgments

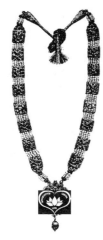

As a physician, I have used the drugs and procedures invented by various people in the world. I've learned how to prescribe them for my patients. In this book, the focus is not on pills, but on skills. I have carefully used my thread to make this book as a garland, selecting the best flowers from Eastern and Western sources. For some of the flowers, I have planted the seeds in our own garden and learned to grow it differently.

In the Reversing Heart Disease Model, Peter Nixon, MD, from London, England permitted us to use the European model, the human function curve. Two American cardiologists, Robert Eliot with his "hot reactor" concept, and Dean Ornish, with his reversing heart disease books and scientific papers have been very useful for my patients. Ramesh Kapadia, MD, from Ahmedabad, India shared his Indian version of Ornish's model. The hyperventilation model of Peter Nixon is further enriched by my biofeedback teachers, Erik Peper, PhD from Berkeley, California, and Robert Fried, PhD from New York. Enas Enas, MD, from Chicago, Illinois helped with the information on heart disease in Indians and Pill Power for the Heart. Diane Ulmer, RN, MS, the author of type A behavior concept, helped me to change my own type A traits, so that I can teach my patients by personal example.

In the cancer healing model, Carl Simonton, MD, and Bernie Siegel, MD, are to be mentioned. The personal teachings of these healers helped to reverse my father's disease. I am grateful to my father, who diligently practiced the healing methods given in this book, and proved their value to the extent that he joined some of my lecture tours as a proponent.

Michael Lerner, PhD, and Waz Thomas from the Commonweal in Bolinas, California have shared their model of a cancer help program with me and my staff.

In the caring love model, Rollin McCraty, PhD from HeartMath Institute, Boulder Creek, California has been very helpful in sharing their research. David J. Mischelevich, MD, of the Circadian Company from San Jose, California helped us with high tech computers for the Holter study of heart rate variability. Jerry Jampolsky, MD, from the Center for Attitudinal Healing in Sausalito, California spent memorable spans of time with me to clarify my model of forgiveness, love, and peace of mind.

In the meditation model, Acharya Govinda from Haridwar, India is responsible for teaching meditation to me and my family. Other significant inputs to our meditation model came from Swami Sachidananda of Yogaville in Buckingham, Virginia, and Rishi Prabhakar of Bangalore, India.

In the atomic model of free radicals and antioxidant counterattack, Kenneth Cooper, MD, from Cooper Aerobic Center in Dallas has been my inspirational source.

My friends Ram Rao, MD, and H.S. Ranganath, MD, have been a constant source of encouragement and positive feedback. Mala Seshagiri, RD, helped edit the chapter on *Mindful Eating*.

In preparation of this book, the staff at our Stress Cybernetix Institute has spent countless hours writing, rewriting, and editing. The team includes: Thomas Browne, PhD (neurotherapist, helped with the chapter on biofeedback); Kathleen Hickey, PhD (helped with conceptualization and editing); M.N. Rao, PhD (appendix on yoga); Matt Martello (computer work and editing); Gloria Passarella (biofeedback). This book is illustrated by the talents of our staff artist, Jay Mazhar. Editorial assistance came from Jyoti Bhat, Anita Bhat, Kusum

Bhat, Joy Bhat, Uma Iyer, Sanjay Adhia, Tania Kapoor, Anna Dabney and Robert Berman. Final production assistance came from Hal Shillito and Mary Lou Hulphers of The Write Graphics. This book was designed by Dilip Gohil of Dilip Gohil Designs, Pleasant Hill, California.

My family has sacrificed relentlessly for making this book a reality. When my mind was focused on the book, my family, pet, and plants experienced countless hours of lack of attention and care. I am indebted to them for their acceptance and tolerance.

Thousands of my patients and seminar attendees all over the world have given me the opportunity to test the tools given in this book. Their feedback has helped to make the tools sharp and user friendly.

SPECIAL NOTE TO READERS

If you have heart disease, cancer, or any other ailment, you should consult your personal physician for guidance in changing your treatment. This book is based on my experience with my patients. Each individual's medical condition is different, and this book is not a substitute for professional consultation.

Naras Bhat (MD)

Concord, California   *Naras Bhat, MD, FACP*

Introduction:

Why Read This Book?

LET'S PRETEND FOR A MOMENT...

Let's pretend the book you're holding is a magic lamp, and you've just rubbed it. The genie materializes and tells you he'll grant three wishes.

You're no fool, so you say, "OK, I'll take wealth, long life and happiness."

Well, the genie is no fool either. He answers, "I'm fresh out of 'wealth' today. But I can add years to your life; definitely improve your quality of life; and who knows, you could become more productive, so wealth might also follow."

Would you go for it? Of course you would.

NOW LET'S GET REAL.

The book is not a magic lamp; and I am no genie. I am a physician with MD, FACP after my name and a wall of medical diplomas, citations and licenses. The disciplines of modern medicine–scientific research and study–are at the very core of my practice.

Yet this book can become your magic lamp. It CAN add years to your life and enhance its quality–whether you are recovering from a heart attack or stroke; or have been recently diagnosed with cancer; or simply want to avoid those possibilities in the future.

Indeed, science-based proof you can improve and lengthen your life is what motivated me to write the book in the first place. In my studies, I found not just that heart disease and cancer are reversible or avoidable; but that the techniques involved are rooted in solid provable research.

WHAT THIS BOOK IS

Allow me one more analogy: That of a vehicle and the human body. This book is your body's "owner's manual," complete with a tool kit for reversing and preventing the two most likely things to go wrong with your body: heart disease and cancer.

Like any owner's manual you have to read it carefully. Allow yourself sufficient study time so you thoroughly understand it. If you wish to learn even more, you'll find a list of key references at the back that will further add to your understanding.

For reversal and prevention to succeed, you must practice with the tools and techniques I describe here. Each has been scientifically tested and verified (with computerized biofeedback monitoring systems) hundreds of times over. Your "tools" come out of stress control and heart disease reversal training developed in seminars, workshops and clinics worldwide. We know that, utilized properly, the tools work.

WHAT THE BOOK IS DESIGNED TO DO.

This book is designed to help you change the way you live your life. We call that "resetting the heart." Impossible? Well, not easy perhaps - few worthwhile things in life are. But it is not all that difficult either, and certainly not impossible - particularly when you keep in mind the alternative.

HOW THE BOOK IS ORGANIZED.

First, as part of the introduction, you'll find a "Picture Tour" – graphs and text that give you an overview of what goes on in the human body, and the tools for making changes. (pages 13–20.)

Second, also part of the introduction, are some Basic Questions (and answers) about Reversal of Disease: (pages 21–36.)

Chapters one, two and three look at the Resetting Approach.

Chapters 4 through 7 cover the first problem, the Biological War that rages inside us.

Chapters 8 through 12 examine the second problem, the War Victims: Stress and Reactivity.

With chapters 13 through 26, you'll find solutions to: 1) Anger Control; 2) Reactivity Control; and 3) Stress Control.

Chapters 27 and 28 give you your heart Resetting Tools; and show you how to use them and provide exercises that will make you an expert in their use.

Finally, we've included an Appendix dealing with a variety of health-related subjects from diet to humor to yoga.

Also, for your convenience, there is an expanded reading list, references, and, of course, an index.

HOW TO READ THIS BOOK

While the book goes from problems to solutions in a natural flow, you need not read it that way. Each chapter is complete, and most include a brief summary ("key points") at the end for easy review. Also, some material is repeated or rephrased. This is to help reinforce your grasp of certain basic principles and ideas we consider to be most important.

For quick results, we recommend you:

1. Browse through the Picture Tour and Basic Questions of Reversal.

2. Go directly to the Resetting Tools chapter, get oriented and start practicing one tool at a time.

3. Read each of the other chapters thoroughly to understand the dynamics of the resetting tools.

4. Use the Appendix for quick reference and "coffee table" discussions.

Here's to continued success in all your efforts to Reverse and Prevent Heart Disease and Cancer!

A Picture Tour

A Picture overview

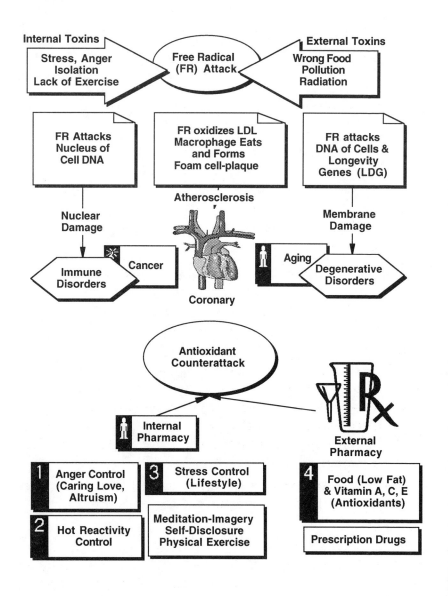

Here at the dawn of the 21st century, we still try to prove all our human experiences scientifically. It is what's given us such modern wonders as jet flight. Until 1903, we didn't know how birds fly. Then the Wright brothers built a model of the first airplane, and discovered that it could only fly if wings were proportionate to the body of the plane.

That same model works for jetliners today. But apply the jetliner wing/body proportion model to a bumblebee, and the bumblebee shouldn't be able to fly at all!

Science leaves part of nature unexplored. **Nature has something beyond models that cannot be *experimented* with, but rather *experienced*.** Yet, the jetliner model does work for human needs.

This book provides models within the border of the scientific horizon. **At the same time it gives you the perspective to experience things beyond that horizon.**

Let's start with the model at left. It shows what goes on constantly in all living humans. Here we demonstrate the principles of opposites in nature: attack and counterattack. **What you're looking at is literally atomic and chemical warfare!**

Attack

The "bad guys" - attackers - we call **free radicals.** They result from two toxin-producing sources. First, **internal:** your own mind–body. Stress, anger, isolation, and sedentary habits all produce toxins from within. Second, **external:** wrong foods and pollution create toxins from outside the body. They all fire up angry atoms, or **free radicals**.

The attacking villains wage war against your body. The front lines are the cell membrane and the cell nucleus.

Nuclear War

Free radicals attack the cell nucleus, causing denaturation of DNA, the master–code of life. This leads to a weak immune system, which in turn may cause allergies, infections, autoimmune disorders, or cancer.

Membrane War

The cell membrane gets oxidized and denatured as its frontiers crumble: skin wrinkles; arteries become coated or clogged (atherosclerosis, coronary artery disease); joints get inflamed (arthritis); glands weaken (diabetes); and vitality is reduced. These are all effects of angry atoms, our free radicals.

Counter Attack

Fortunately, we have two strategies to counter this chemical warfare. They lie in our internal and our external pharmacies. You'll learn how to deploy weapons in both.

Internal Pharmacy

1. **Anger Control:** Develop the "caring love reflex Heartfelt Resonant Imaging (HRI). This is altruism (thinking of others before yourself) to generate chemicals that help you heal and thrive.

2. **Hot Reactivity Control:** Measure, monitor, and modify the pumps and tubes of your mind–body, including heart rate, blood pressure, breathing patterns, restless mind, insomnia, bowel functions, and muscle tension.

3. **Stress Control By Life-style Changes**: Use meditation (imagery) to calm the restless mind. Or, self–disclosure to release emotional tension. Or physical exercise to dissipate pent up toxins and generate healing chemicals.

External Pharmacy

1. **Low Fat Diet**: Starch based, vegetarian diet, with fresh fruit and vegetable snacks eaten in six meals throughout the day. Also supplemental vitamins A (Beta–carotene), C, and E as antioxidants.

2. **Pill Power:** Traditional and alternative medicine. Take advantage of the prescription drugs that medical science has to offer you. Use your personal physician as your coach and guide.

PICTURE TOUR OF TOOLS:
MEASURING TOOLS
Human Function Curve

The Human Function Curve measures your life-style. Notice as your performance increases so does stress arousal. Up to a point, it is healthy tension. Then the down-slope sets in. Performance diminishes with increased tension The mind-body connection is upset. You become exhausted, your mind restless. You can't sleep. Relationships suffer, and you're more susceptible to illnesses such as heart disease. In this book, we repeatedly refer to this human function curve. Can you figure out where you are in the human function curve right now?

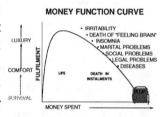

HUMAN FUNCTION CURVE

Money Function Curve

As you earn more money and spend more, life becomes complex and stressful. Once you have enough for survival, comfort, and minimal luxury, you start buying your own death in installments. You become irritable, the "feeling brain" atrophies. You experience insomnia, marital, social, and legal problems. Finally, you succumb to money stress and *"rest in peace"*. Can you locate yourself on the money function curve right now?

MONEY FUNCTION CURVE

Energy Exchange Cross Checks

Your energy efficiency is based on how you relate to yourself and others. On the vertical axis, you relate to your own mind–body and to your higher self. On the horizontal axis, you relate to your close family and society at large. How you

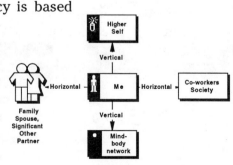

---

give or take energy from each source is based on how you relate to people, either with anger or caring love. Can you measure your energy quadrants right now and see how you are losing or gaining energy?

MONITORING TOOLS

CyberScan™

CyberScan™ is a simple method of **taking a picture of your behavior** repeatedly throughout the day. The procedure is like using a camera. First, you stabilize the camera. Second,

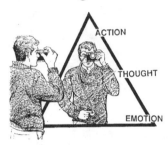

you focus on the object, and take a picture. You stabilize your mind by centering on your belly (belly button, actually). Second, focus on your actions (muscle emotions and relate each with another. You can do CyberScan™ while doing something else because the human mind is a parallel processor. At the end of the day, you review your multiple snapshots and figure out your dominant muscle contractions, thoughts, or behavior patterns. This gives your mind–body intelligence system the insight for self–regulation.

HRI (Heartfelt Resonant Imaging)

The HRI is just like CyberScan™, except you focus on the heart. The objective is to centralize your energy system in the area of your heart and resonate the state of caring love. First,

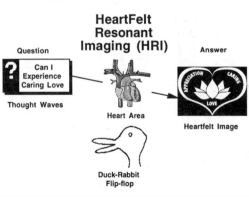

you focus your awareness on your anatomical heart. Second, you ask your heart, "Can I experience caring love towards a person, animal or an object?" Third, your heart always answers "yes," and at that moment you experience caring love. Contrast this state with your head-centered feelings when you are judgemental and not focused on your heart. You learn to flip–flop this heart–centered state with the head–centered state (the duck–rabbit flip–flop). Vertically, it is a rabbit, and horizontally it is a duck.

Energy Quadrants of Emotions

When you do your CyberScan™ or HRI, pay attention to how tense or relaxed you feel. You have basically four energy quadrants: high positive state of pleasure, love, and flow; low positive state of sleep, rest, and meditation; high negative state of fear and anger; and low negative state of guilt, sadness, and repression. The purpose of energy quadrants is to make you aware when you are in any of the quadrants so you can shift to the positive side, just like changing gears in a car.

Energy Quadrants of Emotions

High + Pleasure Love Flow	High - Fear Anger
Low + Sleep, Rest Meditation	Low - Guilt, Sadness Repression

Picture Guide to
Modifying Tools for Resetting the Heart

The modifier tools to reverse or reset your heart fall into two groups: Muscle–to–Mind or Mind–to–Muscle. Become familiar with the fact that there are two directions of nerve traffic: up-going traffic from muscle to mind and down-going traffic from mind to muscle. The tools intervene and reduce the traffic at either end. The principles of major tools are summarized on the next page.

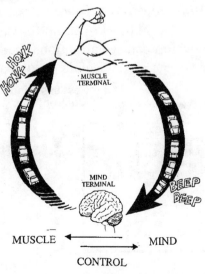

Muscle–to–Mind Tools

Muscle-to-mind tools stretch and reset your muscles to reduce traffic to the brain.

Heart centering by HRI is covered on the previous page.

Belly centering and mindful breathing means breathing with the diaphragm, so the belly bulges with each inspiration.

Resetting the mind's eye is moving the eyeballs deliberately to disconnect the eye–to–brain traffic congestion.

To reset the mind's voice, reduce the tension in voice and speech muscles.

Progressive relaxation contracts and relaxes the body's different muscle groups.

Yoga stretching lengthens the muscles and brings awareness to the body.

Physical exercise relaxes muscles cutting upward traffic.

Ultradian rhythms. Track the body's rest–activity cycle every 90 to 120 minutes at the onset of the daydream cycle.

Mindful eating refers to eating starch based, low fat, plant foods six times a day to keep your insulin and mood level even.

Mind–to–Muscle Tools

These tools open up the narrow focus of one's mind and develop passive attention. Your primary tools are meditation and imagery. A beginner's mind and thought watching helps in being non–judgemental. Self–disclosure of emotions and spirituality help to open the congestion in one's mind.

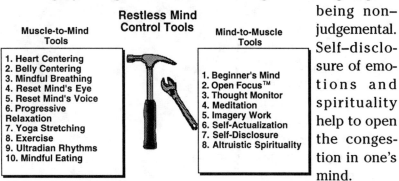

Restless Mind Control Tools

Muscle-to-Mind Tools	Mind-to-Muscle Tools
1. Heart Centering 2. Belly Centering 3. Mindful Breathing 4. Reset Mind's Eye 5. Reset Mind's Voice 6. Progressive Relaxation 7. Yoga Stretching 8. Exercise 9. Ultradian Rhythms 10. Mindful Eating	1. Beginner's Mind 2. Open Focus™ 3. Thought Monitor 4. Meditation 5. Imagery Work 6. Self-Actualization 7. Self-Disclosure 8. Altruistic Spirituality

Meditation Begins When Restless Mind Ends

Basic Questions
of Reversal

Basic Questions of Reversal

SOME QUESTIONS ANSWERED

When you think of reversing heart disease or preventing cancer, you have to answer some questions first:

- What is heart disease?
- What is cancer?
- What is common between heart disease and cancer?
- Why are they important to me?
- What is healing? How does it differ from treatment?
- What do reversal, regression, and reset mean?
- Why reset my heart?
- What is the proven scientific basis of reversal?
- What are the Ornish–Simonton Models?
- How can I do it?
- What is new and proven?
- How can this book help me?

What is Heart Disease?

The most common heart diseases in the civilized world today are coronary artery disease and high blood pressure. In the past rheumatic heart disease involving blockage or leak of heart valves, congenital heart defects, and infections of the heart were the common disorders.

But all heart conditions, if not reversed, turn into failure to pump–**heart failure;** sudden death of part of the heart muscle–**a heart attack**; or electrical irregularity, known as **cardiac arrythmia.**

We'll focus on coronary artery disease and hypertension, classic examples of heart disease. Coronary arteries bring nourishing blood chemicals and oxygen to the heart cells. When these pipes get clogged or kinked, what happens is a heart pain (**angina),** death of the heart muscle (**myocardial infarction**), or sudden death.

The basic abnormality in coronary artery disease is **atherosclerosis** (the Greek words *athere,* porridge, and *scleros* hardening, refer to the porridge–like cholesterol deposits on the inner lining of the coronary arteries). These deposits build up layer on layer, like plaque or tartar on teeth. Plaque makes the artery wall weak and vulnerable. As with a small break in a garden hose, it's the first place to rupture when you suddenly increase pressure.

Inflammation of Coronary Arteries: Coronary artery disease is an inflammation. In any inflammation, the immune system is part of the disease process. That system's cells and chemicals act as a "circulating brain."

Three basic elements produce the coronary artery events: blood cholesterol, damage to the artery wall, and acute inflammation (clotting disorder).

Cholesterol plays the villain–bad guy, and hero–good guy game. The bad guy, LDL (low density lipoprotein), takes over when the good guy, HDL (high density lipoprotein), weakens.

The artery wall gets damaged by the stress of the pressure inside the vessel and the chemical burn of inflammation. Inflammation comes from an acute anger atom carried out of the brain by messenger molecules of terrorists (activated monocytes and macrophages). These terrorists invade the frontier of the artery wall and release chemicals (protease enzymes), causing an acute burning.

As a result of the inflammatory invasion, tourist blood platelets are enraged, so they join with the terrorist macrophages and clump together in clots. The clots clog and block the artery.

Reversal here means reversing the anger atoms; rewriting messages; combating the terrorists, helping the hero to win over the villain; and counteracting the chemical warfare with helper chemicals.

What is Cancer?

Cancer is the uncontrolled, disorderly multiplying of abnormal cells, forming a new growth called a **neoplasm.** The new growth is either benign and localized in a capsule, or malignant and spreading all over the body.

The fundamental problem with cancer is that the innermost core of life (DNA in cells) operates outside the laws of nature. Cell growth can become erratic and uncontrolled like weeds in a garden. Normally, these weeds are contained by the immune system. But during cancer growth, the freedom fighter killers (NK cells) are ineffective. Here again, it's good guys vs. bad guys. Cancer cells are bad guys. NK cells are good guys. The immune system, like the department of defense tries to keep the terrorists out.

Cancer spreads (metastasizes), forming tumors that cause pain, obstruction and destruction of normal tissue. Organs fail, and death results. Reversing cancer is like suppressing weeds in a garden. **You prevent further growth and stop "weeds" from sprouting at the cellular level by changing of the messages to the unit of DNA.**

What do Heart Disease and Cancer have in common?

The common denominator in both are the terrorist molecules called **free radicals.** These molecules attack and damage normal tissues. In both cases, the attack has a past, a present, and a future. The past is whatever structural damage the disease produced, such as blockage of the coronary arteries or swelling by a tumor. The present is the active biological or chemical warfare going on in the tissue. The future is repairing war damage and preventing such warfare.

Research clearly shows that the cardiac events–anginal chest pain, heart attack, heart failure, sudden death–are not the result of past structural damage, but of the current chemical warfare. For example, you can reverse blocked arteries only by 2% with treatment. Yet you can still cut cardiac events by 91%. The same is true for cancer as well.

Iceberg of Degenerative Death

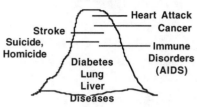

Why Are Heart Disease and Cancer Important?

They are the number one and number two causes of death, respectively. The number three cause of death is a stroke. These catastrophic illnesses are the tip of the iceberg of degenerative diseases. Accidents, suicide, immune disorders, lung diseases, diabetes, etc., make up the rest of the iceberg. **And underlying all these conditions is the disregulation of the mind–body information network.**

Cardiovascular diseases kill approximately one million Americans every year, accounting for 50% of all deaths. Cancer is responsible for 25% of all deaths. One American dies of a cardiovascular disease every 34 seconds. One in four Americans has some sort of heart disease. In America, every year, one and a half million heart attacks occur, 500,000 of the victims end up dying, and half do not even make it to the hospital. Approximately half a million strokes occur each year, and about sixty million people have hypertension. The United States has over 17,000 cardiologists and 1,200 coronary care units. In 1990, 285,000 angioplasties,

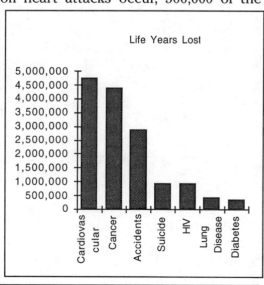

392,000 bypass surgeries, and 1,935 heart transplants were performed in the United States. About 40,000 Americans below the age of 65 need heart transplants and about half of that figure are below the age of 55. The last graph depicts the life years lost due to these diseases.

What is Healing and How does it Differ from Medical Treatment?

Modern medical science has conditioned us to think in terms of *treating* a disease. This book focuses on the *result* of treatment, or **healing.**

Treatment is the use of an outside agent, or an outside force: medication, surgery, radiation, physical therapy, or manipulation. The goal of treatment is to mechanically or chemically repair the symptom and signs of the disease.

Healing is the use of inner power or resources to balance and harmonize the mind–body by restoring its self–regulation and wholeness. The power of healing comes from our internal pharmacy, or internal resources. *The external drugs given by the doctor have to work through the internal pharmacy for healing to take place.*

Healing is bringing the body back to self–regulation using two components: **mindful monitoring** and **self–directed modification** of behavior. This is similar to diagnosis and therapy in medical treatment. Here you will learn how to measure, monitor, and modify self–regulation so that your mind–body can resume its original healing power. All self–directed changes in behavior come from moment–by–moment interventions and modifications. These interventions are the process called re-setting the heart. Read on.

What Does Reversal Mean?

Regression of a disease is changing the structural abnormality in an organ, for example, by recanalizing the arteries, or reducing the tumor size. **Reversal** *leads* to regression. It works in the same way adding a brick helps build, and removing a brick destroys a house in small increments.

The fundamental problem is a chemical war raging at the cellular level, with messages to the war front in the form of anger atoms being dispatched from the angry person's head.

You counter this by sending atoms of love from the heart—one brick at a time.

We use the term, "resetting the heart." Resetting is a moment by moment correction of something that is out of order. In a metaphorical way, it is **a heart transplant every moment**, replacing the old, habitual, hostile heart with a fresh, fragrant, and vibrant lotus of love.

Regression occurs over months and years. Reversal occurs over days and weeks. But it all happens moment by moment.

An easy way to understand the reversal process is by analogy.

The Last Straw on the Camel's Back

A camel's back will withstand a load increase up until the last straw. Likewise, if you have 90% blockage of the coronary arteries, you might think, "no matter what I do, I can't fix the blockage, so why bother?" **But, like a straw, each time you neglect the arteries, you get closer to "breaking the camel's back."**

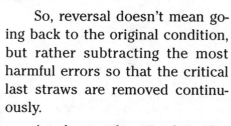

So, reversal doesn't mean going back to the original condition, but rather subtracting the most harmful errors so that the critical last straws are removed continuously.

Another analogy is that of a person moving towards a switch which will set off a time bomb. As long as you keep the person farther than an arm's length away from the switch, no havoc will take place. The reversal program works in the same way. You just keep away from the time bomb switch.

Reconstructing a Broken Egg

If you have a broken egg in your hand, how would you reconstruct it? Surgical procedures to open coronary arteries or remove tumors bring up the same question.

To prevent further breakage, you have to go after the forces that broke it in the first place, and then reverse these forces. This book can help you do just that.

Clogged Drain

If you have a clogged drain, of course you get a roto–rooter to unclog it. That is the role of angioplasty in surgery. You still have to prevent and reverse the cause of the clog, or else it will clog again. The chemical process that clogged the drain has to be reversed or removed.

Why Reset Your Heart?

The heart resetting program outlined in this book applies to everyone. You need not experience a heart attack to reset your life. You don't have to get ill to feel better.

Although, for some people, there has to be a crack to see the light. *For the wise it is observation; for the rest it has to be an experience.* **In the Chinese language, opportunity and crisis are depicted by the same symbol**. Catastrophic illnesses, such as a heart attack or cancer, can be a switch to reset the rest of your life.

This reset is not a philosophical, ethical, or moral statement, but a biological conditioning based on principles of animal and human learning. **The resetting process is a chemically mediated change in behavior.** It is replacing biological and chemical warfare with biological peace and chemicals of love and joy.

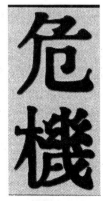

Chinese symbol for opportunity and crisis.

Dr. Robert Eliot, a professor of cardiology, was delivering a lecture on preventing heart attacks and he himself was struck with a heart attack. He writes in his book, *Is It Worth Dying For?*

"My own heart attack has caused me to worry less and less about hardening of arteries and disturbances of the heart rhythms—standard physical precursors of heart trouble— and more and more about stress. They say that insight often follows insult. Few bodily insults are as power-ful as a heart attack. Let yours—or the heart attack of someone close to you—open your eyes to the way you live with stress. If you've had the heart attack and been able to answer the question, Why now? Then you know how to answer the next big question: Why ever again?"

What is the Scientific Basis of Reversal?

Coronary artery disease reversal is scientifically proven to be possible by drug therapy, life-style modification, or a combination of the two.

Scientists first thought that the benefit of reversing heart disease was purely the mechanical widening of the arteries. Research done by Greg Brown from the University of Washington has shown that drug treatment reduced the blocking plaque by only 1%, **yet cardiac events such as angina, heart attack, and sudden death were reduced up to 73%.**

Dean Ornish's life-style modification without drugs reduced the plaque size by 2%, **but cardiac events reduced by 91%.** Blankenhorn's Cholesterol Lowering Atherosclerosis Study (CLAS) showed regression in both animals and humans. The St. Thomas Atherosclerosis study (START) showed 38% of people with a low fat diet had plaque regression compared to 4% in controls. In summary, more than 10 studies (CLAS I, CLAS II, FATS, MARS, STARS, PLAC I, PLAC II, POSH, NHLBI TYPE II, Life Heart Trial, etc.) involving more than 10,000 patients over 10 years follow up have conclusively demonstrated that **coronary artery disease can be reversed by the aggressive use of medication or by major life-style changes, or both.**

Dean Ornish's Lifestyle Study

Dean Ornish did two breakthrough studies focusing on lifestyle changes in four major areas: vegetarian low fat diet, moderate exercise, stress management (yoga, meditation, and imagery), and group support. His research was published in 1990, in the medical journal *Lancet*. An earlier study by Ornish was published in the *Journal of American Medical Association (JAMA)*, in 1983. This study showed that in 24 days of lifestyle changes, the treated group showed average changes as follows:

- 44% increase in exercise duration
- 55% increase in work capacity
- 6.4% more pumping power (ejection fraction) of heart
- 20.5% decrease in cholesterol level
- 91% decrease in anginal episodes.

In both of Ornish's studies, the following points are noteworthy:

1. The chest pain reduction was 91% on average, and occurred soon after (within a few days) joining the program.

2. The age of the patient or severity of the disease was not a deterrent for regression. Women responded more easily than did men.

3. There was a dose response curve. This means that the more of a lifestyle change, the more of a regression.

4. Reversal in blockage was prominent even if cholesterol drop was minimal.

5. Cardiac events, such as angina, arrythmia, and heart attack, reduced significantly even if the anatomical blockage was minimally improved.

6. Lifestyle changes produce noticeable results in as short as 24 days, even without drugs.

7. Lifestyle changes included diet, exercise, stress control, imagery, and group support.

Kapadia Model in India

Ramesh Kapadia, a practicing cardiologist at Ahmedabad, India, successfully duplicated the Dean Ornish Model. He has treated several hundred heart disease victims using the Dean Ornish protocol, and has confirmed the results by the reduction of cardiac events, echocardiography, cardiac stress testing, and biofeedback.

We will give you practical ways to measure, monitor, and modify your lifestyle based on this research, plus two additional tools of anger control and reactivity control of the heart.

Heart Disease Reversal Collaborative Network

As of 1995, thirty-one centers throughout the United States, Australia, and India do cardiac rehabilitation with the specific focus on lifestyle changes. All focus on lifestyle changes. In the past, cardiac rehabilitation was basically exercise oriented. Now this Heart Disease Reversal Collaborative Network is an umbrella association for exchange of information on heart disease reversal programs. Please refer to the appendix for names and addresses of different centers involved in heart disease reversal.

Simonton Cancer Research

Carl Simonton, a physician specializing in cancer therapy, and his former wife, Stephanie, a psychologist, developed breakthrough research in mind–body healing of cancer.

In a 1978 study, they took 159 patients with incurable cancer, whose life expectancy was less than 12 months (according to national cancer statistics). Conventional medical science had given up on them.

Simonton developed a treatment system by consulting the biofeedback leaders from the Menninger Clinic, especially Joe Kamiya and Elmer Green. The treatment consisted of mind–body self–regulation by healing imagery, meditation, biofeedback, group therapy, and active participation of the patient in the process of healing.

After four years, the results (As published in their book, *Getting Well Again*) were remarkable:

- No evidence of disease in 14 (22.2%)
- Tumor regression in 12 (19.1%)
- Disease stable in 17% (27.1%)
- Normal activity level in 51%
- Survival rate 40%
- Average survival rate doubled.

Bernie Siegel Approach

Bernie Siegel from Yale University followed the Simonton method and found that several of his "twelve months to live" patients were permanently cured of cancer, and he called these patients "Exceptional Cancer Patients (ECaP)."

Siegel developed new mind–body awareness in his ECaP patients by asking them the following five questions:

1. **Hope to live:** Do you want to live to be one hundred?

2. **Mind–body connection:** What happened to you a few months to a year before your illness?

3. **"Hidden motive":** What "benefit" did you derive from the illness? How did you disconnect yourself from the "meaning of life?"

4. **Helpless hopeless state:** What does the illness mean to you? How is it a give–up, given up state in your life?

5. **Symptoms and symbols:** Describe your disease in drawings, metaphors, and symbols.

Spiegel Study at Stanford

David Spiegel, a cancer specialist at Stanford University, studied terminal breast cancer patients and found that supportive expressive therapy of intimacy, caring love, and sharing the suffering doubled the longevity of cancer patients.

Mind–Body Healing of Cancer

The current scientific model of mind–body healing of cancer is shown here. Stress and anger release hormones, neurotransmitters, and immune transmitters to suppress immunity. In particular, suppressed NK cells allow cancer cells to grow.

Caring love, hope, meditation, and imagery release healing messenger molecules and the stronger immune system suppresses cancer growth. The body's normal cancer-suppressing internal pharmacy is closed by anger and stress. You can open it up with caring love, self–disclosure, and joy.

Mind-Body Healing of Cancer

Anger Stress Insomnia Drugs	Caring Love Hope Meditation Imagery
↓ Messenger Molecules	↓ Messenger Molecules
↓ Immune Suppression	↑ Strong Immunity
Cancer Growth	Cancer Suppressed

What is New?

The practice of medicine is both a science and an art. It is like using a camera. The latest computerized camera will not take a picture unless you focus the aperture on the right object and click. Our Resetting the Heart Program is the art of applying cutting-edge, information age science to the heart.

Body–Mind Medicine

Medical schools, as well as legal and insurance regulations, still regard the standard of medical care as treating the body as a "mindless machine." That means coronary artery disease treatment is like a plumbing repair of blocked pipes. Never mind that the patient is anxious or depressed. His mind is treated as "disembodied thoughts," with the help of tranquillizers and psychotherapy.

This old tradition in medical practice is called Cartesian duality, based on the 17th century physiologist from France, Réné Déscartes. Déscartescreated the mind–body split entirely for the sake of religious injunctions, so that the sacred body could be dissected in the laboratory without hurting the soul.

Mind–Body Medicine

In the 1980s and 90s, we have the New Age hype of Mind–Body Medicine. The mind has the key to open the internal pharmacy in your body to heal. **The mind and body are parts of the same information system.**

The mind–body hyphen is a bridge filled with messenger molecules called neurotransmitters, hormones, and immune transmitters. Besides the "liquid media" connection, the mind–body bridge is also directly connected by the "hard wire" of the nervous system and the "vibrational whisper" of one cell to another.

Psycho–Neuro–Immunology

The brain is connected to the immune system by the nerves, messenger molecules, and also direct vibration. **The cells of the immune system can be conditioned through training of the mind.** The immune system is the "circulating mind."

During the last decade we recognized psycho–neuro–immunology as the intelligence network of the mind–body. The mind or brain is believed to be the headquarters of this network. Types of brain waves mark the functional dynamics of this information system.

Cardio–Neuro–Immunology

Newer high tech methods of heart-wave analysis have shown that the heart has 40 to 60 times more powerful electromagnetic signals than the brain. The heart, like a large stone thrown into a lake makes big ripples. Comparatively, the brain is a small pebble making small ripples. This stronger heart ripple dominates the weaker ripple of waves from the brain.

This led to the new model called Cardio–neuro–immunology where the heart is the center of the information network. There is an information field around the heart termed the "heart intelligence" or **"intuitive field of the heart."**

Heart Rate Variability

The heart is its own generator of beats. The brain tries to dance to the beats of the heart. Sometimes the brain misses the steps and starts to dance to its own rhythm. This dissonance of beats is what we experience as conflicts in life.

When brain and heart resonate in sync, the two parts of your autonomic nervous system, the parasympathetic and sympathetic (the yin and yang), are in balance.

Heart rate variability is the most sensitive index of this balance, for two reasons: one; the heart is the strongest electrical generator in the body. Its beat-to-beat variation can be captured by the computer screen and studied in detail. Cardiologists use heart rate variability to predict sudden cardiac death in victims of heart attack.

Two; heart rate variability has corresponding changes in cellular DNA and in the immune system. Emotional control tools in this book use heart rate variability research. This is perhaps the high tech world's greatest gift to heart disease and cancer victims. But we can all benefit.

Resetting Cybernetics

Cybernetics refers to control by feedback communication. It's like a home heating system. The furnace works by the feedback of room temperature to a temperature gauge which turns the switch on or off. We use the principle of cybernetics to train our patients. We can sort out mindfelt and heartfelt feelings, as well as killer anger and caring love, by watching heart waves displayed on a computer. With training, one re-learns the harmony of the mind dancing with the heart.

Our Resetting the Heart Program tackles the subject from

microcosm to macrocosm. It traces the yin–yang balance from the atomic level of free radicals and antioxidants to molecular levels of endorphins and catecholamines, to tissue levels of blocking and unblocking. From mind levels of anger and caring love, to global levels of separation or union with the Universal Mind.

Three Arrows Aimed at the Target

Three different arrows target resetting the heart.

1. **Anger Control:** Anger is the killer. Heart disease and cancer are the results of its attack. We will focus on how to replace anger with caring love in a biological way. We verify our method by monitoring one's heart rate and blood chemicals in the research laboratory.

2. **Reactivity Control:** Every action has a reaction that often continues with a domino effect. The body's reacting systems are: the heart (heart rate and blood pressure); heart rate variability from beat to beat; breathing, restless mind and restless sleep; and the connection between gut feeling and feeling gut. You'll learn how to control each of these reactive patterns.

3. **Stress Control:** Stress control involves meditation and imagery (yogic disciplines adapted for today's world), self–disclosure of emotions, rest and activity, and mindful eating.

1

Crossroads:
Victim or Victor?

Some of us know that we have heart disease, cancer, or some other serious illness. Some do not know what we may have or when we may have it. The crossroads approach could apply to any one of us.

Crossroads–Victim or Victor?

A catastrophic illness, such as a heart attack or cancer, brings you to a crossroads in your life. The heart event or cancer is the tip of our degenerative disorder iceberg. We will focus on heart events, such as an angina, as the prototype of this iceberg.

Take a typical man having a heart attack or being diagnosed with a heart problem for the first time. He's now at a crossroads with two possible paths to follow:

#1. The helpless defeat path–where, as on a sinking ship, one can only rearrange the seating.

#2. **The cybernetic resetting of life patterns with a new heart.**

Helpless Defeat Path In A Sinking Ship

Modern science provides heroic interventions that are very good at repairing or replacing parts of the sinking ship. It even pumps out the water that got inside the ship until the last drop of the leak appears dry for a moment. But the hole in the bottom remains to allow water in. **This book will examine how to fix the hole in the ship.**

Changing Seats In a Sinking Ship

The traditional biomedical system provides the victim different alternates like drugs, surgery, and other therapies. All are just seating arrangements.

There are gadgets to measure, monitor, and modify the *body*. We do little to measure, monitor, and modify the *mind*. It's as though the body were a "mindless machine," the parts which need only be repaired or replaced–as in the case of organ transplants.

If the patient complains of stress, anxiety, and sleepless nights, the modern medical system gives you tranquilizers or sends you to a psychiatrist who will treat your mind as though its contents were just "disembodied thoughts." Heroic modern medicine is no doubt a scientific miracle, but still is unable to patch up the hole in the ship. **You must go after the forces that made the hole.**

"Why me?" Guilts

Surging guilt waves ruminate in the mind with questions of "Why me? Why now? What did I do wrong? What will happen to me?" This leads to stress arousal, thoracic breathing (hyperventilation), and disturbed sleep.

Fear of "What will happen to me?"

Fear and anxiety take the form of haunting thoughts like: Will I live? Will I love? Will I work? Will I play? When will the next attack be? This causes a restless mind, loss of energy, fatigue, and sleepless nights. **Sleep is a litmus test of health.** Sleep is a healer, and also a slayer.

Anger at "Difficult People"

The restless mind leads to cynical mistrust, anger, and aggression. It judges everybody as "difficult to get along with." There is a wise saying, "The definition of a difficult person is the other person." A heart victim treats visitors and well wishers with hidden cynicism–increasing isolation and loneliness. Anger kills in slow installments until the time bomb of a heart attack explodes. After the heart attack, the heat of anger and depression melts a person like fire melts ice. Denial covers up anger and frustration.

Depression and Exhaustion

Misplaced efforts, lack of restful sleep, loneliness, isolation, and the feeling of a loss of control all lead to depression which ends up as defeat, despair, hopelessness, and helplessness. This is the result of the loss of control and the loss of vital energy. The underlying devastating forces are the **lack of both caring love and altruism in life**. Collectively, all these changes are known as **the lack of meaning in life.**

Grabbing Straws while Sinking

The down-slope for a heart victim is graphically described by British cardiologist, Peter Nixon, in his Human Function Curve. The curve is an inverted U. Heart attacks occur on the curve's down-slope when the body's reserves are dried up under the heat of anger and stress.

As the down-slope of human function continues, victims grab straws in sheer desperation. Yet the "sinking ship" process continues. Breathing becomes more thoracic (hyperventilation). Sleep is increasingly non-restful. Physical and mental exhaustion set in. Hostility, depression, and learned helplessness drive the victim into seclusion and isolation.

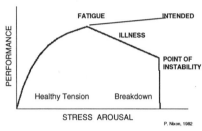

HUMAN FUNCTION CURVE

Cybernetic Reset Buttons

The other pathway that we offer applies cybernetic reset buttons. There are three distinct approaches:

1. **Anger Control** and resolving mental conflicts. This automatically rekindles the biology of altruism.

2. **Reactivity Control** of tense muscles of the body and restless mind control.

3. **Stress Control** through four proven lifestyle changes: meditation and imagery, self-disclosure, physical exercise, and a low fat diet with antioxidant vitamin supplements. The coronary artery disease reversal program of Dean Ornish and the cancer healing program of Carl Simonton, two scientifically validated approaches, use these lifestyle changes.

But the most important reset buttons to press immediately for a new life pattern are the first two: heartfelt feelings leading to altruistic egotism and reactivity control.

Heartfelt Resonant Imaging (HRI)

Have you ever stopped to think what the opposite of love is? It's not only anger and hatred, but also simple apathy. This is because people forget how to experience and express caring love. We'll train you to use caring love as a tool.

Your heart only knows how to care and love. Your brain may rationalize and hate. But all you have to do to find your heartfelt feelings is just close your eyes, focus on the area of your heart, and ask your heart what your heartfelt feelings are. Your *heart* will always say it loves the person. Resonating these *heartfelt* feelings with the brain heals you.

Heartfelt feelings are non-judgmental with an approach of mindfulness and a beginner's mind. On the other hand, mindfelt feelings are conditioned by analytical, rational thinking and are usually judged by the hidden agenda of "what's in it for me?"

BIOLOGICAL ALTRUISTIC EGOTISM

Hans Selye, the father of Stress Medicine, coined the term altruistic egotism in his book, *Stress Without Distress*. Egotism is self-centeredness. Altruism is "other centeredness." **Altruism means that you are also included in my agenda.** The word altruistic egotism is not an oxymoron, but rather a paradox. A paradox is something that is amazing but true. To quote Selye, altruistic egotism is not "love thy neighbor as thyself" (for that is impossible), but to "*earn* thy neighbor's love." In Sanskrit this attitude is called *seva*, (*sa* = the other person, *eva* = included). This means to include the other person in your personal agenda.

There are thousands of medical articles to show that altruism heals the heart and prevents further heart attacks. But what is altruism? Many heart attack victims create an artificial "schedule" of altruistic behavior by feeding the homeless or volunteering in church over the weekend after a week of hostility at work or at home. We define altruism in the

---

chemical and biological sense. Altruism is a return to being a *human being* by release of endorphins and serotonin in the brain. This is the biological resetting of human beings–not by taking external drugs, but by calling on one's internal pharmacy.

A moment of Heartfelt Resonant Imaging creates a state of endorphin release in the brain because you are experiencing caring love. This endorphin state links your contact to other people with a sense of altruism. This conditioning is like having a product advertisement flashed at you after a romantic scene. You enjoy the product because of its association with love.

It is also like the famous Pavlov dogs. When Pavlov rang a bell just before feeding his test dogs, they soon associated the bell with eating and would salivate. Finally, just the bell ringing made them salivate whether there was food or not.

We were all capable of loving anyone and everyone as a child. With the Heartfelt Resonant Imaging technique, you rediscover love for the second time in your life.

Larry Sherwitz from the University of San Francisco has shown that the more a person uses personal pronouns, such as I, me, myself, and mine, the greater his risk of heart problems. With biological altruism, you replace the "I-ness" with "You-ness" and "What Can I do for You?" You can train yourself in this the same way Pavlov trained his dogs.

Reactivity Control

Reactivity of the heart is the marker of reactivity of the rest of the mind-body. Every moment of your behavior is a reaction to the external and internal environment. Reactivity in your mind-body is manifested in the pumps and pipes of your body.

Pumps: Heart, lungs, urinary bladder, gall bladder, and muscles of the body.

Pipes: Blood vessels, tubes of gut, urinary system, and the reproductive system.

The most important aspects of reactivity to be monitored in order of importance are:

1. **Heart:** Heart rate variability and pulse pressure.

2. **Lungs:** Hyperventilation or over breathing.

3. **Brain Arteries:** Insomnia at night and a restless mind during the day.

4. **Gut Tubes:** Constipation, irritable bowels.

5. **Muscle Tensions:** TMJ (temporomandibular joint) disorder, shoulder pain, back pain.

In our clinic, we retain reactivity of the heart by biofeed-back-monitoring of heart rate variability, and beat-by-beat change of blood pressure. Reduced and erratic heart rate variability is a sign of a "brittle" heart and we know scientifically an ominous premonition of sudden death.

Anger makes the heart rate variability erratic. Caring love makes it smooth and regular. This laboratory research was used to designed the Heartfelt Resonant Imaging (HRI) tool to control anger.

Hot Reactors are people who react with increased heart rate and blood pressure to stress arousal. Robert Eliot, a cardiologist who researches hot reactors, has a laboratory test for measuring heart rate and blood pressure in response to mental stress or physical stress. In a doctor's office, hot reactors are diagnosed by 24-hour Holter monitoring of the heart and 24-hour ambulatory blood pressure monitoring. The newer Holter monitors measure heart rate variability over 24 hours.

Diaphragmatic Breathing

Hyperventilation is measured in a doctor's office by a machine called a capnometer. You can pay attention to your own breathing and catch yourself breathing thoracically by observing more of chest movement as opposed to abdominal movement. Thoracic breathing typically causes pain in the shoulders and between the shoulders due to the use of accessory muscles in breathing.

You reset your breathing reactivity by learning diaphragmatic breathing. That is, breathing abdominally, through your belly.

Diaphragmatic breathing helps in several ways. First, it is an excellent centering tool. Second, prolonged expiration switches to a parasympathetic mode of healing. Third, it conserves the buffer, and reduces stress arousal and insomnia. It mobilizes the energy center in the navel called the jewel *chakra* (*manipura* chakra) and equalizes the mind with the heart.

We teach diaphragmatic breathing in two different ways. First is the two hands method with or without computer monitoring. Put your hand on your belly and make sure that it is going up and down while inhaling and exhaling. Also, you determine whether you are breathing diaphragmatically or not. The second way is to reset your heart by HRI. Resetting your heart commands the brain to reset the breathing pattern.

Restless Brain

A restless brain is the result of poor oxygen supply and chemical changes in the brain in response to stress-causing hyperventilation. A restless brain leads to a restless mind during the day and insomnia at night. Restless sleep at night prevents healing and makes you ill, in addition to setting you up for a heart attack or cancer.

We will address the specific aspects of controlling insomnia at night and a restless mind during the day. Meditation and imagery, diaphragmatic breathing, progressive muscle relaxation, and eyeball desensitization are some of the methods used to control a restless brain.

Irritable Gut

Irritable gut is due to the calcium, potassium, and magnesium changes in the gut muscles in response to stress and over breathing. Observing the gut function and monitoring the connection between "gut feeling" and "feeling gut" is an important aspect of reactivity control.

Muscle Tension

The most common muscle to tense up is the jaw muscle due to the "biting instinct" or "death grip." This clenching leads to TMJ (temporomandibular disorders). Back pain, shoulder pain, fibromyalgia, and chronic fatigue are some of the other manifestations of muscle reactivity.

DEAN ORNISH–CARL SIMONTON LIFESTYLE CHANGES (STRESS CONTROL)

The four lifestyle changes–meditation and imagery, self-disclosure, physical exercise, and a diet with vitamins–are the four basic components of stress control. Dean Ornish's reversing heart disease program and Carl Simonton's cancer healing program focus on these four factors.

Meditation and Imagery

Meditation and imagery go hand in hand. When you meditate, you alter your state of mind. This new state of mind is conducive for imagery. This book shows you the meditation methods we use in our heart clinic. **Our meditation method can be used in one minute or five minute segments of time, eliminating the most common excuse, "I don't have enough time to meditate."**

The heart disease victim constantly ruminates on past problems or future doom. When you catch yourself doing this, immediately get centered and breathe out three times diaphragmatically. Then, focus on the heart area and create healing images. We train people to use healing imageries every time something negative happens. In our clinic, we train people to meditate using biofeedback monitoring of their brain waves.

Self-Disclosure

You learn self-disclosure of emotions in two steps: self-actualization of your own mind-body dynamics, and sharing this information with someone else.

Self-actualization gives you insight into how you are different from others in six different respects: perceptual types, mindfelt and heartfelt feeling levels, physiological signature levels, gender differences, money style, and explanatory style. In self-disclosure, you share self-actualized feelings with someone in a "three-T" session: time, touch, and talk. The feelings and perceptions of an individual dovetail with another's to develop empathy and intimacy.

Physical Exercise

You have to balance rest and activity to keep the mind-body tuned. Sleep is a healer as well as a slayer. This means that if you get enough rest, then sleep is a healer. But if you sleep too much and don't get enough exercise, or you can't get enough sleep because of insomnia, sleep is a slayer.

Diet and Vitamin Supplements

The goal of any diet is directed at degeneration or regeneration of the mind-body. The healing diet is a low fat, high fiber, vegetarian diet with antioxidant supplements.

MEASUREMENT IS SCIENCE

We use the human function curve to measure stress and performance. This curve is a graphic visualization of your own mind-body's reactivity response to chemical changes in your body. Your goal is to learn the different stress reactions and observe the reactivity of the pumps and pipes in your body. On the up-slope is health, with effort and performance proportionate to each other. Markers of the up-slope are healthy fatigue with recovery and restful sleep. Breathing is calm and diaphragmatic most of the time. Gut functions are regular, and muscle tension is minimal.

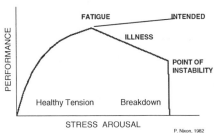

HUMAN FUNCTION CURVE

FATIGUE · INTENDED

ILLNESS

POINT OF INSTABILITY

PERFORMANCE

Healthy Tension · Breakdown

STRESS AROUSAL

P. Nixon, 1982

Life is pleasurable and experienced as a balanced "flow." On the down-slope, anger, irritability, and insomnia occur. The heart beats faster, blood pressure rises, you over breathe with your lungs, the gut becomes irritable, and your muscles tense up.

Our approach teaches you how to measure your recovery using the human function curve.

Crossroads of a Heart Event

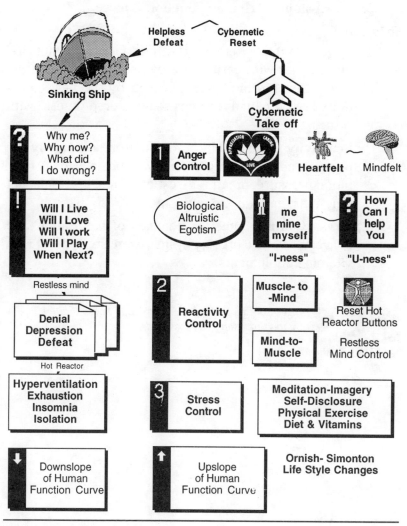

CROSSROADS OF HEART EVENT SUMMARY

Problem

1. **Illness:** Helpless Defeat.

2. **Guilt and Fear:** Why me? What will happen now?

3. **Restless Mind:** Denial, Depression, Defeat.

4. **Hot Reactivity:** Hyperventilation, Exhaustion, Insomnia, Isolation.

5. **Down-slope of Human Function Curve.**

Solution

1. **Anger Control:** Remove the heart-brain conflict. Replace anger with caring love by heartfelt resonant imaging. Develop biological altruism by the new conditioned reflex which replaces self-centered "I-ness" with "U-ness."

2. **Reactivity Control:** Measure, monitor, and modify the pumps and pipes of your body, especially heat rate, blood pressure, breathing, restless mind, insomnia, gut functions, and muscle tension.

3. **Stress Control:** Lifestyle changes of meditation and imagery, self-disclosure, physical exercise, and diet with vitamin supplements.

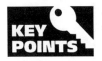

Anger Control, Reactivity Control, and Stress Control are the three steps of Crossroads.

2
Learned Helplessness

Learned Helplessness

You can understand what happens in coronary artery disease or cancer by looking at the model of learned helplessness and learned optimism. This model is based on sound scientific studies done on animals and human beings, mostly by Seligman at the University of Pennsylvania.

People with a positive attitude have an optimistic explanatory style in life. People who are usually negative have a pessimistic explanatory style of life. At times of setback, illness, loss or an error, the pessimist and optimist lifestyles will differ in three distinct aspects: **permanence, pervasiveness,** and **personalization**.

Permanence is the belief that the setback will be forever. Pervasiveness is the belief that the setback will occur again and again for the rest of the person's life in an all-encompassing way. Personalization is attributing the failure to personal inadequacy.

Optimism: The optimist thinks that setback or failure is temporary and there is a specific reason for it. He thinks that the fault is not entirely his own, and he will take the challenge to recover and learn from the incident.

Pessimism: The pessimist assumes a permanent and universal cause for his setback. He thinks he can never recover, and he will fail in all of his endeavors. He attributes the cause for the setback to his personal failure.

Hope: is defined as perceiving and explaining the setback as temporary and specific to that particular situation.

Hopelessness: is perceiving and explaining the setback as permanent and all pervasive.

Learning: is a change in behavior by experience. When a pessimist tries something and fails and when the experience is repeated, he stops trying altogether. This is called **learned helplessness** because he resolves that no matter how much he tries, he cannot succeed.

The most self-defeating aspect of learned helplessness is when you conclude this state of failure is permanent and pervasive, and not just limited to the specific area where you failed.

Rats and Electric Shock

Researcher Madeline Visintainer, a student of Seligman, divided rats into three groups. The first group was given electric shock from which an escape was possible by pressing a lever. The rats mastered a way to escape. The second group was given mild 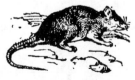 electric shocks from which they had no way to escape. The rats became helpless. The third group received no shock at all. Tumor cells were injected to each group. Normally 50% of rats would die of a tumor in about a month. Of the mastery group, 70% rejected the tumor, proving strong immune systems. Of the helpless group, only 27% rejected the tumor, proving weakened immune systems. In the non-shocked group, 50% rejected the tumor. However, the helpless group lost interest in all activities, playing and eating, indicating a generalization or pervasiveness of their helpless state. The self-efficacy group showed interest in all activities, play, and eating. A similar experiment was done on pigeons, and these birds would not fly away from electric shock.

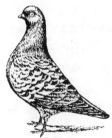

The Helpless Dogs

In another experiment, dogs were confined to a cage and exposed to inescapable electric shock. After several such exposures, the dogs learned to behave in a helpless manner, and they learned to accept the shock. Even if the barricade was removed, the dogs wouldn't run away. The dogs' immune systems were suppressed. Now, if a person dragged the dogs 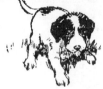 away from the shock several times, the dogs would relearn how to escape.

Battered Women's Syndrome

A woman who is being battered gets into a trap of learned helplessness, just like rats, pigeons, and dogs. She thinks that the situation is permanent, pervasive, and personal. Like the pigeons, rats, and dogs, she doesn't try to escape. Rather, she learns to accept her situation.

Nursing Home Residents

Langer and Rodin of Yale University studied nursing home residents. First floor residents were given the choice to select the breakfast menu, the type of movies to watch, and the freedom to water plants. Second floor residents were given a fixed menu for breakfast, predetermined movies, and plants with no opportunity to participate in watering them. The researchers evaluated the results after eighteen months. The first floor people thrived, and were happy. The second floor residents became helpless and unhappy. They died faster than the first floor people.

EVERYDAY EXAMPLES OF LEARNED HELPLESSNESS

Learned helplessness occurs in our daily life. The basic problem is that one major or several minor setbacks in life lead to a vicious cycle of frustration and the inability to escape. An easy analogy is of a river rapid dragging you into a whirlpool, and no matter how a good a swimmer you are, you cannot escape. Common examples are chronic insomnia, test anxiety, and athletic "choking."

Chronic Insomnia

In chronic insomnia, one major, or several minor stress episodes cause hyperventilation during the day and waking up at night due to lack of body buffers. The insomnia then feeds itself to create a more restless mind, reactive chemistry, and an altered immune system. One loses a sense of control and feels helpless.

Test Anxiety

A student taking examinations offers another example of learned helplessness. First, the student performs poorly in one or more subjects. Then, he or she generalizes the problem into every subject and every situation. The student thinks that because he/she didn't do well in a few subjects that he/she does not have the "brains" to do well in other subjects.

The student gets into the pervasiveness, permanence, and personalization trap. To escape, you get involved in something that you are able to do comfortably with challenge and commitment. For example, if you are weak in geography, do something you are good at, like mathematics or sports. The successful performance in mathematics or athletics will rejuvenate your immune system and you will be back on the road with your original vigor.

Athletic Choking

Athletic choking happens when self-centered criticism and stress arousal leaves you feeling unable to improve performance. Again, the solution is to switch to something you can do better. If, for instance, you are stuck with helplessness in tennis, try swimming or golf for a few days to recover your immune system from the whirlpool effect.

New Biology of Helplessness

Extensive research into the biological effects of helplessness in animals and humans leads us to the following conclusions.

1. The helpless state leads to immune suppression (depressed T-cell and the NK cell activity and decreased immune globins), which may lead to infections, and cancer. The helpless state releases cortisol and testosterone-like hormones, increasing atherosclerosis and coronary artery disease.

2. Helpless people resolve that "nothing I do matters, so I shouldn't do anything," leading to unhealthy behavior.

3. Helpless people's explanatory style is negative, so they experience more "catastrophic" events in their life and thereby increase the vicious cycle of helplessness.

4. Helpless people stay away from others because their ability to love is dampened. They don't have the capacity for pleasure.

5. It is possible to turn the pessimist around by "retraining" one's explanatory style and engaging in tasks where the experience of success in increments will pull one out of the helpless state and into self-efficacy.

6. Learned helplessness and depression merge into each other.

7. There is a tug of war between your mindfelt feelings of helplessness and heartfelt feelings of love. Caring love remains suppressed, which makes you more helpless biologically and socially.

One fascinating aspect of the helpless state is that you can come out of it by doing any activity that you are able to do with commitment, challenge, skill, and control. For example, if you have a setback in college due to test anxiety and learned helplessness, you can take up tennis and build your self-worth. Your intelligent immune system will sense it and you can come out of your test anxiety.

In the next section, you'll learn how to make optimism and success replace pessimism.

LEARNED HELPLESSNESS

1. **Setback in life** (rapids leading to a whirlpool) such as a heart attack, a loss of a loved one, or major errors in finance are causes.

2. **Whirlpool effect**, inability to escape, and the loss of control. Losing a sense of effectiveness leads to distorted thinking patterns with feelings of permanence, pervasiveness, and personalization.

---

3. **Pervasiveness becomes a chain-reaction.**

   (a) Helpless thoughts lead to feelings of hopelessness, depression, and despair. This leads to isolation and withdrawal from society.

   (b) The immune system gets depressed with poor T-cell and NK cell activity, leading to frequent infections, susceptibility to cancer, and autoimmune diseases.

   (c) A tug of war between heartfelt and mindfelt feelings occurs. The mind constantly judges and seeks perfection. This is a set up for heart problems or illnesses.

4. **Feelings of total ineffectiveness** occur with anxiety, fear, and distress. Along with it comes a lack of pleasure, loss of a sense of humor, a meaning in life, of control in everything, and most importantly, the inability to experience and express caring love towards people.

Learned helplessness is a biological state of chemical reactivity and immune system suppression. This state can be changed by engaging in any *activity that consistently builds the sense of self -worth.*

Learned Helplessness

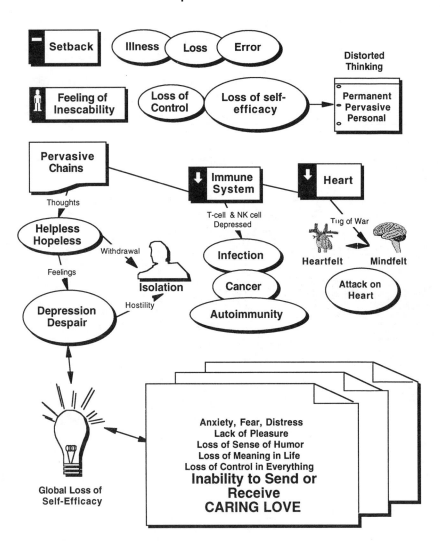

3

Learned Optimism–
Self–Efficacy

Learned Optimism

Learned helplessness often comes after a series of setbacks or one major setback, like a heart attack or cancer.

Learning to become an optimist is the same as learning to regain control in life. A sense of control increases connectedness to people in a meaningful way.

Cancer patients and heart attack victims go through three phases of recovery: control, connectedness, and *meaning* in life. Learning control and self reliance is a behavioral change. This follows four basic requirements.

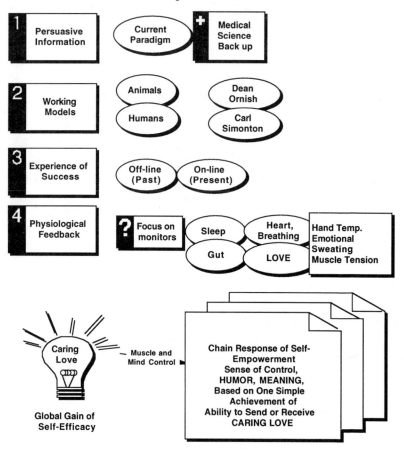

1. PERSUASIVE INFORMATION

We are rational thinkers. Today, health–related information has to be scientifically proven and backed up by medical research. It should also be consistent with current examples. We know cell injury by free radicals causes all diseases. Any behavioral change should have the ability to stop this damage.

Another example is Kyzen, the Japanese management system of a total quality–control. It's based on process control and the moment of truth. Process control pays attention to the process rather than the outcome. The moment of truth pays attention to every moment in a dynamic way.

Our cybernetic approach of stress control focuses on the present moment to rebuild self–worth. Cybernetics is control by feedback of information.

2. WORKING MODELS

Our studies of helplessness and loss of control tell us that learned optimism is practical and efficient. We are also guided by Dean Ornish's reversing coronary artery disease and Carl Simonton's cancer healing in designing our cybernetic resetting of heart attacks and cancer. These two models of healing are scientifically proven to reverse heart disease and even cancer.

3. EXPERIENCE OF SUCCESS

Humans trust their own past successes to form their belief systems. Yet they need on–line immediate feedback of present success. The human brain has a control center called the limbic system. This center learns to move towards a behavior by anticipating pleasure, and moves away by anticipating fear or anxiety. The experiencing of success is essential to maintain this feedback system. Our tools show you how to measure, monitor, and modify your experience, on–line at the moment, and off–line later.

---

4. PHYSIOLOGICAL FEEDBACK

We verify the beneficial results of our cybernetic tools by focusing on one or more physiological sensors. In our laboratory, we use biofeedback monitors to show people the change in heart rate, breathing, hand temperature, emotional sweating, carbon dioxide level in expired air, and muscle tension. You can monitor your physiological changes in the "pumps and pipes of the body," e.g. quality of sleep, gastrointestinal functions, muscle tension, symptom reduction of various illnesses, and, most importantly, your ability to love and connect to other people.

Remember, the helpless state is a psycho–neuro–immune condition in which your immune system learns to give in and give up. You can turn this system around by doing anything that gives you a sense of commitment, challenge, and control.

We found in our laboratory research the easiest way to escape learned helplessness is to learn the control of your own physiology by using a biofeedback monitor. This is done by watching the computer monitor. You see your physiological changes. It becomes a fun game rather than a threatening challenge. The feelings you experience resets the immune system and reduces the whirlpool effect.

Even without biofeedback, you can learn the skill of Heartfelt Resonant Imaging in a day and start using it. The method of HRI and anger control is simple to learn, and within a week of consistently practicing it, you can escape the helpless state. The altruistic biological state gives a boost to your immune system and you feel better overall.

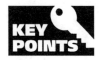

The key point of learned optimism is to engage in some skill–building task that gives immediate feedback of the success so that the suppressed immune system can wake up. The best way to do this is to learn a way of monitored self–regulation, with or without biofeedback, yoga, meditation, or imagery.

4
Common War Front–
Radical Attack

Common War Front– Radical Attack

Bad News

Scientists have figured out that every disease in your body is due to an atomic war by villains called **free radicals.** It is estimated that one free electron radical can knock out 30,000 other electrons before it stops.

Good News

Scientists have also found the counterattack heroes, **antioxidants**. These heroes can be fostered inside your body or they can be taken in as food and vitamins.

The smallest building block of the human body is an atom. Health and illnesses are based on the structures and functions of these atoms. Your organs, like the brain, heart, muscle, etc., are made of tissues or groups of cells. The cells have a central nucleus or control center, and an outer membrane or cell wall.

The cells are made up of molecules which are made of atoms. Modern science has found diseases at the atomic level . A constant attack goes on in your body by terrorist "bad guy" atoms (free radicals) on normal atoms. This attack can be rescued by the freedom fighter "good guy" atoms (antioxidants).

Injured Tiger

Scientists have concluded there is a single cause for aging, heart disease, atherosclerosis, strokes, arthritis, allergy, and immune disorders. The villain is oxygen, the same element that makes fuel burn, oil turn rancid, paint dry up, and iron rust. It is not oxygen in its native form, but in a ferocious form called a **free radical**.

A free radical is not a living organism like a virus or bacteria. It is an atom. The problem with free radicals is that they contain injured oxygen atoms. These oxygen atoms have unpaired electrons. They are like an injured tiger launching a frenzy of attack.

Free radicals are electrically and chemically unstable. **They are "biochemical bad guys."** They have an unpaired electron, which makes them "ferocious," attacking normal cells and damaging proteins, fats, DNA (the genetic master code), and RNA (the messenger of cells).

The concept of free radicals is schematically depicted. At

Schematic Model of Free Radicals

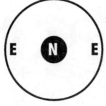 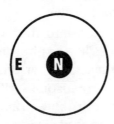

**Paired Electrons
Normal Atom**

**Unaired Electron
Free Radical**

the center of each atom in your body is the nucleus (N), made of protons and neutrons. The electrons (E) are paired and balanced in a normal cell. This is the *yin–yang* balance of nature at the atomic level. When one of these electrons (E) falls out of orbit around the nucleus, the other becomes lonely, unstable, and wild, attacking normal cells. The chemical warfare by free radicals can be summarized as **membrane or nuclear wars.**

Membrane Wars

Free radicals react by attacking normal fatty cell membranes and producing *lipid peroxidase enzymes (LP)* which damage the cell. Free radicals attack unsaturated fat in the cell membrane and create LP's. These LP's damage the inner lining of blood vessels by oxidizing the LDL (bad cholesterol) and inhibiting the protective enzyme, *Prostacycline synthetase*. This damage is manifested as arteriosclerosis (hardening of arteries), diabetes, cataracts, arthritis, premature aging, and coronary artery disease. The tissue damage done by free radicals is similar to the browning of a freshly cut apple or the rusting of metal. The damage to the membrane manifests itself as degenerative diseases such as:

- Diabetes
- Cataracts
- Arthritis
- Wrinkled Skin
- Premature Aging
- Coronary Artery Disease
- Strokes
- Peripheral Artery Disease
- Inflammatory Bowel Disease

Free radicals shoot deep into the nucleus of a cell and destroy the DNA. DNA looks like a spiral staircase made of two parallel ropes that wind on each other. Stored inside the staircase chain are 23 pairs of chromosomes with more than 100,000 genes. These genes carry the "blue prints" of information to make other cells of the same kind. Each cell in the human body is challenged on an average by 1,000 to 10,000 attacks on its DNA every day. Fortunately, a repair enzyme called *DNA polymerase* continually repairs the damage. The immune system keeps a "surveillance" on this action. When cells are not copied exactly like the parent cell, the immune system senses this and destroys the imposter cells.

Genetic experts estimate that each DNA molecule contains the equivalent of 500,000 pages of typed information. Can you think of a system that records information trillions of times a day with hardly any errors? Our biological computers correct the errors, if any, immediately.

Occasionally, the correction system fails, and one such error will lead to cancer. Scientists estimate that everyone gets cancer six times in his or her lifetime. It is the efficiency of the immune system that keeps the cancer checked. **The entire process starts at the level of atoms as a free radical attacking the DNA of the cell.**

WHAT INCREASES THE FREE RADICALS?

Excessive free radicals are produced in the human body by two factors: internal chemical toxins from lifestyle factors and external chemical toxins from environmental pollution, food, and drugs.

Internal Toxins

The internal chemistry of your body is changed by emotions and physical exercise.

Lifestyle Factors: Emotional stress, fear, anger, guilt, and sadness release stress chemicals into your body, which alter its metabolism and release increased numbers of free radicals. Exercise is a double edged sword – too little or too much (overtraining) exercise increases the number of free radicals in your body.

External Toxins

Environmental Factors: Nuclear radiation, x–rays, pesticides, insecticides, cigarette smoke, sun exposure, exhaust fumes, ozone depletion, and other chemicals increase free radicals in your body.

Food Factors: High fat foods lure free radicals into your body. Animal products that contain a lot of heme–type iron, certain food preservatives, chemicals, and drugs also contribute. High oxidant foods like animal products, especially red meat, welcome free radicals. Recent research shows that people who eat animal products have a high heme–iron level in their blood, which increases the risk of coronary artery disease.

WHAT DECREASES THE FREE RADICALS?

There are two ways to reduce free radicals: through your internal pharmacy and external pharmacy.

Internal Pharmacy

There are protective mechanisms in the body against free radicals. Among them, a naturally occurring enzyme called *super oxide dismutase (SOD)*, *catalase*, and *glutathione peroxidase (GSH)*. These enzymes neutralize free radicals and prevent the formation of LP's which damage the cell wall. Each individual enzyme produces a different level of this internal pharmaceutical, depending on heredity and lifestyle.

Positive emotions like love, peace, and joy increase these enzymes' activities, and reduce free radicals. Social connectedness, self–disclosure of emotions, and caring love increase antioxidant enzymes, enhancing the immune system.

Relaxation and Diaphragmatic Breathing: A relaxation response is opposed to a stress response. It eliminates free radicals. Specifically, diaphragmatic breathing clears the blood of toxins like free radicals. Meditation is also a good antidote.

External Pharmacy

Scavengers: Natural foods **(fruits and vegetables)** without preservatives and with high levels of vitamins are the best insurance against free radicals. Three vitamins are particularly effective scavengers: vitamin A, C, and E. Remember them by the mnemonic, **ACE.** They engulf free radicals. Bioflavonoids (pigments in fruits and vegetables), coenzyme Q10, zinc, and selenium also facilitate the scavenger action against free radicals. They're in fresh fruits and vegetables. Cooking, heating, canning, and preserving destroy the enzymes.

Antioxidant Theory:

New antioxidant theory states that *the free radical's missing electron is replenished by antioxidants.* If an antioxidant does not "help," a free radical takes an electron from vital cell structures, damaging the cell and eventually leading to diseases.

WHY TAKE VITAMIN SUPPLEMENTS?

The "apple a day" principle is not enough to keep you healthy. Up until the 1980s, vitamins were not recommended if you ate a balanced diet. Vitamins were used for prevention of deficiency diseases like scurvy, beriberi, and rickets.

In the 1990s, the evidence for antioxidant supplements is overwhelming. *The National Institute of Health*, *The American Journal of Cardiology*, and *The New England Journal of Medicine* have all endorsed antioxidant supplements for people who eat a "normal American diet." **Only 9% of Americans get the recommended antioxidants in five servings of fresh fruits and vegetables per day.** Birth control pills and certain drugs increase the need for certain vitamins. Even if food requirements are met, the remaining factors of air pollution and stress arousal require much more free radical removal for the immune system to prevent heart disease, cancer, cataracts, premature aging, and Alzheimer's disease.

The following studies are well-documented support for vitamin supplements.

Beta Carotene (Provitamin-A)

A Harvard Physician study showed a 44% reduction in heart attacks and a 49% reduction in strokes for the groups given 50,000 units of beta carotene every other day. In a study of 87,245 nurses over 8 years, there was a 40% reduction in stroke risk and a 22% reduction in heart attacks in those who took beta carotene. Beta carotene decreases the incidence of stomach, cervical, and lung cancer.

Vitamin C

In a California study, a vitamin C intake of greater than 300 mg per day showed men having a 42% less mortality rate and women a 10% less mortality rate as compared to those with a low vitamin C intake. High vitamin A and C reduced the occurrence of cataracts by 39% in a study of 50,000 nurses.

Vitamin E

A vitamin E intake greater than 100 IU per day reduced heart attacks by 46% in women and 26% in men in a large study of 130,000 nurses. Several large scale epidemiological studies in the U.S. and Europe proved people with low vitamin E level in their blood have the highest incidence of heart disease. The amount of damage caused by a heart attack in rabbits can be reduced by vitamin E.

Coenzyme Q10

Coenzyme Q10 improves energy utilization of the heart and helps improve cardiomyopathy and congestive heart failure. It decreases blood pressure and enhances the immune system.

Mineral supplements:

Multivitamin/multimineral preparations with zinc reduced infection–related sick days in the elderly by 50%. Magnesium reduces the incidence of death from heart attack and arrhythmia; helps prevent coronary spasms, and lowers blood pressure. Boron and calcium lend musculoskeletal support.

Reasons for supplemental vitamins summarized:

1 Western food habit: **Less than 9% of people living in the western hemisphere have a balanced diet with at least five servings of fruits and vegetables a day.**

2. Processed food: **Processed food is stripped of natural enzymes and vitamins.**

3. Environmental pollution: **Depleted soils, water supplies contaminated with heavy metals and toxins, and air polluted with chemical toxins and radiation.**

4. Stress Chemicals: **External toxins add to a stressful lifestyle. The result is an overwhelming release of toxic stress chemicals in the body.**

Practical Tips

The damage caused by free radicals can be minimized by increasing antioxidant heroes and decreasing the free radical villains.

Benefits of Counter Attack on Free Radicals:

1. Protection from heart disease

Antioxidants prevent or reverse heart disease regardless of changes in the cholesterol level, because the oxidative process of LDL cholesterol is reversed.

2. Protection from cancer

3. Prevention of cataracts
4. Delay of premature aging
5. Stronger immune system
6. Protection from Parkinson's disease
7. Clearing of inflammations such as arthritis

ANTIOXIDANT ACTION PLAN

A. YOU CAN ACTIVATE THE INTERNAL PHARMACY BY:

1. **Stress control:** Focus on diaphragmatic breathing, meditation, and restful sleep.

2. **Conflict resolution and caring love:** Control anger and learn to remove the conflict between your head and heart. Disclose your feelings to someone and increase your social connectedness. In summary, learn the skill of biologically entering into the chemical state of altruism.

3. **Doing moderate physical exercise:** During exercise, maintain a level of less than 80% of your maximum heart rate in order to achieve aerobic fitness. Walking, swimming, bicycling, tennis, etc. are good exercises. Overtraining and exertion above 80% of maximum heart rate increases the free radical count in your body. Ideally, you should exercise in the target heart rate zone for 30 continuous minutes three times a week or twenty continuous minutes four times a week. The target heart rate is calculated by the following: Your maximum heart rate is 220 minus your age. Sixty–five to 80% of this number is your target training zone. Another simple rule of thumb is, if you can maintain a comfortable conversation during exercise, you are in the target zone.

B. TAKE ADVANTAGE OF THE EXTERNAL PHARMACY

1. **Learn to cook and eat the antioxidant way.** Fresh fruits and vegetables are the best sources of antioxidants. A lot of exposure to harmful oxygen, heat, and light reduces the antioxidant power of fruits and vegetables. Fresh vegetables should be stored in the vegetable crisper section of your refrigerator. Reheating cooked vegetables reduces their antioxidant levels.

Microwaving, steaming, or stir–frying your vegetables is better than deep frying, boiling, or simmering them.

A simple approach is to try eating fresh vegetables and fruits with each meal. Eat six times a day. Eat at least one serving of fresh fruit and vegetable with breakfast, lunch, and dinner. Additionally, eat a mid–morning, mid–afternoon, and a bedtime snack of fresh fruits and vegetables. This six–times–a–day meal plan maintains your insulin level and mood balance, and further reduces the free radicals in your body.

FOOD SOURCES OF ANTIOXIDANTS

Vitamin A (as Beta Carotene)

Vitamin A occurs as beta carotene in yellow and dark green vegetables, such as carrots, pumpkins, sweet potatoes, collards, yellow corn, kale, spinach, turnip greens, tomatoes, broccoli and squash, to mention a few. Beta carotene is also present in many types of fruits – cantaloupe, mangoes, papaya, and apricots are a few examples. Fully formed vitamin A is found in animal products, such as liver, butter, and eggs, but this form of beta carotene is more harmful than helpful to your body. The recommended daily dose ranges from 10,000 to 50,000 IU.

Vitamin C (Ascorbic Acid)

Vitamin C occurs in all citrus fruits: oranges, tangerines, grapefruits, etc. Other sources are broccoli, cauliflower, brussels sprouts, strawberries, cantaloupe, and kiwi. The recommended daily dose ranges from 500 to 3000 mg, depending on gender, age, and activity level.

Vitamin E (d–alphatocopherol)

New research has shown that natural vitamin E is preferred over synthetic sources. Natural vitamin E is extracted from vegetable oils such as soy. Look for the label d–alpha tocopherol. This label indicates that it is a natural source. If there is a "dl" prefix to alpha tocopherol or alphatocopheryl, it indicates a synthetic source.

The Cooper Clinic experts recommend natural vitamin E in your diet. Food sources of vitamin E are wheat germ, almonds, hazelnuts, mayonnaise, corn oil, cottonseed oil, and sunflower seed oil. Egg yolk and butter contain vitamin E, but these food sources are not recommended because of their high fat content. The recommended daily dose ranges from 200 to 1,200 IU, depending on gender, age, and activity level.

We recommend the following antioxidant inventory:

List favorite antioxidant fruits and vegetables for each family member and take turns surprising each other with a gift of their favorite snack during the day.

2. **Take antioxidant supplements.** The daily recommended antioxidant supplement for preventing deficiency diseases is much higher than the RDA (Recommended Daily Allowance) of vitamins. The least one can do is take 10 times the RDA of vitamin A, C, and E. The prescription for antioxidant supplements is based on three variables: gender, age, and degree of physical and mental stress.

3. **Minimize exposure to air pollutants.** Avoid radiation, direct sunlight, ultraviolet rays, and smoke. Alcoholic beverages should also be avoided.

"Bank Balance" of Antioxidants

Free radicals are like withdrawals from a bank account. Antioxidants are like deposits into the account. Each credit or debit can be accounted for, moment by moment, in minutes, hours, or days.

Credit: Caring love, joy, peace, meditation, diaphragmatic breathing, moderate exercise, good sleep, eating fresh fruits and vegetables, and taking vitamin A, C, E supplements are all credits to your antioxidant account.

Debit: Anger, frustration, stress arousal, thoracic breathing, overexertion, insomnia, red meat (and other animal products with toxins), high fat diet, and exposure to environmental pollution are debits from your antioxidant account.

Basic Rules of Antioxidant Intake

1. Pay attention to the gender, age, and physical activity variables of your antioxidant recommendation. Men need more vitamin C than women. Increased physical activity and overexertion, as well as obesity, require a higher dose of antioxidants.

2. Take your vitamins with meals for better absorption, and preferably three times a day for constant blood levels.

3. Use natural vitamin A/beta carotene and natural vitamin E/d–alphatocopherol/d–alphatocopheryl.

4. Pay attention to expiration dates. Expired vitamins may not only be less effective, but could be toxic.

5. Learn the difference of units. Vitamin C is usually in milligrams, vitamin A and E are in International Units (IU).

6. Eat at least six servings of fruits and vegetables per day, even if you are taking antioxidant vitamins. Science may discover new vitamins, but you can't go wrong by eating mother nature's package of plant foods.

Rx   Anti-oxidant
Vitamins- Daily

Age (yrs.)	Sex	5-12	12-50	50 Plus	Overexertion Weight >200lbs
Vitamin A (Beta carotene)	M	10,000 IU	25,000 IU	50,000 IU	50,000 IU
	F	10,000 IU	25,000 IU	50,000 IU	50,000 IU
Vitamin C	M	500 mg	1500 mg	2000mg	3000mg
	F	500 mg	1000 mg	1000 mg	2000mg
Vitamin E	M	200 IU	400 IU	600 IU	1200 IU
	F	200 IU	400 IU	600 IU	1200 IU

1. Free radicals are produced by external toxins such as pollution and the wrong food and internal toxins of life-style, particularly anger and stress arousal.

2. The antidote to free radicals is antioxidants.

3. Antioxidants are increased by external pharmacy of the right food (fresh fruits and vegetables), and vitamins, A (Beta-carotene), C, and E, and internal pharmacy such as caring love, stress control, meditation and imagery.

5
Membrane War– Heart Disease

Membrane War – Heart Disease

Coronary artery disease is the most serious, and it can take different forms:

1. **Sudden Death:** According to the American Heart Association, about 250,000 sudden cardiac deaths occur in the United States every year. Most occur in the morning, especially on Monday, as job stress begins after a weekend break.

Usually there are warnings. But not always. It occurs in known heart patients and patients with high blood pressure. It can happen to those without known coronary artery disease.

Research has shown two types: The first is death of heart muscle by blockage from a sudden kinking spasm or clogging by a clot. The spasm or clogging cuts off blood supply and oxygen to the heart muscle. It becomes irritable and sends out an electrical storm of irregular heart beats.

Sudden Cardiac Death

Coronary Artery Blockage by Spasm or Clot

Rupture of Heart Muscle by Adrenaline Toxicity

Oxygen Deprivation

"Chemical Burn"

Coagulation Necrosis

Contraction Band Lesions

Electrical Storm

Ventricular Fibrillation

Clotting is somewhat different, but the results are the same.

The second kind of heart attack involves stressful contraction rupture of heart muscles - not kinking or clogging of the arteries. Acute stress reaction releases massive amounts of adrenaline and noradrenaline. Heart muscles contract so severely, they rupture. The rupture breaks the electrical continuity of heart impulse and leads to the same electrical storm or Ventricular Fibrillation (see graph). In one study by Giorgio Barolli of Milan, about 86% of all sudden cardiac deaths were due to such ruptures. Heart researcher Robert Eliot looked at NASA space scientists who, between 28 and 35 years of age, had suffered sudden cardiac death. He found all were under high stress from job uncertainty and overwork.

---

2. **Congestive Heart Failure:** Congestive heart failure is a condition that occurs because the heart muscle is unable to pump blood due to damage or overwork. The failing heart is unable to circulate the blood which the body needs. As the blood flowing out of the heart slows down, the blood returning to the heart gets congested. Excess fluid leaks from veins into tissues causing swelling in the legs and abdomen, swelling of the lungs with shortness of breath and inability to lie down flat. The effort tolerance is limited and the person feels quickly fatigued. Coronary artery disease is the most common cause of congestive heart failure. Death of the heart muscle leads to scarring, and weak muscles make the heart dilate. The pumping power of the heart muscle is reduced.

3. **Cardiac Arrhythmia (Irregular Beats):** The heart has its own pacemaker generating an orderly rhythm. The heart beat has to be conducted along the conducting tissues. Lack of blood supply and oxygen to these tissues leads to electrical aberrations called arrhythmia. Some of the irregular beats are benign and harmless, while others are hazardous and may cause dizziness, fainting and even sudden death.

4. **Angina:** When the heart muscle does not get enough blood supply or oxygen, it cries in pain. This is called angina. Angina occurs when the heart muscle's demand for oxygen exceeds the supply. The need for oxygen is increased in situations of physical exertion, mental stress (particularly anger and frustration), exposure to cold temperature, and after a large fatty meal.

Angina has several forms. Often it is experienced as a dull, heavy pressure in the center of the chest. The pain has typical radiation to the neck, jaw, left shoulder or left arm. Shortness of breath, sweating, weakness, faintness or light–headedness may occur. Angina is often triggered by exercise and excitement, and relieved by rest.

5. **Variant Angina (Prinzmetals angina):** Angina occurs due to spasms of the coronary artery by emotional stress

(especially anger), and this often occurs at rest rather than with exertion. This type of angina has a strong component of hyperventilation or over breathing, which alters the acid–base balance and chemical equilibrium of the blood and leads to cardiac arrhythmia. It is possible to have a coronary spasm, heart attack, or even sudden death with perfectly normal coronary arteries. It is estimated that as high as 15–30% of heart attacks may be due to coronary artery spasms.

6. **Unstable Angina:** As the name indicates, unstable angina refers to pain provoked by a lower level of exercise, pain at rest, pain of different duration and failure to obtain relief from nitroglycerin type of coronary dilators. This type of unstable state may lead to a heart attack or myocardial infarction.

7. **Silent Ischemia:** Not all people with myocardial ischemia or lack of blood supply to the heart experience pain. This condition is diagnosed by abnormal electrocardiograms (EKG) or Holter monitoring.

8. **Heart Attack:** The heart muscle responds to a lack of blood supply by angina, silent ischemia, or sudden death of a muscle called myocardial infarction or heart attack. Most heart attacks are painful, some may be silent. Heart attacks occur due to a rupture of atherosclerotic plaques or formation of thrombus (clot). The consequences of heart attacks are based on how many cells die and in which location the damage occurs. **Heart attacks are usually manifested by chest pain, radiating pain, sweating, nausea, and shortness of breath.** Heart attacks kill at least 300,000 Americans every year, before they reach the hospital. One in ten hospitalized heart attack victims die within three days. The overall mortality rate of a heart attack victim is 30%, and 20% will suffer another heart attack within four years.

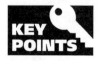

1. Coronary artery disease (CAD) is due to cell membrane damage by free radicals and deposit of oxidized LDL cholesterol.

2. CAD manifests as chest pain, irregular heart beats, pump failure of the heart, heart attack or even as sudden death.

Heart Disease and Cancer

6
Nuclear War–Cancer

Nuclear War–Cancer

Cancer is a typical example of biochemical warfare affecting the cell nucleus. The word cancer refers to more than 200 diseases that originate in any cell or organ in the body. All cancers have one thing in common: they produce abnormal cells capable of irregular, uncontrolled growth and which invade normal tissues. The message for this abnormal cell growth is carried in the DNA part of the cell nucleus.

What is DNA?

Each cell has a central station called the nucleus. The crucial part of this nucleus is DNA. DNA stands for deoxyribo-

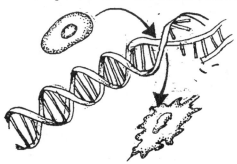

Change in DNA programming and cancer.

nucleic acid, found in the nuclei of all cells. Each DNA molecule carries information that could be typed on 500,000 pages of manuscript. It is the blueprint to build new cells and tissues. Steven Spielberg's movie, *Jurassic Park*, suggests a dinosaur could be developed from a DNA message. The same DNA, when attacked by free radicals, loses the original architecture of cells, and can grow into cancer.

Programming of DNA

Humans have about 100,000 genes. All genes are not inherited destiny. About one-third of them are "housekeeping genes" that change their mood according to your own habits and emotions.

The new science of psycho-neuro-immunology deals with the mind-body connection. The links between mind and body are called messenger molecules. These messenger molecules can bring good or bad news from one part of your body to another. This news can help or damage the DNA. Anger and frustration disturb the DNA structure. Caring love winds the DNA back into its natural state.

When a normal cell's DNA is damaged, the genetic master code changes into a cancer code called an oncogene. The carcinogenic (cancer producing) factors of chemical toxins, diet, stress, and lack of exercise increase the free radicals which attack the cell's nucleus and change the genetic master code. The cancer process goes through the following stages:

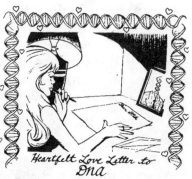

Heartfelt Love Letter to DNA

When you are in a state of caring love, you send a love letter to your DNA.

1. Carcinogen factors turn on the oncogene.

2. The precancerous cell now multiplies rapidly.

3. The precancerous cell turns into multiple cancer cells.

4. The cell's DNA programming is permanently altered and a tumor growth occurs.

5. Cancer spreads through bodily fluids, such as blood and lymph, or by direct invasion of neighboring tissues.

The tumor presses on the tissues and causes pain, obstruction, or destruction of otherwise normal tissues. Eventually, the nutrition and metabolism of normal tissue is affected, leading to infection, hemorrhage, or failure of these tissues.

Cancer leads to abnormal chemistry of the body, including change in pH or acid base balance; promotion of cancer growth but not normal cell growth; suppression of the immune system; elevated metabolism; chemicals causing apathy and depression; and grabbing of nutrients from the blood.

How and When Do You Know of Cancer in You?

A tumor has to be the size of a pea for it to show up in an x-ray or a physical examination by the doctor or you. By then, it has existed for quite some time, possibly years. Cancer starts as one abnormal cell dividing into two, into four, eight, sixteen, thirty-two and so on. It may take one to ten years for this duplication to become a tumor with thousands of cells and large enough to be detected. This duplication is normally suppressed by the body's immune system. If that is weakened, cancer growth continues, uncontrolled.

Some of the myths of cancer: cancer is invincible; it is always incurable; a cancer patient is out of control of his or her own illness; and a cancer patient has always had a physical or mental trauma before the event.

The fact is that cancer is a disorder of the immune system. It is precipitated and aggravated by any insult to the immune system, including anger and stress. Cancer patients enter into a state of learned helplessness. Research by Simonton and Siegel has shown that mind-body healing methods such as meditation, imagery, and nutritional therapy are very effective in cancer healing.

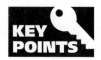

1. Cancer is due to nuclear damage of a cell by free radical attack denaturing the structure of DNA.
2. New research has shown that the programming of housekeeping genes can be changed by changing mind-body communication.

Heart Disease and Cancer

7

Risk and Disease

Risks of Coronary Artery Disease

More than 500,000 people die of coronary artery disease every year in the United States. What makes you prone to develop coronary artery disease depends on risk factors. There are two kinds of risk factors: uncontrollable and controllable. These are shown in the picture below.

Uncontrollable factors are age, gender, heredity, race, ethnicity and previous heart attacks. The controllable risks are stress (type A behavior and hot reactors), social isolation, a sedentary lifestyle, smoking, cholesterol, hypertension, obesity, diabetes, hyperinsulinism, *yin–yang* imbalance and the 21st century lifestyle.

Coronary Risks

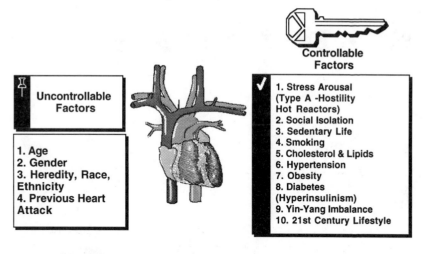

Controllable Factors

Uncontrollable Factors

1. Age
2. Gender
3. Heredity, Race, Ethnicity
4. Previous Heart Attack

1. Stress Arousal (Type A -Hostility Hot Reactors)
2. Social Isolation
3. Sedentary Life
4. Smoking
5. Cholesterol & Lipids
6. Hypertension
7. Obesity
8. Diabetes (Hyperinsulinism)
9. Yin-Yang Imbalance
10. 21st Century Lifestyle

UNCONTROLLABLE RISK FACTORS

Age and Gender

The process of aging increases the risk of heart disease. For men above age 45 and for women above age 55, the risk of heart disease increases progessively. Four out of five heart attacks happen to people above age 65. The female hormone, estrogen, increases the good cholesterol, HDL, and decreases the bad cholesterol, LDL. After menopause, the risk for women is the same as it is for men.

Family History (Heredity)

If you have an immediate relative with coronary artery disease, you have a 25% higher risk of getting it. There is a tendency for diseases that contribute to heart disease to run in the family: high blood pressure, diabetes, and obesity.

In Asian Indians, additional factors of inheritance are added risks: high Lp (a), hyperinsulinism, apple type obesity, and low HDL cholesterol with high triglyceride level. If you have a history in your family of branches falling due to heart attacks, prune some of the controllable risk factors.

Previous Heart Attack(s)

If you have already had a heart attack, the emotional turmoil that it has caused becomes another factor that increases the risk. Negative emotions, such as denial, defeat, and depression, make the situation worse. In our Resetting the Heart program, we see a heart attack as an opportunity to change your lifestyle.

CONTROLLABLE RISK FACTORS

Stress and Hostility

The most important controllable risk factors are hostility and stress. Let's look at how they affect three types of personalities: types A, B, and C.

Type B is assertive and balanced. Type C is passive and suppresses emotions. Type A is aggressive and anger–prone.

Type A behavior has three parts: hurry sickness, excessive competitiveness, and hostility. Hostility divides into cynical mistrust, anger, and aggression. Of these, according to the Duke University study by Redford Williams, **hostility is the most toxic risk factor.**

The study showed that as hostility increases, the subjects

had a five times higher death rate from a heart attack. Hostility increases blood pressure and releases harmful chemicals like adrenaline, noradrenaline, cortisol, and testosterone, which damage the blood vessels of the heart.

Hot Reactors

People with high reactivity of heart to stress are called "hot reactors" by heart researcher, Robert Eliot. If you challenge them with physical or emotional stressors, such as arithmetic problems, video games, or putting their hands in cold water, they respond with high blood pressure, increased heart rate, and increased amounts of blood pumped from the heart.

The combination of a racing heart and vigorous pumping against the overload of high pressure in the tubes is called a "double product." This double product leads to excessive wear and tear on the cardiovascular system.

Social Isolation

Hostility and depression in a type A personality reduces their social acceptability. They live a life of loneliness and isolation. So they lose the confidence to express their emotions.

Smoking

Smoking increases the risk of getting coronary artery disease by 250%. Quitting smoking reduces your risk by 70% in a year.

Yin–Yang Imbalance

Our nervous system has two branches: the voluntary (somatic) and involuntary (autonomic). The autonomic branch is divided into two opposite parts: parasympathetic (yin) and sympathetic (yang). The yin and yang balance each other in dynamic equilibrium.

This balance works from the basic atomic level: free radicals vs. antioxidants; the chemical level: catacholamine vs. endorphins; with emotions: anger vs. caring love; and up through the social level: connectedness vs. isolation. When this balance is lopsided, it can lead to disorders like heart disease and cancer. It even shows up in your heartbeat; healthy and flexible heartbeats have unequal intervals between them. This is called heart rate variability. Recent research shows that **heart rate variability is the most sensitive indicator of the *yin–yang* balance or imbalance.**

When a heart is unhealthy, heart rate variability becomes low and erratic. Anger and frustration cause abnormal heart rate variability. Caring love and compassion make it flexible.

Cholesterol

Half of all Americans have a cholesterol problem. So, cholesterol gets a lot of attention. The cholesterol problem increases the risk of coronary artery disease by a factor of 2.4. In one year, 300,000 heart attack deaths are attributed to cholesterol problems. Look out for:

1. High total cholesterol, more than 200mg.
2. High bad cholesterol (LDL), more than 130mg.
3. Low good cholesterol, less than 35.
4. High cholesterol/HDL ratio, more than 4.5.
5. High LDL\HDL ratio, more than 3.5.
6. High triglycerides, more than 150.

Extensive research among people from India who settled in Western countries, such as the United Kingdom and North America, show that in addition to conventional risk factors, they face these additional cholesterol related risks

1. High Lipoprotein (a).
2. High Apolipoprotein B.
3. Low Apolipoprotien A1.
4. Low LDL\Apolipoprotein B Ratio.
5. Low Apo A1\Apo B Ratio.
6. High TPA inhibitor Level (pAI–1).

Little Big Monster

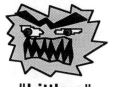

"Little a" Monster

The lipoprotein (a), also called "little a," is a little, yet big monster causing a lot of havoc. High lipoprotein (a) is associated with a 10 times higher atherosclerotic and heart disease risk. If the little a is more than 30mg/dl, the risk of arteriosclerosis doubles. Add increased LDL, and the risk rises three to five fold. "Little a" is a genetic problem and dietary changes do not alter the little a lipoprotein. Similar in structure to LDL, it is now believed this lipid protein promotes blood clots and prevents disintegration of formed clots. Niacin is known to reduce lipoprotein (a) level.

We can summarize the blood lipid risk factors using the good, bad, ugly, and deadly lipids as opposing vectors. The terminology comes from the cardiologist Enas A. Enas, a world authority on coronary artery disease among Asian Indians.

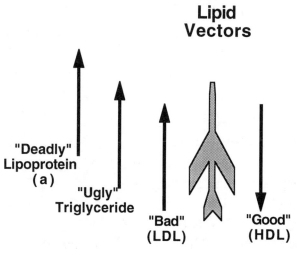

Lipid Vectors

"Deadly" Lipoprotein (a)

"Ugly" Triglyceride

"Bad" (LDL)

"Good" (HDL)

Michael Brown and Joseph Goldstein of the University of Texas received the Nobel Prize in 1985 for a fascinating discovery related to the receptors of LDL in people with high cholesterol.

Some are born with a deficiency of LDL receptors, and the body tries to compensate for this defect by producing an excess of LDL "bad cholesterol." Others indulge in high LDL producing behavior or overeat on fat, have a sedentary lifestyle, and are stressed.

Heart Disease and Cancer

All have a reduction of LDL receptors as a compensatory mechanism. In both cases, there is a vicious cycle going on between reduced LDL receptors and high LDL in the blood. You have to break the cycle where you can: with lifestyle changes, cholesterol lowering drugs, or both.

The National Cholesterol Education program regards cholesterol as the most important risk factor. Cholesterol causes atherosclerosis (plaque deposits hardening arteries) by oxidation. This oxidized LDL cholesterol is the problem. And it's relatively new information. So a brief history.

We discovered cholesterol in atherosclerotic plaques in 1910. By 1952, we'd found oxidized lipids. In 1961, a special type of white blood cells (macrophages) was located in plaques. Ten years later, foam cells (macrophages filled with lipid) were discovered. By 1980, Steinberg's theory of oxidized LDL causing plaque was well accepted. In 1991, Steinberg chaired a world assembly of the National Heart, Lung and Blood Institute. They concluded that free radicals attacking the LDL, and oxidizing causes plaque formation.

Now we know bad cholesterol or LDL is not really bad until it is oxidized. And free radicals cause the oxidation. The free radicals are set free by internal and external chemical toxins. Stress is a major internal toxin. Certain foods are major external toxins (e.g., red meat, high fat diet).

High Blood Pressure

If you have hypertension, your relative risk is 2.1. Which means high blood pressure will increase your chance of heart attack by 210%. Every year, 195,000 cardiac deaths in the U.S. are related to high blood pressure. Blood pressure increases the load on the heart and makes the heart over–work. Arteries harden in response to high blood pressure. With each pulse beat, the pressure pushes against the artery wall and causes damage. In hot reactors, heart rate and blood pressure increase in response to stress arousal.

Sedentary Life

The relative cardiac risk of a sedentary lifestyle is 1.9, which means there's a 190% increased chance of heart attack. Since 60% of Americans do not exercise enough, 205,000 cardiac deaths every year are related to a lack of exercise.

The Paffenberger study of 16,036 Harvard graduates showed people who exercised the equivalent of nine miles walking per week had the lowest death rates. The Cooper Clinic study by Blaire and Associates showed just getting up from your couch and doing any exercise, however mild, decreased coronary artery disease risk.

Exercise and Your Heart

Physical exercise helps your heart in three different ways:

1. **Fights Atherosclerosis:** Atherosclerosis results from an increase of cholesterol and other lipids; damage to artery lining, and clotting disorder. Exercise reduces all three components.

Exercise helps reverse atherosclerosis by decreasing the LDL cholesterol and increasing the HDL cholesterol. It also decreases blood pressure and blood clotting factors, such as platelet stickiness. New research shows exercise decreases the tissue plasminogen activator (tPA) inhibitor and the tendency to form blood clots inside the body. The net result is, exercise opposes atherosclerosis (hardening of arteries) and thrombogenesis (clot formation), both of which lead to a heart attack.

2. **Stronger Heart Muscle:** Exercise improves collateral circulation and the heart's pumping power. It increases the circulation's effectiveness by improving the way tissue utilizes oxygen. Exercise balances the yin–yang components of the heart beat.

3. **Risk Factor Reduction:** Exercise increases the sensitivity of tissue insulin receptors. Higher fluctuations of insulin contributes to fat deposits in tissues and arteries, the increase

Exercise & Heart

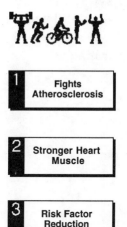

| 1 | Fights Atherosclerosis |

| 2 | Stronger Heart Muscle |

| 3 | Risk Factor Reduction |

| ↓ | Cholesterol Blood Pressure Clotting System |

| ↑ | Collaterals Pump Power Circulation Yin-Yang Balance |

| ↓ | Insulin Level Obesity Stress Chemicals |

of blood pressure, and mood swings. Hence, low insulin levels reduce obesity. Exercise clears the stress chemicals, such as adrenaline and cortisone, from the blood.

The graphic depicts how exercise helps your heart.

Diabetes

Diabetics are two to four times more likely to die of heart attacks than non–diabetics. Diabetes increases the chance of atherosclerosis and also heart rate variability. Hyperinsulinism is an early warning of adult onset diabetes.

Obesity

More than one third of Americans are obese. Abdominal obesity or apple type rather than pear type (obesity in the hips) increases the risk of heart problems. A ten percent gain

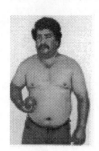
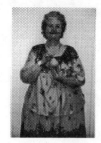

in body fat increases the chance of a heart attack by 25%.

Apple and Pear

The far left photo shows apple type central obesity. The one at near left shows pear–shaped hip obesity.

INSULIN RESISTANCE (HYPERINSULINISM)

Reaven, a Stanford Scientist, described a syndrome called insulin resistance or hyperinsulinism. The essential defect is lack of sensitivity of insulin receptors in the tissues. The basic features of insulin resistance is shown in the graphics.

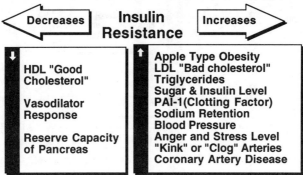

Insulin excess is bad because it increases bad cholesterol and triglyceride while decreasing good cholesterol. This leads to fat deposits, hardening and narrowing of blood vessels including coronary arteries. Blood clotting is increased by synthesis of plasminogen activator inhibitor -1 (PAI-1), which is the opposite of t-PA given during a heart attack to dissolve the clot. Insulin increases sodium absorption from the kidneys which leads to hypertension. Insulin increases sympathetic arousal and anger. Insulin resistance stimulates the pancreas to secrete more and more insulin just like whipping a tired horse to run faster.

VECTORS OF INSULIN SECRETION

Insulin level in the blood is affected by external pharmacy and internal pharmacy.

High fat, refined sugar, and processed food increase insulin levels. Natural, low fat, starch based, high fiber food decreases insulin level. Any fat antagonizes insulin action including olive oil or fish oil. Research shows that fat is more responsible for diabetes than sugar. A University of Kentucky study compared 65% fat in diet and 5% fat with one pound of sugar per day. After two weeks, all the subjects on the fat diet turned

Insulin Vectors

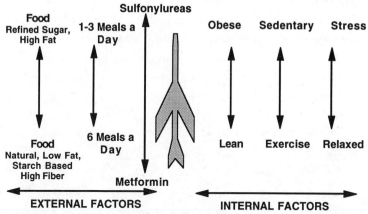

into mild diabetics. In the Pacific island of Nauru, the natives ate complex carbohydrates and their diabetes incidence was negligible. The phosphate mining attracted Americans, whose high fat diet was adapted by natives. The diabetes incidence increased to 35%. Eating infrequent meals leads to roller-coaster swings of insulin levels. Eating at least six meals a day balances the insulin level.

Sulfonylurea type (glipizide and glyburide) antidiabetic pills stimulate pancreas and increase insulin levels. Metformin increases glucose utilization without increasing insulin levels.

Obesity increases insulin level in a vicious cycle. Sedentary lifestyle increases insulin resistance. Regular sustained exercise, 20-30 minutes, twice a day is a good antidote to insulin resistance. Stress arousal releases adrenaline, noradrenaline, and cortisol which antagonize insulin action.

When you eat refined sugar, the insulin level quickly rises, tryptophan, an amino acid, enters the brain, and brain serotonin rises to give a sense of pleasure. After 30-40 minutes, the effect is gone, and you crave the sugar again. Complex carbohydrates slow down this roller coaster process, and the pleasure is sustained longer. Sugar substitutes, such as saccharin and aspartame give you a sweet taste without subsequent rise of the pleasure chemical, serotonin. This leaves an after taste with an unfulfilled gratification.

Amino acids can be sweet, but they do not act as sugars to raise serotonin levels. So there's no pleasure effect.

Fructose sugar does not require insulin for metabolism. When you eat fructose in fruits, berries, honey, and vegetables, you bypass this insulin need. In America, fructose is easily available as a sweetener. Fructose does give you a mood elevation after 15 minutes, but without the need for insulin. So we recommend fructose sugar as a sweetener.

Other Risk Factors

Over the years, medical science has discovered more than 270 risk factors for heart disease. Consumption of animal protein, regardless of fat content, is a risk factor for heart disease and cancer. A meat–based diet is methionine–rich and folate deficient. That increases blood levels of homocysteine and the risk of atherosclerosis. Other problems with a meat–based diet are: high uric acid, high fibrinogen, high toxins, cholesterol and fat, and low fiber content.

Some recently discovered risks of heart attacks are: frequent dental infections, respiratory infections by chlamydia, male type baldness, elevated serum iron, depression, and anxiety disorders. We'll amend the list as science finds new evidence. For now, let's pay attention to the major risks above.

Relative Impact of Risk Factor Modification

Risk factors don't follow the mathematical rule of 1 + 1 = 2; but the geometric rule of 1 + 1 = 5 or more. Medical schools classically teach that if you decrease the bad cholesterol or increase the good cholesterol, you'll have a major impact on coronary artery disease.

But take it one step further. These and other factors all tie into stress control at the final common pathway of a free radical attack. **That is why we propose stress control as the most important factor.**

CANCER RISK FACTORS

There are four accepted risk factors for cancer: toxic overload, nutrition, stress, and exercise.

Toxic Overload

There are five million registered chemicals in the world. Mankind comes in contact with 70,000, of which 20,000 are known to be carcinogenic (cancer producing). Each year Americans alone use 1.2 billion pounds of pesticides on crops, dump 90 billion pounds of toxic waste in 55,000 waste sites, and nine million pounds of antibiotics are fed to farm animals.

The University of California in Berkeley estimates each of 60 trillion cells in the human body gets hit 1,000 to 10,000 times by toxins, which potentially lead to breaks in DNA.

One of the most common toxins causing cancer is tobacco. According to the **National Institute of Cancer, 30% of cancer deaths are due to tobacco use.**

Nutrition

The human body is built of food from the outside. Food can start cancer growth, and the breakdown products of food can also be carcinogenic.

Food can contain antioxidants that neutralize the effect. Fruits and vegetables are known to contain large amounts of these antioxidants. **According to the National Cancer Institute, 35% of cancer deaths are due to dietary factors.**

Stress

According to the research by Candace Pert at the National Institute of Health, the human mind–body creates an internal pharmacy of messenger molecules to heal or kill.

Stress releases these chemicals in the form of neurotransmitters, hormones, and immune transmitters. The final common pathway is an attack on the cell DNA by free radicals that alter the DNA messages, producing cancer or heart disease.

Exercise

One out of three Americans get cancer, but only one out of seven Americans that exercise get the disease. Exercise improves cell oxygenation, the immune system, sugar–insulin balance, circulation and lymph flow, and reduces stress chemicals and toxins.

Radically Common Risk Factors

Medical science has advanced from the cellular and molecular level to the atomic level. For example, MRI (magnetic resonance imaging) is at the atomic level of medicine–sending radio waves

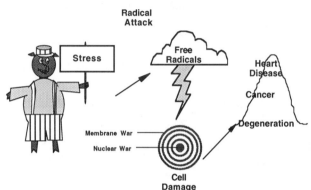

to the cell proton and asking atomic level questions about the state of the atom. This is like earlier chemistry and celllular-based diagnosis–only better.

Similarly, we now have a better understanding of risk factors in coronary artery disease at the atomic level. Some examples:

Physical and mental stress creates free radicals at the atomic level. These free radicals oxidize the LDL cholesterol and cause membrane damage on the lining of the coronary artery. **This is called membrane war.** The free radicals attack the cell nucleus and change the genetic master code (DNA).

This affects the immune system, which can cause infections, autoimmune disorders, or cancer. **This is nuclear war.** Its end result is degenerative disorders, and the tip of that iceberg happens to be heart disease and cancer.

ANGRY ATOMS

Injured free radical atoms get the message of anger from messenger molecules. Current research shows stress of expressed or suppressed anger is the fire that ignites the inflammation of heart disease and the havoc of cancer.

How Anger Attacks the Heart:

1. There is a brain–heart conflict. The brain says "get angry." The heart says "love." This tug–of–war between the brain and the heart creates stress.

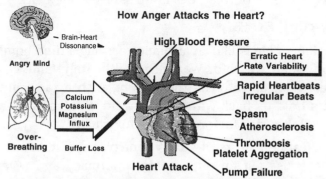

How Anger Attacks The Heart?

2. You over–breathe, which leads to alkaline blood and the loss of bicarbonate buffer in the urine. Calcium, potassium, and magnesium go into the cell and cause neuromuscular irritability all over the body. But in the heart, there are particular changes:

A. Blood pressure rises due to constricted blood vessels.

B. Heartbeats become irregular. The smooth variability of heart rate between inspiration and expiration becomes erratic. This is a sensitive index of the yin–yang balance of your body. **In fact, for people who have low and erratic heart rate variability, the chance of sudden death is increased two to five times.**

C. The coronary artery can go into spasms, which can cause anginal chest pain or heart attacks.

D. The free radicals increase in the body and oxidize the

LDL cholesterol (bad cholesterol) and reduce the HDL (good cholesterol). This leads to atherosclerosis.

E. Adrenaline makes the platelets stick together, which can cause thrombosis: another way to develop a heart attack.

F. The rapid heart, high blood pressure, and decreased blood supply to the heart due to spasms of the coronary artery weakens the pumping power of the heart. This is pump failure: heart attack is usually due to a blood clot that does not dissolve right away.

THE TIME BOMB

Human life is like an airplane carrying a time bomb set to go off when we land. We will all ultimately land. But some forces push us towards the landing with a tail wind, while others hold us back with a head wind. **Controllable and uncontrollable risk factors push us forward.**

Lifestyle factors of stress control, social connectedness, and exercise act on our internal pharmacy and reverse the journey towards the time bomb.

The external pharmacy of food, vitamin supplements, and prescribed or abused drugs can act in either direction. You have the choice to make. You can change your landing time by skill power of lifestyle changes or pill power of drugs.

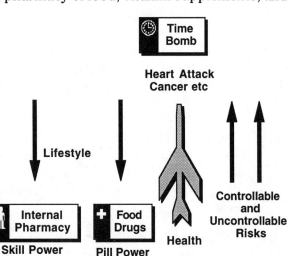

21st Century Lifestyle

In the process of civilization, we have come through three distinct waves of growth: agricultural era, industrial revolution, and now, the third wave, the information explosion. The 21st century lifestyle is focused on problem solving and information processing.

21st century life has impacted health and illness by three factors:

1. **Eating Habits:** People eat processed foods high in fat, refined sugar, animal protein, and salt. Eating is infrequent, irregular and hurried. Eating excess of fat is the most important dietary risk for health in general and heart disease in particular. Most of the fat in the Western way of life comes from animal sources. For example, a typical Chinese diet contains only 7% animal protein compared to 70% in American diet. Heart attacks kill only 4 of every 1,000 Chinese men compared to 67 of every 1,000 American men!

2. **"Motion Sickness":** Desk–top work, automation and television has led to a sedentary life. Another aspect of motion are the "new nomads"—people changing their place of residence in pursuit of promotion and novelty in life. This has cut off the root connections with nursery school friends and high school sweethearts. Transcontinental migration and intermixing of people has led to aculturation, transculturation and unflocking of "birds of the same feather." In the agricultural era, human tribes moved just like the migrating birds of "the same feather, flocking together." New research has shown that lack of ethnic support increases the incidence of ill health including coronary artery disease.

3. **"Emotion Sickness":** Modern life is lived under pressure to do more and more in less and less time. People, as time managers, are having a two–dimensional focus of matter and motion, ignoring the third dimension of emotion. In the pursuit of power and control, preference is given to *achievement* over

affiliation. The net result is a robotic workaholism with suppression of emotional values. Constant vigilance and competition leads to a fight–or–flight reaction hundreds of times a day. As cavemen, we had that reaction only when a saber toothed tiger–like hazard appeared.

Paradigm shift is the shifting sand of values. A product, procedure, or concept rapidly gets over–ruled by a new one. Material based values become obsolete rapidly. If you buy a refrigerator today, next month somebody proclaims it is defective. *Experimentally* it can apprear true, but *experientially* it has to be assimilated. *Logically* it can be obsolete, but *biologically* there is a lag phase to cope. The opposite of material based values is principle based. Caring love is an example. Its "currency value" never becomes obsolete. The 21st century paradigm shift focuses mostly on material values.

ASIAN INDIANS AND THEIR RISKY HEART

Taj Mahal, one of the world's wonders, is a landmark of India– home to one–fifth of the world's population. This is also where vegetarianism, yoga, and meditation took root.

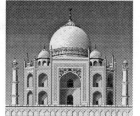

But here's the paradox: premature coronary heart disease (CHD or CAD) before age 40 is 5 to 10 times more common in Indians.

A study of Coronary Heart Disease in Indians led by Enas A. Enas, MD from Chicago, Illinois looked at 2000 Indian physicians and their spouses living in the U.S. Doctors, especially cardiologists, constituted the majority of this group. The study confirmed high incidence of insulin resistance, abdominal obesity, and lipid disorders (especially low HDL, high triglyceride, high Lp–(a)) in Indians.

From 1970 to 1980, amongst UK based Indians, the CHD increased by 6% in men and 13% in women compared to a decrease of 5% in men and 1% in women of British origin.

At the same time, there was a 23% decrease in men and 36% decrease in women of CHD in other non–British people living in the UK. **Premature CHD below age 40 is 10 times**

Coronary Heart Disease Risk in Asian Indians

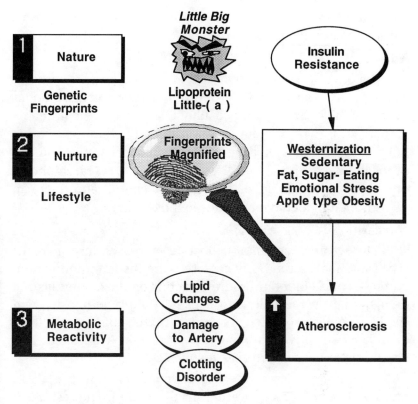

more common in Indians. The Kaiser Permanente study in California showed that Indians in general have 4 times higher hospitalization for CHD compared to whites and other Asians. In New Delhi, India, a study showed that men had 4 times and women had 10 times higher CHD rate when compared to the Framingham study. Similar statistics are confirmed in a South Indian study at Vellore, India.

A new study comparing Indians settled in West London, UK to their siblings in India found that the **westernized Indians had higher metabolic disorders and CHD incidence.**

The whole spectrum of CHD risk in Indians is an example of how a high stressed, mechanized, sedentary, fat–eating lifestyle leads to CHD. The above graphics summarizes these concepts.

The problem of heart disease in Indians is both due to nature and amplified by nurture.

Nature

Genetically, some people are exempt from early atherosclerosis. The susceptible group is born with genetic finger prints of high Lp (a) and insulin resistance. The little big monster (Lp (a)) problem starts from early childhood and is not altered by diet or drugs. The insulin resistance, on the other hand, can be altered by lifestyle. New research shows one–third of human genes are "housekeepers," and they can be retrained by behavior change just like training a dog.

Nurture

The western sedentary lifestyle increases insulin resistance and makes the body secrete more insulin. High insulin increases one's blood pressure by acting on the kidney. Insulin deposits fat on the belly and causes apple type obesity, and the LDL cholesterol stick in arteries. High insulin comes from decreased sensitivity of insulin receptors in tissues. Fat and simple sugar eating increases insulin secretion.

Emotional stress releases adrenaline, noradrenaline, and cortisol, which counteract insulin action. The result is a demand for more insulin. This insulin resistance, lipid disorder of low HDL and high triglyceride, apple type obesity, and premature coronary artery disease is what we call the Reaven Syndrome, named after the Stanford scienist.

Metabolic Changes

The metabolic changes of westernization lead to three different factors promoting atherosclerosis:

1. **Lipid Changes:** The good cholesterol (HDL) level falls. Bad cholesterol (LDL) and triglyceride increase. LDL–to–HDL ratio increases.

2. **Damage to Artery:** The pulse pressure rises due to rapid heart rate and blood pressure. This damages the lining of the arteries on which the immune cells (macrophages) deposit oxidized LDL cholesterol.

3. **Blood Clotting Disorder:** Clotting is increased by increased fibrinogen and sticky platelets. **A sedentary life style is the major culprit.** The clot dissolving enzymes become weaker. Recent research has shown that Asian Indians have increased plasminogen inhibitor and reduced plasminogen activity. Plasminogen helps to dissolve blood clots. Most of the heart attacks are due to sudden blood clots, or coronary thrombosis.

Yet more than 50% of Asian Indian who are heart attack victims or who have heart disease, show cholesterol levels 20 to 40 mg/dl lower than Whites. The National Cholesterol Education Program recommends a cholesterol level of less than 200mg/dl as ideal. This is too high for Asian Indians, particularly if their Lp(a) is higher than 30mg/dl, or in the presence of apple type obesity, low HDL, or hyperinsulinism. Average normal cholesterol level in China is 162; Japan,166; rural India,180; urban India,196. Indians usually have a low HDL level. For this reason, the ratio of cholesterol divided by HDL is a better indicator of risk. The ratio should be less than 4.5.

Lessons from the Indian Paradox

The Indian paradox of high CAD and *not that high* cholesterol level indicates there could be other risk factors yet unknown. But urbanization, mechanization, and westernization have changed the "native" lifestyle of Asian Indians, making their heart more vulnerable to attack.

The Japanese have one of the lowest incidence of CAD. Recently, the workaholic Japanese have been dropping dead at work with a heart attack, called *Karoshi*.

Leonard Syme, Unversity of California, Berkeley, studied heart attacks among Japanese living in Japan, in Hawaii and in California. Heart disease incidence was higher for those in California than for those in Hawaii. But the Hawaiian Japanese had a higher incidence than those living in Japan. "Westernization" clearly has a price.

Italians moving to America also showed increased heart incidence in a surprising way. When they first moved to a small town in Pennsylvania, they had half the number of heart attacks of neighboring communities. But as "Americanization" replaced their old–country values, the heart attack rate equaled that of the other communities. Again, the lack of ethnic support and alienation of your own culture raised the risk of heart trouble.

Risk Factor Reduction

What steps you take to reduce risk factors depends on your situation. If you don't suffer from heart disease or cancer, you of course want to prevent it (primary prevention). If you have any one of those conditions, you want to stop its progression (secondary prevention).

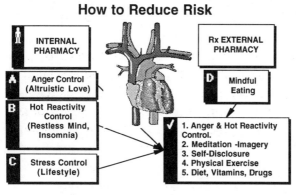

How to Reduce Risk

Secondary prevention of heart disease targets reducing total cholesterol and triglyceride below 150mg/dl, and LDL below 100mg/dl. The total cholesterol–HDL ratio should be below 4.5. Most methods of preventing heart disease also apply to cancer prevention.

If you have a family history, or one of the major risk factors, take it seriously. Start the reversal of your risk factors.

Heart Disease and Cancer

Here is an axiom from Enas:

"Waiting for chest pain to diagnose heart disease is no different than waiting for labor pains to diagnose pregnancy."

Action Plan for Risk Reduction

You can reduce your risk factor by changing the external pharmacy (pill power), or internal pharmacy (skill power), or both.

The external pharmacy includes prescription drugs, food and antioxidant vitamins. Follow your physician's advice in using your prescription drugs. The risk reduction diet is starch–based, low fat, low salt, high fiber, vegetarian diet eaten 6 times a day to balance the insulin and mood. Vitamin A (beta carotene), C and E as antioxidants are recommended.

Skill power has the edge in risk reduction. The internal pharmacy is opened up by anger control, hot reactity control and stress control. Meditation and imagery, self–disclosure and physical exercise are effective tools to modify the internal pharmacy to heal.

The risk control has two *inter–dependent* areas to measure, monitor and modify. One is the chemical values such as

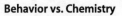
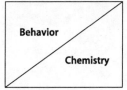

cholesterol, blood sugar and catecholamines. The other is your behavior. You ask your physician to measure and monitor your good, bad, ugly and deadly cholesterol patterns; *this book will guide you how to work on the diagonal of behavior.*

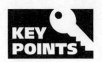

1. Anger Control by learning the art of altruistic love.
2. Hot Reactivity Control by controlling restless mind and insomnia. This helps to control blood pressure and heart rate.
3. Stress Control by lifestyle modification. This includes meditation and imagery, self–disclosure, and physical exercise.

8

Cybernetic Model of Stress Arousal

Heart Disease and Cancer

Cybernetic Model of Stress Arousal

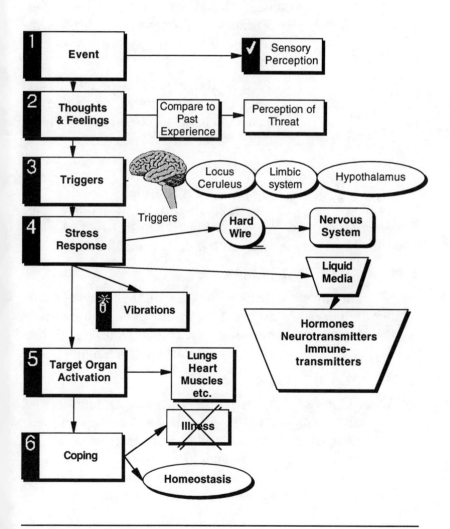

Cybernetic Model of Stress Arousal

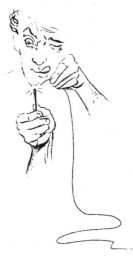

Under stress with misplaced effort

Stress is misplaced effort. It's like overexerting and tensing up to thread a needle. If, instead of using the hands and fingers precisely, you tense up, you are misplacing your effort. Physiologically, the misplaced effort causes unwanted arousal of the sympathetic branch of your nervous system.

Based on original research by Walter Cannon and Hans Selye, (modified by Herbert Benson and George Everly) the stress model has six stages.

1. STRESS EVENTS:

Something happens outside the mind–body or within it. Outside events can be physical, chemical, or biological in nature. Inside changes are either real or imagined.

2. THOUGHTS AND FEELINGS:

We compare with past experiences and belief systems, to decide whether or not the event is a threat. Once we appraise it as a threat, emotional arousal occurs. This activates our brain's limbic system, the emotional headquarters of the mind–body.

3. NEUROLOGICAL TRIGGERS:

Three different brain structures (locus ceruleus, limbic system, and hypothalamus) act as neurological triggering centers. These release chemicals called neurotransmitters. The locus ceruleus releases norepinephrine, causing the fight or flight response to stress. Repetitions of the stress and response turn on the other centers.

This is called ergotrophic tuning and limbic hypersensitivity. Once the triggering mechanism is aroused, it stimulates the nervous and chemical pathways to produce the stress response.

4. THE STRESS RESPONSE:

This has three distinct pathways: the **"hard wire"** or neuromuscular system; the **"liquid media"** of the neurotransmitters, immune transmitters, and hormones; and the **"vibrational whisper"**- electromagnetic waves. Through a subtle form of these waves, etheric and astral waves, the mind–body communicates with the mind–body of other people. This is sometimes called "universal mind."

The **hard wire** system has a muscle and a mind terminal. The nerve signal traffic congestion in one affects the other. You control your voluntary muscles (neuromuscular system), and through this system you can control your mind. The involuntary or autonomic (acting on its own) part of your nervous system has two parts: the **sympathetic branch of the nervous system,** mind–body functions which react to stress, and the **parasympathetic nervous system,** mind–body functions which respond to relaxation or meditation.

Your body swims in a **liquid media** of **neurotransmitters**, such as acetylcholine and endorphins; **immune transmitters,** such as interferons and interleukins; and **hormones,** such as adrenaline and cortisone. The mind meets the body at the level of these messenger molecules, which jump from one nerve cell to the other to pass on information between each of the subsystems of the mind–body.

Nature has its own primordial rhythms. The sun's energy is transmitted through the earth's rotation to your mind–body in rhythmic oscillations. These primordial waves connect us all through an invisible "satellite" of Universal Mind or Universal Intelligence. When you're stressed, your natural waves are in turbulence. When you meditate and relax, your mind–body's energy waves come into sync with nature's rhythm.

5. TARGET ORGAN ACTIVATION:

This is our predisposition to respond to stress with certain weaknesses that are our **signature responses**.

One person may always experience a migraine headache. Another may experience stomach "butterflies." A third may sweat profusely. Nearly everyone develops improper breathing during stress, either holding the breath or over breathing (hyperventilation).

6. COPING MECHANISM:

You can manage stress by avoiding it. Or you can reduce the intensity of stress by making internal bodily changes. These internal adjustments are called "homeostasis," (meaning "bringing back to balance"). Without homeostasis, mind-body disregulation or illness occurs.

Cybernetic Approach to Stress

Through cybernetic measuring, monitoring, and modifying components at various levels, we can control stress with do–able tools.

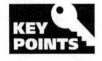

1. Stress arousal is produced by the interpretation of events.
2. The trigger response in the emotional control center of the limbic system leads to hard wire, liquid media, and vibrational messages to target organs.
3. Coping with the stress leads to restoration of balance. Otherwise, illness occurs.

9

The Yin and Yang of the Mind–Body

The Yin and Yang of the Mind-Body

Yin and Yang
or Prakriti and Purusha in Nature

In Chinese and Taoist thinking, **yin and yang represent opposites in nature,** as the eternal dynamics of the universe. A parallel in Hinduism is *prakiriti,* feminine nature, and *purusha*, masculine nature. *Yin* and *yang* are complementary to each other, like day and night.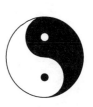

Opposites in nature help us understand the balance in life. An excess of *yang* energy leads to a Type A personality marked by hurrying, competition, and hostility. An excess of *yin* energy leads to a Type C personality noted for suppression of emotions, helplessness, and hopelessness .

Medical science treats male prostate cancer with female hormones, and female breast cancer with male hormones. However, the problem today is, the loss of *yin* hampers healing. For optimal health, *yin* and *yang* have to be in dynamic balance.

The right-brain and left-brain is another example of *yin* and *yang*. Roger Sperry won a Nobel prize in the 1970s for the discovery of these two functional sides of the brain. The right brain attributes are: intuition, imagery, music, art, emotion, relaxation, meditation, and healing. The left brain attributes are: analysis, verbal language, science, mathematics, and stress arousal.

The yin and yang principles come under three headings: the parasympathetic and sympathetic system, yin and yang functions of the body, and stress and relaxation.

PARASYMPATHETIC AND SYMPATHETIC BALANCES

The autonomic part of the nervous system has two opposing branches: parasympathetic (yin) and sympathetic (yang).

When you arouse the sympathetic, pupils dilate; saliva dries up; the heart beat increases; bronchial tubes open up; gastrointestinal function slows down; glycogen breakdown

The Yin and Yang of the Mind–Body

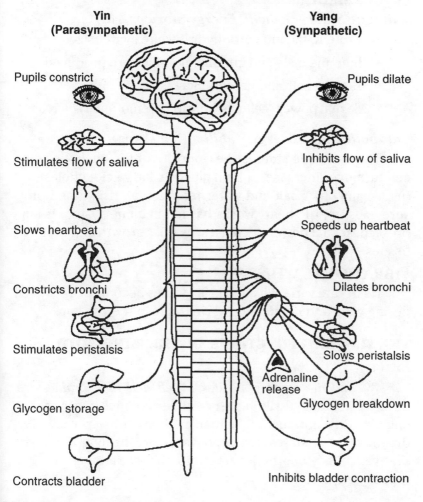

Yin (Parasympathetic)	Yang (Sympathetic)
Pupils constrict	Pupils dilate
Stimulates flow of saliva	Inhibits flow of saliva
Slows heartbeat	Speeds up heartbeat
Constricts bronchi	Dilates bronchi
Stimulates peristalsis	Slows peristalsis
	Adrenaline release
Glycogen storage	Glycogen breakdown
Contracts bladder	Inhibits bladder contraction

---

increases in the liver; and bladder contraction is inhibited.

During parasympathetic stimulation, the pupils constrict; saliva pours out; the heart beat slows; the bronchial tubes constrict; intestinal movement increases; bile is released; and the bladder contracts.

HARD WIRE:

The neuromuscular traffic increases during yang and decreases during the yin state.

LIQUID MEDIA:

Anabolic State – Growth, Energy Storage (Yin)

- Protein, fat and carbohydrates are synthesized.
- Immune cells and immunoglobulins are produced.
- Bone repair and growth increases.
- Sexual power (cellular, hormonal, emotional) increases.

Catabolic State- Energy Mobilization (Yang)

The catabolic state is the opposite of the anabolic state; cell turn over increases, blood glucose, fatty acid, cholesterol (especially LDL), salt and water retention all rise. Blood pressure goes up, the heart works harder, immune system is suppressed, sexual power decreases, as does growth and repair of tissues.

VIBRATIONAL WHISPER:

Heart rate variability and brain waves become disregulated during yang and regulated and rhythmic in the yin state.

THE YIN-YANG FUNCTIONS OF THE MIND-BODY

Brain

We find the same opposites in left and right brain sides: intuitive vs. analytical; imagery vs. verbal; music, art vs. science, math; emotional vs. factual; meditative vs. aroused; daydream vs. alert states; receptive vs. active; healing vs. degenerative; parasympathetic vs. sympathetic; rapport visit vs. report visit, etc.

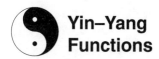

Yin–Yang Functions

FUNCTION	*YIN*	*YANG*
BRAIN	**RIGHT BRAIN**	**LEFT BRAIN**
	Intuitive Imagery Music, Art Emotional Meditative Alpha-theta Daydream Receptive Healing Parasympathetic Tropotrophic "Rapport Visit"	Analytical Verbal Science, Math Factual Aroused Beta Waves Alert Active Disregulated Sympathetic Ergotrophic "Report Visit"
Heart	Heart Rate Variability is Smooth and Regular	Heart Rate Variability is Low and Erratic
Anger Vs Love	Caring Love (Endorphins)	Hostility (Catecholamines)
Reactivity	Diaphragmatic Breathing Muscles Relaxed Restful Mind	Thoracic Breathing Muscles Tense Restless Mind
Stress Arousal	Eustress (Appropriate for the Situation) Upslope of Human Function Curve	Distress (Misplaced Effort) Downslope of Human Function Curve
Metabolism	Anabolism (Regeneration)	Catabolism (Degeneration)

The Yin and Yang of the Mind–Body

Heart

Heart rate variability is the interval between two consecutive heart beats. This interval varies from one pair of beats to another. The heart rate variability of the yin state is smooth and regular. The heart rate variability of the yang state is low and erratic.

Anger vs Love

Caring love is a yin state with release of endorphins. Anger and frustration is a yang state with release of adrenaline and noradrenaline (catecholamines).

Reactivity

As we breathe, our diaphragm muscles are appropriately tensed or relaxed for the task at hand; the mind is restful in the yin state. Breathing is thoracic; muscles are tense; and the mind is restless in the yang state.

Stress Arousal

The yin-yang contrasts are seen here, too: good stress vs. distress; appropriate vs. misplaced effort; and up-slope of human function curve against down-slope of human function curve.

Metabolism

In the yin state, metabolism is anabolic or regenerative for the tissues. In the yang state, metabolism is catabolic or degenerative for the tissues.

STRESS AND RELAXATION

The graphics on the next page show the opposing features of stress and relaxation in different systems of the body. The heart acts as the master commander of these changes. The breathing pattern, brain waves, muscle tension, gut function and metabolism follow the footsteps of heart and dance in sync.

Stress and Relaxation Response Compared

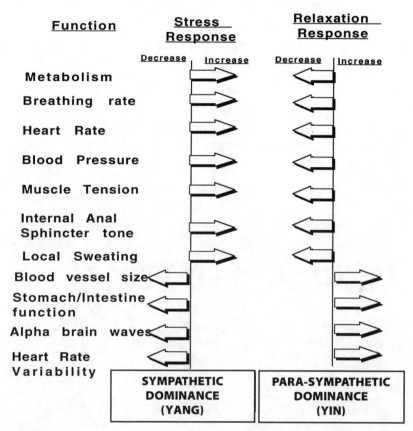

Function	Stress Response		Relaxation Response	
	Decrease	Increase	Decrease	Increase
Metabolism		→	←	
Breathing rate		→	←	
Heart Rate		→	←	
Blood Pressure		→	←	
Muscle Tension		→	←	
Internal Anal Sphincter tone		→	←	
Local Sweating		→	←	
Blood vessel size	←			→
Stomach/Intestine function	←			→
Alpha brain waves	←			→
Heart Rate Variability	←			→

SYMPATHETIC DOMINANCE (YANG)	PARA-SYMPATHETIC DOMINANCE (YIN)

KEY POINTS

1. Life is a wave. The peak of the wave is yang (male principle, purusha), and the bottom of the wave is yin (female principle, prakriti). Anger, frustration, and the information processing mode of life lacks balance unless we include an equal amount of caring love, intuition, and connectedness to our life.

2. This yin-yang balance restores the healing chemistry. Healing chemistry is a balance of endorphins and catecholamines (adrenaline and noradrenaline)

3. The anatomical heart is the master oscillator of yin-yang waves.

10
Addiction to Stress

Addiction to Stress

The sign of addiction is a feeling of helplessness to break a habit. At first, you believe you have control over your actions. Over time, that sense of control is replaced by a feeling that the response has control over you. As a Japanese saying has it, a person takes a drink. Then the drink takes a second drink and third drink. Then the drinks take over the person. A self-feeding cycle develops, with a feeling of powerlessness. Much the same thing happens with the "stress addict."

Stress creates a vicious cycle; it leads to more stress, in a circular, self-feeding (as well as self-defeating) process. This feedback loop is particularly true in our breathing response to stress.

When you are stressed, you over breathe, or **hyperventilate**. This may not be dramatic, like the heaving chest of a runner after a race, or the rapid, gulping breaths of a person in fear. On the contrary. You may just unconsciously and continuously breathe more than the 15 times per minute normal breath rate.

When you over breathe, you breathe out an excessive amount of carbon dioxide, which causes the blood to become alkaline. The body tries to counteract this imbalance by sending a signal to the kidneys, leading to bicarbonate excretion through urination (the bicarbonate causes the alkaline state in the blood). When you pass the bicarbonate out of your body, you do not have enough reserve bicarbonate in the blood-stream (called a "buffer") to counteract the surging acidity in the blood.

Unfortunately, bringing on the relaxation response by it-self, does not counteract physical addiction to stress. When you try to relax after hyperventilating, and your breathing begins to return to normal, you retain carbon dioxide, and your blood now becomes acidic due to the low buffer reserve.

Addiction to Stress

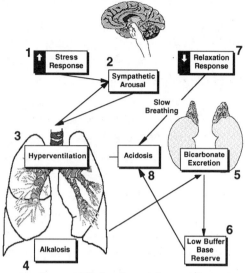

Stress addiction is a vicious cycle.

This, in turn, causes the hyperventilation to begin again, forming a vicious cycle. This is how you become addicted to stress.

Let's trace the addiction to stress in the above graphs.

1. **Stress Perceived:** First, you perceive a threat, leading to the state of sympathetic arousal.

2. **Sympathetic Arousal:** The sympathetic nervous system stimulates the body through nerve impulses and the release of messenger molecules, such as hormones.

3. **Hyperventilation:** You breathe at a rapid rate, blowing out carbon dioxide from the lungs.

4. **Alkalosis:** The low carbon dioxide makes the blood alkaline.

5. **Bicarbonate Excretion:** The kidney gets the message that there is too much bicarbonate and excretes alkali in the urine.

6. **Buffer Deficit:** There is a deficit of body buffers in the blood.

7. **Relaxation Attempt:** Now, if you try to relax, the breathing slows down and leads to relative acidity in the blood.

8. **Acidosis:** There is not enough buffer to counteract this acidity. Hyperventilation is the only alternative for the body to regain balance. Thus, the vicious cycle starts again.

This faulty breathing contributes to a restless night's sleep and waking up in the middle of the night (typically between 1:00 and 3:00 AM), with a racing, restless mind and excessive perspiration. In the daytime, breathing-induced restlessness produces the workaholic's compulsive urge to be doing something.

This acid-base imbalance causes an influx of calcium, magnesium, and potassium into the cell from the blood stream. That leads to excitability, tense muscles, and a restless mind. The heart becomes irritable, creating a rapid heart beat, an erratic breathing pattern, and spasms in the coronary arteries. They may trigger an actual heart attack. This connection of heart problems to hyperventilation is further explained in the section on reactivity of the heart.

How to Break the Chain of Stress Addiction?

The solution lies at various steps:

1. Remove conflicts in your mind so that the stress arousal is minimized.

2. Learn mindful breathing, and to consciously relax with various relaxation exercises. Diaphragmatic breathing conserves the buffer system. As you consciously build up an energy reserve with purposeful relaxation, you deposit "energy dollars" into your reserve.

With repetition, you change your unconscious, habitual breathing pattern from hyperventilation and thoracic breathing to one of slow, diaphragmatic breathing. You not only learn an antidote to chronic stress, but you break the pattern of physical and chemical breath-induced stress arousal.

Also, in times of acute stress, if you have built the foundation of mindful breathing, you can deliberately go into diaphragmatic breathing to calm yourself for whatever actions you need to take. These principles are explained step by step in the Cybernetics Tools section.

Automatic Reactivity

Addiction to stress leads to a chemical state of automatic reactivity. That means your body continues to be tense and your mind restless without control. It's like being on a treadmill or tread-wheel.

The solution is to deliberately slow down at every step, using the muscle-to-mind approach, rather than allow a restless mind to keep up with the momentum. In this book, we will be using these muscle-to-mind tools first to regain control.

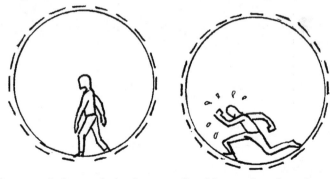

At left, you push the tread-wheel at a comfortable speed, and stay in control. At right, you push the tread wheel so fast that you become a slave to your own action and cannot get out of the vicious cycle.

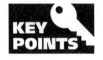

Stress arousal becomes an addiction because of ongoing chemical changes. Chronic hyperventilation and buffer loss in the body is the hallmark of stress addiction.

11

What is Relaxation?

What is Relaxation?

Relaxation is the antidote to stress and reactivity. Physicians prescribe bed rest, but unfortunately, many simply toss and turn in bed, and can not relax even while *trying* to rest. In fact, some get more tense when you tell them to relax.

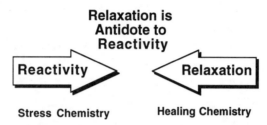

Relaxation is Antidote to Reactivity

Reactivity > < Relaxation

Stress Chemistry   Healing Chemistry

The commands, "don't worry, relax," and "take it easy," are often annoying because they don't tell you *how* to relax.

The opposite of relaxation is reactivity. You relax when you reduce the reactivity of the mind–body. Mind–body reactivity is a chemical state. This state increases nerve impulse traffic from muscle to mind and mind to muscle.

Relaxation is "letting go." At the muscle end, it is the lengthening of muscle fibers by letting go of the contracted tension. At the mind end, it is the letting go of worrisome thoughts. When relaxed, the body's metabolism, heart rate, blood pressure, breathing rate, and muscle tension are decreased. Also, the mind develops an "open focus" with passive attention to thoughts.

The principle of letting go is illustrated by the way they catch monkeys in India. The monkey's hand is just big enough to enter the bottle neck, but if the monkey holds on to the banana, his hand cannot come out. **A monkey's greed and pride does not allow him to "let go."**

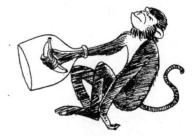

IMMEDIATE RELAXATION RESPONSE–
THE ANTIDOTE TO ACUTE STRESS

In an acute stress response, there is a sudden tensing of the muscles of your body. You're up on the balls of your feet, ready for action.

For example, if I yell at you by calling you by your first name, you develop a startle response within 100 milliseconds. Immediately, you release hormones, specifically adrenaline and noradrenaline, your hands and feet start sweating, your heart beats fast, and you hold your breath or over breathe thoracically. Your mind becomes restless and you develop an angry or fearful emotion.

The antidote is creating an immediate relaxation response. You do this by getting centered (thinking of your belly button), deliberately breathing from the diaphragm, and letting the air out slowly. You can focus your awareness on your heart and do the HRI as an additional step to relax.

Awareness of Control Signal

A sense of muscle tension is your **control signal**. Tension is when muscles contract. Relaxation is when they lengthen. You have control over your skeletal muscles–this is why they are called voluntary muscles. When your muscles are tense, they send nerve impulses to your brain, and make your mind tense. When your mind is tense, it sends more nerve impulses to your muscles to make them even more tense. Such reverberating neuromuscular circuits create a state of tension in your mind–body.

Relaxing involves two steps: 1) learning to recognize tension; 2) relaxing that tension and experiencing the contrast between the two states. For example, clench your jaws tightly. Feel the tension in your jaw muscles. Now, relax and let go, and notice the difference. The tension you feel in your jaw is the control signal. It indicates the degree of tension in a muscle. Next, clench your jaw with less force perhaps 50% less tension. Then 25%, 10%, and so on.

That's how you develop sensitivity to more and more levels of subtle tension. Pretty soon, you'll become aware of your tense jaw throughout the day as the tension begins. You'll learn to relax it by letting go of the tension before it "locks in." The goal is to sensitize yourself to subtle tension.

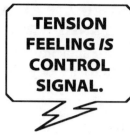

TENSION FEELING *IS* CONTROL SIGNAL.

You also want to understand how the mind and body connect with respect to tension. Close your eyes and imagine you are holding a hammer in your hand. Now picture yourself hitting a nail with the hammer three times. The first time, picture doing it spontaneously. The second time, pay attention to the control signal of tension as you hammer the nail. Can you experience the tension? The third time, use this heightened awareness to verify your sensitivity to the tension.

Misplaced Effort vs. Differential Relaxation

Differential relaxation is the optimal contraction of only those muscles required to accomplish a given task. In the above example, if you tense the whole body rather than the hammer-holding hand, you have a condition of **misplaced effort**. A child doing homework anxiously writes a report by tensing his/her whole body, rather than just tensing the writing hand. In this case, develop an awareness of such misplaced effort, and differentially relax the unwanted tense muscles.

Benson shows you can practice differential relaxation during physical exercise. He compared two groups of people exercising on a bicycle ergometer at equal speed for thirty minutes each. One group exercised spontaneously. The second group focused on a sound (mantra) or prayer while exercising. The second group decreased their metabolism by 11%. In another study, he found similar open–focusing produced the runner's euphoria after one or two miles of running, as compared to the control group having such euphoria after four or five miles.

How Do You Relax Muscles?

If I ask you to relax a muscle, you probably would not know how to do it. If I ask you to contract or tense your muscle, you probably could do it right away. As you contract your muscle, feel the control signal of tension in the muscle. Now let go, and feel the contrast of relaxation. The muscle contraction follows the **principle of a pendulum.** When you push a pendulum from midline to one side, it comes back, overshooting to the opposite side. Similarly, the contracted muscle relaxes to a state better than base line.

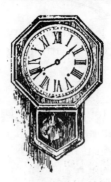 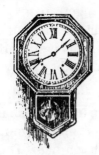 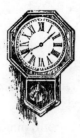 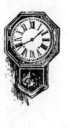

Heart synchronizes the body by "pendulum effort."

This is how progressive contraction and relaxation of muscles leads to a state of relaxation. This also demonstrates how the principle of physical exercise helps you relax. The largest pendulum is the heart. It is the major oscillator in the body. If you relax your heart, everything follows suit. Other oscillators in the body synchronize with the heart, and thus operate more efficiently.

STRETCH THE MUSCLE FIBERS TO RELAX

How Do You Relax the Mind?

When you are vigilant and restless, your mind is narrow focused. All the nerve traffic is congested in one channel. You can distribute the traffic into multiple channels by opening up your focus. For example, a stockbroker spends his working day narrow focused, watching the stock table. When he comes home,

---

he reads the newspaper with narrow focus and remains tensed up. Now, if his child comes and asks a question, he becomes grouchy because his mind–body chemistry is in a reactive mode. The easiest way to open your focus is to relocate your head–centered thinking to body–centered thinking. Imagine that you are in your heart area or belly button area. Shift your "I–ness" from the highness of your head to your body. The moment you shift your awareness from head to body, you get open focused. You can do this while reading, talking, or doing any activity in a parallel fashion. This is the principle of attaining passive attention in yoga and meditation.

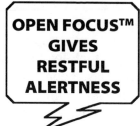

OPEN FOCUS™ GIVES RESTFUL ALERTNESS

Set Point of the Neuromuscular System

The tense–muscle, tense–mind feedback loop keeps telling the brain's control center (limbic–hypothalamic center) to keep the body's "thermostat" on high. The room (our body) remains very hot if the thermostat is set at 100 degrees Fahrenheit. The furnace works hard, burning energy. The room contents stay hot.

In this analogy, the heating system is the sympathetic nervous system and the cooling system is the parasympathetic nervous system.

Let us take the heating analogy further into the dynamics of a fireplace. Put a log in a burning fireplace. The log gradually gets so hot that a minor spark can ignite it. This state of maintaining a highly ignitable temperature is called **kindling.** Your control center (limbic–hypothalamic system) reaches such a kindling state by repeated "fires" (stress arousal). These repeated fires (acute stress response) will vary in magnitude.

The set–point of the thermostat (where it is activated) gets turned up by three mechanisms: 1) the hard wire of the neuromuscular circuits, 2) the chemical fuels of high adrenaline–like

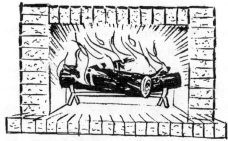
Stress chemicals heat up the control center like a "kindling log."

hormones, lactic acid from tense muscles, and a low buffer system (over breathing), and 3) the vibrations of worries or anxious thoughts. These keep the kindling phenomenon burning. **The goal of relaxation practices is to dampen this kindling.** Furthermore, you can do this dampening piecemeal. Sprinkle on "coolant" by taking deliberate relaxation mini–breaks throughout the day.

Relaxation is not an exercise in the active sense of the word — that is why you cannot make yourself relax or try not to worry. **You can only remove the conditions that provoke or perpetuate the stress arousal, one by one.**

REGULAR RELAXATION PRACTICES– THE ANTIDOTE TO CHRONIC STRESS

Chronic stress occurs when the acute arousal does not return to the baseline. This leads to **nonspecific sensitivity and irritability of the neuromuscular system** along with **free–floating anxiety**. This anxiety occurs without any rhyme or reason because the neuromuscular system is on overdrive. You can reverse this nonspecific charging of your arousal system with regular relaxation drills. This is like putting money into an energy savings account. You can save periodically to increase the bank balance and maintain a surplus reserve.

Sleep and Relaxation

Sleep is the most common mode of relaxation. However, in our stressful society, few enjoy a completely restful sleep. So, supplementary relaxation drills are necessary. Benson shows that sleep reduces the metabolic rate by 8%. The meditative state, on the other hand which reduces it up to 16%. For this reason, a meditative or alpha–theta state gives you a better return of energy dollars for the time invested.

Relaxation is Cyclical

Rest and activity is a law of nature. Your mind–body has to go through the cycle of rest and activity. Every 90 to 120 minutes, your mind tries to day dream as a process of switching from left brain activity to right brain activity. If you counteract this natural phenomenon, you tense up.

Relaxed Work or "Flow"

When you engage in an activity with challenge, commitment, and control, you are in a state of "flow" with nature. In this state of flow, you forget yourself and get engrossed in the task at hand. For example, when you enjoy the breathtaking view of a meadow, you, the view, and the process of seeing become one and the same in a state of flow.

What's on TV?

In the modern lifestyle, most people spend their leisure in front of a television. According to research, 95% of the media focuses on negative news and violence. Children who watch TV often are known to develop more hostility.

Watching TV is shown to increase stress hormone levels in the blood. On the contrary, watching a caring love documentary of Mother Teresa improves the immune system and heart function. Norman Cousins healed his incurable disease by watching comic movies on TV.

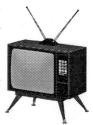

KEY POINTS

1. *Relaxation is "letting go."*
2. *You relax your muscles by stretching the muscle fibers after you contract them.*
3. *You relax your mind by changing the focus from narrow to open.*
4. **The heart is the major oscillator muscle in the body. By relaxing it and opening it, both anatomically and metaphorically, you relax your mind–body.**

12

Mind-Body Dialogue

Mind-Body Dialogue

Mind-Body Language via Messenger Chemicals

A new interdisciplinary science explores how various subsystems of the mind-body communicate with each other. This new science goes by the name of **psycho-neuro-immunology** or "PNI" for short. Breaking the word down, it means mind/spirit/soul (psyche), nervous system (neuron), and immune system (immuno) interaction. After this name was coined in 1981 by Robert Ader, researchers discovered that the endocrine (hormone) system is also part of this grand mind-body network.

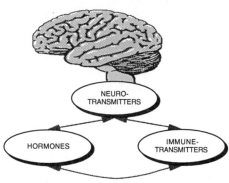

Mind and body are connected by three kinds of messengers.

In studying the interrelationship of these subsystems, researchers found that they communicated with each other via **messenger molecules** or information substances. The messenger molecules have unique shapes that can fit into appropriate receiving areas (receptor sites) in the outer layer of the cell tissue of the brain, nervous system, endocrine glands, lymphatic tissue, and white blood cells. Once connected in this lock-and-key manner, the information can be transferred to activate or tone down the overactivity of the system receiving the information.

The messenger chemicals are mostly manufactured in the brain, particularly in the emotional control center of the limbic system. However, all parts of the total system create messengers.

These information substances fit into three categories: **neurotransmitters** (including neuropeptides), **neuroendocrines** (hormones), and **immune transmitters.**

We refer to these messenger chemicals as the "**liquid media**" of the mind-body. Since nerves also play a part in this communication network, we call them the "**hard wire**" or direct connection of the mind-body. Although not yet addressed, there is a third form of mind-body communication: subtle vibratory energy that also carries messages. We call this the mind-body's "**vibrational whisper.**"

The theory of PNI explains how stress creates mind-body reactions and how actions such as relaxation, meditation, and laughter heal the mind-body.

Although PNI explains how the mind-body communicates via messenger molecules, it doesn't address the content of these messages. We do know that the primary way the mind and body send and receive messages is via the symbolic underlay of "self-talk."

Mind-Body Communication

Your mind is continuously talking to itself as if somebody has turned on a radio talk show. The contents for this **automatic self-talk** come from either your memory bank or newly acquired "real time" perceptions and messages from your sensory organs. At any given time, your mind is either in the mode of self-talk or in the mode of mindfulness. When you are in the mindfulness mode, you see the reactive "self-talk messages" from the body as they occur. This is called **receptive communication** with the body. You can change this self-talk and direct it to your choice of topic. This is **expressive communication** with the body.

Most of your behavior is directed by verbal commands, which come either from others or yourself. In all cases, the final command has to be rephrased or repeated mentally in the form of self-talk. For example, when I ask you to scratch your nose, you have to translate this as, "Okay, now I am going to scratch my nose," and then you do it. Further, the self-talk is translated into nonverbal symbolic images in your mind-body. This symbolic language is called preverbal, because this is how your mind-body talk occurred before you learned your mother tongue as a baby.

Self-talk can be positive affirmations or negative self-criticisms. Becoming mindful of self-talk and reframing the negative thoughts forms the basis of cybernetic healing. However, most of the self-talk is automatic and based on the chemical state your body is in at that time. This chemical state is based on three factors: emotions, body motions, including breathing, and foods and chemicals you ingest.

Mind-Body Symbols

Mind-body communication is a two-way system that occurs as symbols. These symbols simulate your perceptual images. For that reason, they are called **imageries**. Receptive imageries include both **day dreams** and **night dreams.** It is possible to make a "hard copy" of your mental imageries by drawing a picture.

Physician Bernie Siegel asks his cancer patients to draw such a picture of themselves and their illness. Expressive, self-directed imageries include daydreaming fantasies; "scheduling" for night dreams by contemplating a subject prior to going to sleep; and creative visualization for healing or personal growth. **The most negative form of expressive imagery is common worrying**, in which you continuously create self-deprecating images. These symbols are continuously transmitted between the mind and body via the messenger molecules-body chemicals understood by both the mind and body.

Metaphoric language is the verbal equivalent of imagery. Psychologists measure an individual's optimism-pessimism scale on how they use metaphors. Ever since childhood fairy tale time, you've used them.

You can use positive metaphors to heal or self-derogatory metaphors to hurt yourself, because any metaphor you use leaves a marker in your mind-body's intelligence network.

An affliction, such as a fever, heart attack, or cancer, is the body's way of sending a symbolic message to the mind to draw attention to the disregulation of the mind-body.

Although self-talk implies verbal speech, humans actually get and give only 8% of their information through words. The rest comes through body language, such as the breathing rate, inflections, and gestures. They are at a level of internal body awareness. So it is important to learn the body's symbolic coding or internal road map. With this knowledge, you can intercept stress arousal before it happens. This is the benefit of both awareness training and biofeedback.

Communication imagery is enhanced in **altered states of consciousness** such as sleep. Another is the meditative or alpha-theta brain wave state. In meditation, your right brain is dominant, allowing imagery to operate. Meditation allows you to receive symbols from and send symbols to your body. In this manner, the meditative state is like entering an imagery theater. Once you enter the imagery theater, you can watch the show given to you from your body. Or your mind can be the director and create your own show. Furthermore, you can remain in this imagery theater for the length of one breath (two to three seconds) or for as long as a movie.

The mind and body are two ends of the same bridge. For convenience sake, and to show their interdependency, we hyphenate them. This mind-body communication goes on continuously, and to understand it, you can tap into this "hard wire" telegraph, taste the "liquid media" messenger molecules, or listen to the "vibrational whisper."

This tapping into your internal intelligence can be momentary in the form of mindfulness, or extended by entering into the meditative state (alpha-theta state). In either case, you match your mind's "vibes" with your body. When you synchronize the vibes of your mind with the vibes of your body, you are aware of the "state" you are in. This is "awareness of awareness" or state dependent learning.

Mind-Body "Appointments" in Nature

Sleep, night dreams, and day dreams are regular "appointments" for mind-body communication. As you enter sleep (hypnagogic state) and exit sleep (hypnopompic state), your mind-body enters into a meditative state. Once in this state, symbolic dialogue takes place. The day dream cycle that occurs every 90 to 120 minutes is a regular cyclical phenomenon and at this "appointment" time, the mind-body heals from stress and strain.

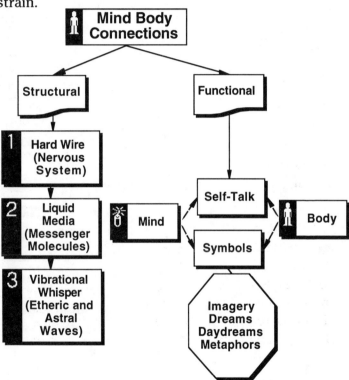

This summarizes the structural and functional aspects of mind-body connections. On the structural side, there are three connections: hard wire, liquid media, and vibrational whisper. On the functional side, there are the self-talk and exchange of symbols. Most of mind-body dialogue occurs underneath your consciousness in the form of imagery, dreams, daydreams and metaphoric symbols. If you create negative imageries and symbols in your mind, your body listens to them and acts accordingly. You can superimpose positive imageries whenever your automatic mind brings a negative imagery. This is the value of imagery work and meditation.

Heart Disease and Cancer

This self-healing process is called the ultradian healing response. If you counteract this healing appointment with coffee or drugs, you are swimming against the tide. If you meditate for a few moments at this time, you are enjoying a swim with the tides of nature.

Blueprint for Healing:

The mind-body has its own blueprint for healing. We use the mnemonic, **PISA**, to teach the optimal states for accessing this blueprint for healing.

Positive Experience includes hope, sensual pleasures (sight, sound, smell, taste, and touch), pleasure of mindful eating, and experience of flow. In a state of flow, you forget yourself and get engrossed in an enjoyable task.

Imagery is either receptive (body to mind) or guided (mind to body).

Self-disclosure is sharing your feelings by sharing time, touch, and talk with a partner.

Altered state is the opposite of a regular wakeful state. This includes sleep, mindfulness, meditation, and biofeedback. In an altered state, your brain waves are in an alpha-theta or delta range, as opposed to beta waves of normal wakefulness.

P	**Positive Experience**	Hope (Spirituality) Sensual Pleasures Mindful Eating "Flow"
I	**Imagery**	Receptive Guided
S	**Self-disclosure**	Time Touch Talk
A	**Altered State**	Sleep Mindfulness Meditation Biofeedback

1. The mind and body exchange messages through self-talk or symbols.

2. Altered states of consciousness, such as sleep, dream, meditation and biofeedback, are conducive for effective mind-body dialogue.

3. Healing dialogue occurs during positive experience, imagery, self-disclosure, and altered states.

13

Emotions of a Heart Event

Emotions of a Heart Event

When someone says, "don't give me a heart attack!," or "that news almost gave me a heart attack," you know the emotional impact that person is experiencing. Heart attack–related emotions fall into before, during, and after any cardiac event.

The causes of a heart event can be divided into two domains:

1. Problem focused

2. Emotion focused

The problem focused factors include high blood pressure, smoking, cholesterol, obesity, sedentary lifestyle, diabetes, etc. The emotion focused factors are emotional reactivity with the self (intrapersonal factors) and with others (interpersonal factors).

The intrapersonal factors include:

1. Hostility and Hot Reactor State.

2. Disconnection with heartfelt feelings (loss of meaning in life); loss of altruism.

3. Loss of control; helplessness, hopelessness.

4. Emotional trauma that is the last straw which breaks the camel's back.

5. Anxiety Disorders.

The interpersonal factors include:

1. Isolation and lack of social support.

2. Job strain.

3. Social or political pressure.

We've studied emotions of the heart event before, during, or after.

BEFORE THE HEART EVENT

We know a good deal about hostility as a pre–heart event factor in type A behavior. Hostility has three components: cynical mistrust, anger, and aggression. A Duke University study showed doctors and lawyers with high hostility scores have a higher incidence of heart disease. Hot reactivity, or increased heart rate and blood pressure, is how a person's body overreacts to anger and stress. Repeated anger–induced injuries to the heart, "primes" the heart to overreact to even minute episodes of anger. This is due to release of anger related hormones, such as adrenaline and noradrenaline.

To understand the action of emotion on the heart, study Peter Nixon's model of the human function curve.

Human Function Curve

The curve is in the shape of an inverted U with an up–slope, peak, and down–slope.

The up–slope is healthy, with performance commensurate with stress arousal. More stress arousal yields better returns. The individual thinks this relationship will continue unlimited in a straight line. But the peak is the point of fatigue. After that, returns diminish as more and more effort is put in. This leads to the down–slope. There is a point of instability, point P, at which one sits and waits for a heart event. Stress hormones, adrenaline, noradrenaline, and cortisol, grease the downslope. These hormones trigger rage and anger, or defeat and despair. On the down–slope, human relationships are very superficial and not associated with caring love or affiliative spirit. This is the state of a workaholic with insomnia who has a never ending urge to

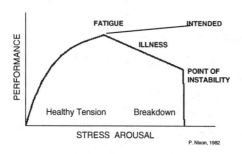

HUMAN FUNCTION CURVE

FATIGUE INTENDED
ILLNESS
POINT OF INSTABILITY
Healthy Tension   Breakdown
PERFORMANCE
STRESS AROUSAL
P. Nixon, 1982

keep doing something.

The hallmark of the down–slope is restless sleep at night, and a restless mind during the day.

The down–slope is a state of vital exhaustion. The difference between healthy fatigue and the down–slope is that during healthy fatigue, you recovery to the base line of energy, In vital exhaustion, there is no recovery.

Vital Exhaustion

About six months to a year before a heart event, the victim feels his or her battery gradually lose its charge. Most people recall three stages before their heart attack.

First: a high stress life for several years.

Second: a lack of meaning, social connectedness, and joy in life for months before the event.

Finally: a few days to weeks before, there is an acute emotional shock, which may or may not be related to the chronic stress factors.

Why this lack of meaning in life? The victim is usually a workaholic, always chasing material things in life, while suppressing heartfelt feelings of caring love, affiliation, and altruism. He/she enters a state of continuous vigilance because of a demand to achieve more and more in less and less time. Human relationships are suppressed.

We find two levels of feelings in our lives; mind level and heart level. Mindfelt feelings are judgmental, and always try to separate things out by answering the question "what is in it for me?" Heartfelt feelings are non–judgmental, and they find unity and caring love in everything.

Life is filled with "report visits" of information processing, problem solving, and earning money. The "rapport visit" of unconditional love, concern, and caring for others, if at all present, appears in a superficial, perfunctory manner. The zest and joy of life is gone.

Loss of Control

Loss of control is felt at many levels. When control in life seems to pass from one's self to others, one becomes more hostile towards those who have it. Personal loss of control is felt at muscle and mind levels. Skeletal muscles become tense and fatigued due to stress arousal. Blood vessel muscles overreact with constriction, which leads to increased blood pressure. The heart muscle overreacts with increased heart beats and erratic heart rate variability.

Heart rate variability is the most sensitive index of yin–yang (parasympathetic–sympathetic) balance. In fact, erratic or low heart rate variability indicates a "brittle heart" ready to break at any moment. Twenty–four hour monitoring shows heart rate variability is a sensitive predictor of sudden cardiac death in patients recovering from a heart attack.

At the mind end, loss of control manifests itself in a restless mind during the day, and restless sleep at night. Emotions are suppressed. The human nature of caring love and compassion withers. There is a disparity between mindfelt and heartfelt feelings. A tug of war goes on in the mind between mindfelt and heartfelt feelings.

Emotional trauma, either major stress load or minor hassle, acts as the "last straw." Many heart attack victims can recall an acute anger episode or catastrophic emotional event just before the heart event.

Lack of social support is the major pivotal factor before and after a heart attack. Family, friends, and coworkers help to dissipate the pent up energy of stress. But, the workaholic's self–centeredness keeps people at a distance and the resulting isolation is a springboard to a catastrophic illness.

People with **high anxiety** have a higher incidence of sudden death from a heart attack. In a long term Harvard study (for 32 years) the researchers asked subjects:

1. Do strange people or places make you afraid?
2. Are you considered a nervous person?

3. Are you constantly keyed up and jittery?
4. Do you often become suddenly scared for no good reason?
5. Do you often break out in a cold sweat?

Each "yes" answer is one point. Men who scored more than two in the scale had a four times higher incidence of sudden cardiac death.

Isolation from society is the hallmark of a cardiac victim. The victim feels lonely in spite of cocktail parties and social get–togethers. For, at the emotional level, there is no companionship. There is an excess of preoccupation with the self. This self–centeredness keeps the stress arousal high because there is no vent for the pent up emotional steam.

Larry Sherwitz, University of California, San Francisco, studied frequency of personal pronouns, "I, me, mine, myself" in thinking and its correlation with heart events. The study showed such excess of "self–referral" went along with a higher incidence of heart events and complications.

Job strain often comes wth high psychosocial demands and low decision latitude. This kind of job takes hard work, but affords very little control, autonomy, or decision over the course of events and tasks. Three research studies make the point:

1. Peter Schnall and his group from Cornell University found that hard work with a poor sense of control produces a high risk of heart attack.
2. A study of 2,000 San Francisco bus drivers showed that latitude of control at the job related to hypertension.
3. The Framingham study showed women with high job demands had a higher incidence of heart disease.

In summary, a sense of loss of control is the key factor. The underlying emotional issue is conflict between mission in life and mission on the job. The mission at the job is often money centered, and the mission in life is always affiliated with caring love.

DURING THE HEART EVENT

The most common response to a heart attack is denial of reality. "Why me? Why now? This cannot happen to me. This is not in my life plan."

Denial helps in the beginning to reduce the fearful stress arousal and thereby reduce the adrenaline–like hormones over-stimulating the heart. But, at the same time, denial may prevent early medical help and lead to catastrophe. In fact, over 60% of deaths due to heart attack occur before reaching the hospital.

There is underlying anxiety and fear. The anxious mind ruminates:

1. Will I live?
2. Will I love?
3. Will I work?
4. Will I play?
5. When is the next attack?

There is anger directed toward self and others in an attempt to answer: Why did this happen to me? Why me? What did I do wrong? This automatically leads to guilt and blame and further reactivity of the heart.

Hospital Anxiety

A heart attack victim goes through various emotional problems in the hospital. Nurses play a major role in recovery. The mechanical, "scientific," robotic attitude of some; bells and whistles of heart monitoring systems; pain and suffering of the illness, disturbed sleep, side effects of drugs, and overall feelings of guilt–all of these lead to extreme anxiety, sometimes called "hospital psychosis."

This is when the "human touch" of caring nurses, concerned doctors, and loving family members help in recovery. A patient needs to be talked to as a person with a heart attack, rather than talked about as a heart attack of certain clinical characteristics (e.g. the left main block patient in room 32).

The role of the family physician, nurses, and family members in extending "caring love" is the crucial point in resetting the heart. It is important to note that when people visit the patient and extend their heartfelt feelings, they heal themselves as well as encourage the patient to heal.

However, the moment of truth is when the patient starts appreciating and extending caring love towards every person involved in his or her care.

The "Mother Teresa Effect" of healing is bidirectional– it heals the victim *as well as the care giver.*

AFTER THE HEART EVENT

After the event, the most common feeling is convalescent depression and irritability. The negative feelings of fear, anger, and guilt consume a lot of energy and this leads to depression. There is some sense of grief due to loss of functions of the body and limitations in lifestyle. Depression leads to defeat, despair, isolation, and a helpless hopeless state. There is a progressive deterioration of balance of the mind–body. Breathing is mostly thoracic and this leads to blow out of carbon dioxide and buffer loss. The outcome is restlessness during the day and inability to sleep at night. This down–slope of the human function curve can lead to progressive deterioration.

The feeling of a "broken heart" continues in the heart attack victim's mind. The key issue is loss of control and meaning in life. Anxiety increases angina and vice versa in a vicious cycle.

The depression may start at the hospital or after returning home. Some people show depression, such as pain, fatigue, and sleep disturbances. Others show mental signs.

Resetting the Emotions

Beat the iron when it is hot. A heart attack is the ideal point in time to change one's lifestyle and emotional style. The heart attack hits the person like a lightning bolt, and this can be used as the ultimate reset button to start a new way of life. It is the crack that lets the victim see the light which can illuminate the rest of his or her life.

Moment of Truth

The moment of truth is a concept from the Japanese management system of Kyzen (Kaizen). **The moment of truth is the moment when contact makes an impact**. In a way, the feeling of having had a "brush with death" leads to a shamanistic awakening of the spirit inside. But, we found at this moment, the patient does not have the knowledge, skill, or guidance to undertake essential steps in changing his or her lifestyle.

With our cybernetic resetting tools (especially accessing heartfelt feelings and changing the "I–ness" from the head to the anatomical and metaphorical heart) one can make the best use of this "moment of truth" repeatedly, so that before leaving the hospital, one can transform the tool into a skill which is part of one's lifestyle thereafter. **You can start re–setting your heart immediately—whether you've had a heart attack or are just afraid of one.**

The emotional roller coaster of heart events is summarized in the following graphics.

On the down–slope of the string of events, there is denial, depression, and defeat leading to helpless hopelessness. We introduce heartfelt resonant imaging. This resets the heartfelt feelings, which automatically helps to reduce the reactivity.

Additionally, we train patients to reduce heart reactivity by biofeedback training of heart rate variability, hand temperature training, emotional sweating response, diaphragmatic breathing retraining, and muscle relaxation training.

The emotion control and reactivity control leads to self–sufficiency and resets the self–regulation of mind–body. **This is learned optimism. You are retrained to adopt an optimistic attitude in life.**

We train our patients to send and receive love using computer feedback. This energizes the mind–body by removing misplaced effort and reconnecting social support. Prayer by relatives and friends adds to the support. Our self–disclosure technique using the time, touch, and talk, helps increase intimacy and replaces isolation with loving companionship.

The heart disease victim is repeatedly ruminating about his problems. We overlay this with imagery of the healing heart, opening of coronary arteries, and heartfelt feelings of caring love. A simple procedure is to close your eyes, breathe out three times, and focus your awareness on your heart and create healing imageries.

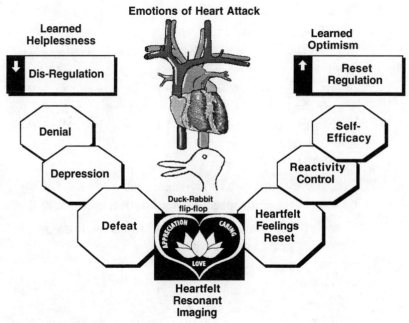

Emotions of Heart Attack

Learned Helplessness

Dis-Regulation

Denial

Depression

Defeat

Duck-Rabbit flip-flop

Heartfelt Resonant Imaging

APPRECIATION CARING LOVE

Learned Optimism

Reset Regulation

Self-Efficacy

Reactivity Control

Heartfelt Feelings Reset

LEARN FROM SABRE

We encourage our patients to memorize **SABRE** (named after Peter Nixon's model from Europe).

S for Sleep, we teach progressive relaxation, meditation, and restless mind contro to regain control over sleep.

A for Arousal control by meditation or relaxation response and our complete set of tools for stress control.

B for Breathing mindfully and diaphragmatically.

R for Rest and Activity. Maintain the rhythm of life by pay-ing attention to the ultradian healing response of rest every 90–120 minutes.

E is for Esteem built up by heartfelt feelings, self–actual-ization, and self–disclosure.

MEASUREMENT IS SCIENCE

The scientific approach involves measuring, monitoring, and modifying the cause and effect relationship. In this book, we are using tools in each area.

Measuring Tools

1. We use the **human function curve as a main measur-ing tool** to track the emotional roller coaster of a heart event. The goal is to keep the person on the up–slope where the in–put gives proportionate returns in life. We constantly remind patients of the down–slope disorders and train them to return to the up–slope using our self–regulatory tools.

2. The Money Function Curve measures one's relationship to money as contrasted with affiliative motives in life.

3. Cross check of energy exchange measure human rela-tionships and energy exchange.

Monitoring Tools

1. Mindful snapshot method (CyberZen) to monitor be-havior in the area of actions, thoughts, and emotions.

2. Heartfelt resonant imaging to monitor the head and heart conflicts and heal by caring love.

3. Energy quadrants monitor the energy cost of emotions.

Modifying Tools

The modifying tools include meditation, stress control, mindful eating, self–disclosure, and physical exercise. HRI is a powerful tool to develop altruism in a biological way.

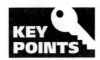

1. Heart events, such as an angina, irregular heart beats, and a heart attack, often lead to the cascade of emotions: denial, depression, and defeat.

2. The victim of these heart events is at a crossroads to deteriorate or escape from helplessness.

3. The steps to escape from helplessness are: heartfelt resonant imaging, anger control, reactivity control, and stress control leading to self–efficacy. The tools to achieve this self–efficacy are given in the chapter Resetting Tools.

14

New Biology of Emotions

New Biology of Emotions

The fields of behavioral science, biochemistry, and physics have all given us a new understanding of our emotions. Here, we summarize this new knowledge under these headings:

1. **What is Emotion?**
   - Iceberg Model of Behavior
   - Five Cardinal Emotions
   - Anger and Love Icebergs

2. **Why Do We Need Emotion?**
   - Experience of Emotion
   - Two Worlds of Experience
   - Centering of Emotional Experience
   - Mindfelt and Heartfelt Feelings

3. **Chemical Basis of Feelings**

4. **Neuromuscular Basis of Emotions**
   - Muscle-to-Mind and Mind-to-Muscle Traffic

5. **Power of Emotional Energy**
   - Physiology of Energy
   - Tomkin's Model of Nerve Traffic
   - Intrapersonal Energy: Emotional Quadrants
   - Interpersonal Energy: Vectors of Emotional Energy

6. **Evolution of Human Emotion**
   - Triune Brain
   - Conditioned Response

FIRST, WHY LEARN ABOUT THE NEW BIOLOGY OF EMOTIONS?

Would you rather degenerate AND DIE IN INSTALLMENTS, or live and THRIVE WITH PLEASURE? Base your decision on the following considerations:

- **ANGER KILLS,**
- **WILL IT KILL *ME*?**
- **CARING LOVE SAVES,**
- **CAN IT SAVE *ME*?**

We will help you answer these questions in the next two chapters. In this chapter, we examine foundations to answer these questions.

What is the New Biology?

The new biology of emotions extends from microcosm to macrocosm. At the atomic level, anger and stress create a free radical attack, which we counter with antioxidants. The antioxidant level goes up with positive emotions of love and pleasure.

At the molecular level, endorphins are chemicals of love. Catecholamines (adrenaline-like chemicals) are chemicals of anger.

At the electrical level, heart rate variability is smooth and regular with emotions of caring love. It is erratic with anger and frustration.

At the body level, the immune system gets suppressed by anger and becomes stronger with love. Healing from deadly diseases, such as heart disease and cancer, is possible by positive emotions of caring love, altruism, and spirituality.

1. WHAT IS EMOTION?

Emotion is evolving motion. It is a tendency to act, and it requires energy. Emotion is the basis of human behavior.

The iceberg model of human behavior helps clarify the concept.

ICEBERG MODEL OF HUMAN BEHAVIOR

Human behavior has three components: action or muscle contraction; thought; and emotion. The iceberg tip is action or

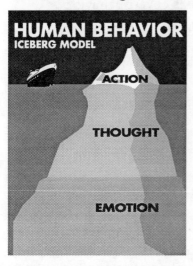

muscle contraction. This is **overt behavior**, the part which we see. But under the surface is **covert or hidden behavior**: thoughts and emotions. We cannot see the expression of covert behavior. Yet the person we observe experiences these thoughts and emotions. Covert behavior is also associated with muscle contraction. However, this level of muscle contraction can only be proven by amplification systems, such as biofeedback recording equipment.

Actions: Action is the contraction of a muscle. When your hand moves, the muscles contract. You and others see it. When you smile, others get feedback from the contracting muscles in your face, and they know you are happy. At the same time, you get internal feedback feeling happy.

Thoughts: Thoughts are like electrical sparks. These sparks travel from nerve cell to nerve cell, similar to the way electricity travels through wires. Your thoughts become images or pictures in your mind's eye when you focus on these thoughts for one to three seconds. These images release chemicals in your brain and body, called **neurotransmitters.** The neurotransmitters mix with other chemicals, called **hormones** and **immunetransmitters,** and thus produce the **"liquid media soup"** of your body. All of your cells swim in this soup. So, every thought has a neuromuscular part and a chemical part in your body.

Emotions: There is always an emotion going on in your

mind and body. Every emotion has its own neuromuscular component and chemical component. **Emotions are there to experience and express feelings.** When an emotion is expressed, others know how you feel. When an emotion is experienced, you know how you feel. Visible expression of emotion is overt. The subtle experience of emotion is covert behavior.

Changing the Components of the Behavior Iceberg

The way you change actions, thoughts, and emotions differs. You change actions by repeating the correct action. This **retraining**, when you repeat a new action, new cell to cell connection pathways (synapses) take place in the brain. This is neuro-associative learning or neurolinguistic programming (NLP). You can do the repetitions covertly in your mental imagery or overtly in action. The NLP remembers the sequence. For example, Vic Braden, a tennis master, says if you use a forehand grip for serving, and want to change to a continental grip, repeat the new grip in your mind or in action at least a 1000 times, and you will change your habit. Repetition is the basis of dog training, learning to type, or any muscle-based activity.

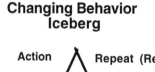

Changing Behavior Iceberg

Action
Repeat (Retrain)

Thoughts
Reframe

Emotion
Replace

You change thoughts by **reframing them**. You question the thought and reframe the interpretation of the thought. By repeating this several times, you have established a new pattern of thoughts. This is **cognitive restructuring**. It's like bringing a defense lawyer to argue in your favor and against your negative thoughts. You then correct your distorted and judgmental thoughts. Heart-centered thinking automatically takes away the negative frame of thought.

In the graphic, change from a horizontal frame to a vertical frame changes the duck into a rabbit. The simple process

Heart Disease and Cancer

Duck-Rabbit Reframing

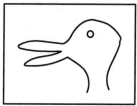 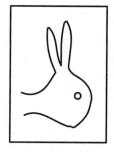

of reframing a thought or idea changes your perspective. For example, traditionally people believed that milk was good for your body. Now, cholesterol awareness has reframed that idea and suggests you avoid milk. Advertising uses reframing to change your belief system.

Emotions do not listen to logic or retraining by repetition. Emotions are changed by **replacing** the old emotion with a new one. This is called *desensitizing*. When you replace an emotion with another, you are overlaying old chemistry a new one. **This is how you replace anger with caring love.** The easiest way to control anger is to replace it with caring love in your mind-body right away. This skill can be learned by using the HRI method described elsewhere in the book.

FIVE BASIC FEELINGS

We have two primary emotions or feelings-fear and love. Fear is a negative emotion because you move away from it. Love is a positive emotion because you move towards it. The reason for fear is self-protection, which leads to the "fight or flight" reaction. This means you either combat or run away from

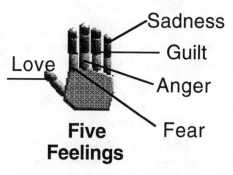

the object of fear. The reason for love is affiliation and satisfaction, which gives pleasure and joy. You can further divide fear into three other negative emotions: anger, guilt, and sadness.

ICEBERG OF ANGER AND LOVE

The iceberg model shows that the visible tip misleads if you do not know the vastness of the base on which it sits. The Titanic sank because the captain underestimated the iceberg's unseen base. The iceberg of anger has three parts: the tip is aggression, the middle part is cynical thoughts, and the base is anger.

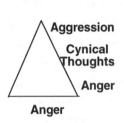

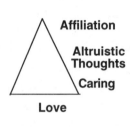

In the iceberg of love, the tip is the action of affiliation and the middle is altruistic thoughts (the concept that "you are also included in my agenda"). The base is the feeling of "I care for you."

2. WHY WE NEED EMOTIONS

We need emotions for survival, protection, and adjustment to the environment. Emotion has two purposes: experience and expression of life. The experience of emotion has two different worlds.

TWO WORLDS OF EXPERIENCE:

You live outside your skin and inside your skin.

The Outside World

You perceive your external world with your five basic senses: sight, sound, taste, smell, and touch. You also have a sixth sense, the sense of position in space called proprioception. Your outside world includes people, things, and events.

The Internal World

The world inside your skin is your own mind-body, and you perceive it differently. This awareness of one's internal state is called **interoception**. The internal state is a combination of all of your muscle contractions. These muscles include your skeletal or voluntary muscles, smooth muscles or involuntary muscles, and muscles of the heart.

You can easily explain your external perceptions with the verbal statements such as "I heard the dog barking," "I saw the dog running," "I smell coffee," etc. **You cannot easily explain your internal sensations because they are not object oriented.** But, you can recognize your own internal sensations by orienting yourself to them.

When you orient yourself to your internal sensations, you have to position yourself in a **vantage point**. For example, you can be head centered, heart centered, gut centered, breath centered, etc. to experience what is happening in your own mind-body. You **anchor** yourself to a vantage point to experience your internal world. The three common anchor zones are:

1. Head.

2. Heart.

3. Belly and Breathing.

Heart as a Reference Point

Modern life has trained you to center yourself in your head, because that is where you identify your thoughts.

You can also center yourself in your heart, and evaluate the experience of the moment. If you have a problem in a certain part of the body, most of your attention centers on it. A sore thumb for example. You center on it, no matter whatever else you try to do.

In heart centered thinking, you deliberately focus your awareness in your anatomical heart area. An emotional state is like a house with multiple windows. What you see inside the house is based on the window of reference. Thus, you can have the heart or the head as a reference point. The basic difference is that the heart is non-judgmental. The head is judgmental.

Interoception of Emotions

Internal perception of emotions includes "muscle sense," or sense created by the muscles. Muscles fall into three groups: (1) Skeletal or voluntary; (2) Smooth or involuntary; (3) Heart.

New Biology of Emotions

You can consciously increase or decrease skeletal muscle tension. The smooth muscles of different tubes in the body (gut, lungs, urinary tract, blood vessels, etc.) create stretching and distending sensations. The heart makes you aware of pulsating sensations.

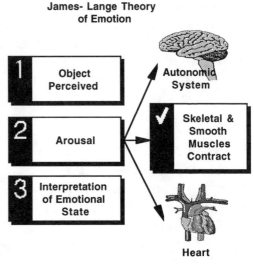

The **James-Lange Theory of Emotions** summarizes how your body perceives emotions, as seen in the diagram.

1. Object perceived: the sensory organs see, hear, smell, touch, or taste; the mind creates an imagery of these sensations.

2. Arousal: there is immediate arousal of the body components.

3. The autonomic nervous system is stimulated.

4. Muscles attached to bones (skeletal) and muscles around the tubes of the body contract.

5. The heart beats harder and faster.

6. All of these events are perceived as an emotional state.

PERSPECTIVE OF CENTERING

The human mind tries to orient itself to a center and anchor experiences to that center. You center in two directions: externally to the outside world and internally to your mind-body or internal world. Internal centering is either focused on the head or the heart.

Let us study the external world centering. There are two distinct motivational areas in which to center your mind at any given time:

1. Achievement-motivated.

2. Affiliation-motivated.

Your achievement-motivated centering is mostly related to money, work, material possessions, or name and fame. One problem with this type of **materialistic centering** is that your mood or mind-body balance fluctuates according to the "market value" of your material possessions. The common example is the depression of your mood when your stocks' prices drop.

	External World	Internal World
Achievement	Money	Head
Affiliation	Love	Heart

Your affiliation-motivated centering is your relationships with people. This is the way you relate to your spouse, parents, children, co-workers, friends, enemies, society at large, animals, and plants. This is **principle-based centering** rather than money-based centering.

If you use caring love, appreciation, and compassion as the basic center of your life, you do not have to worry about devaluation or appreciation of these values. The value is not based on outside factors, but on your internal chemistry. You can learn to call on this internal chemistry by following certain simple rituals explained later as heartfelt resonant imaging.

HEARTFELT AND MINDFELT FEELINGS

Heartfelt feelings only know how to love. Mindfelt feelings know how to love and hate.

The tendency to protect your personal turf keeps your mindfelt feelings on top of your mind even if it is against the wishes of the heart. Thus, the two feelings, heartfelt and mindfelt, can

Head Centered or Heart Centered
1. Judgmental or Non-judgmental.
2. Report or Rapport.
3. Adrenaline or Endorphin.
4. Heart Rate Smooth or Erractic.
5. Yang or Yin.

either agree with each other, a condition called **resonance**, or disagree with each other, a condition called **dissonance**.

It is dissonance that causes conflict and stress in your life. Heartfelt feelings are felt from the vantage point of the anatomical heart. Mindfelt feelings are felt from the vantage point of the head.

Differences between Mindfelt and Heartfelt Feelings

Making Judgments: Mindfelt feelings are judgmental–always trying to decide "what is in it for me? Is it good or bad for me?" Heartfelt feelings are non-judgmental. Mindfelt feelings result from mind-talk or inner dialogue with one's intellect. Heartfelt feelings are undistorted perceptions. We call it "mindfulness."

Report vs Rapport Transactions: Mindfelt feelings seek factual reports or information. The motive here is to achieve something. Heartfelt feelings are rapport-based and the motive here is to affiliate with others.

Mindfelt feelings try to describe in a verbal language, while heartfelt feelings try to experience in a pre-verbal, non-linguistic way. Mindfelt feelings often equate to knowledge, intelligence, and problem solving. Heartfelt feelings often equate to wisdom and intuition.

Chemical Messengers: Mindfelt feelings are often fear, anger, guilt, and sadness. These states are accompanied by stress chemicals: adrenaline, noradrenaline, and cortisol. Heartfelt feelings are often caring love, appreciation, compassion, and pleasure. These states are accompanied by endorphins, serotonin, phenylethylamine, and oxytocin.

Electrical Resonance: The heart and brain produce their own electrical waves. These waves are in sync during heartfelt feelings, and out of sync during mindfelt feelings.

Yin-Yang Balance: Mindfelt feelings create a sense of vigilance and stimulate the yang system of stress arousal. Heartfelt feelings stimulate the yin system and calm down the stress arousal. The yang is the sympathetic branch of the nervous system. The yin is the parasympathetic branch of the nervous system. It is a well-established scientific fact that heart rate variability reduction heralds sudden cardiac death, and we can trace this to the weakening of the parasympathetic system.

3. CHEMICAL BASIS OF FEELINGS

We release different chemicals during different emotions. We produce endorphin, phenylethylamine, and oxitocin with love. We produce adrenaline, noradrenaline, and cortisol in periods of frustration and anger.

New Biology of Addiction

You know addiction behavior is harmful to you, but you cannot stop it. Addicts have a low brain serotonin level and their brain wave is deficient in the alpha-theta range. New research shows these chemical and brain wave abnormalities can be rectified by alpha-theta brain wave feedback therapy.

4. NEUROMUSCULAR BASIS OF EMOTIONS

Muscle-to-Mind and Mind-to-Muscle Traffic

Impulses travel along the mind-body's information super highway from muscle to brain and brain to muscle. The "up" traffic from muscle to brain is called sensory, because it takes sensory messages to the brain. "Down" traffic from brain to muscle is called motor, because it carries action orders to muscles. Traffic congestion can occur at either terminal.

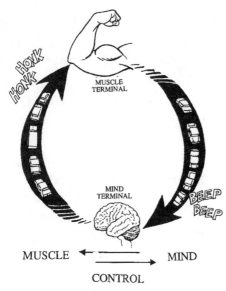

Traffic congestion at the mind end results in a **restless racing mind** with a narrow focus of attention. Traffic congestion in the muscle end causes **muscle tension** with shortened muscle fibers.

To relieve the traffic congestion at the mind terminal, you have to open your attention focus so that traffic gets distributed to multiple channels. To relieve the traffic congestion at the muscle end, you have to stretch those muscles by movement, exercise, yoga, or progressive relaxation.

Breathing connects the muscle and mind terminals with a common bridge. You can use breathing to alter the traffic congestion at either end. Also, synchronizing your awareness to the rhythm of your breathing relieves the traffic congestion at both the mind and muscle terminals.

5. POWER OF EMOTIONAL ENERGY

Physiology of Energy

Emotions drive energy flow. Energy comes from combustion of glucose, fat, and protein in the presence of oxygen. This is like burning gasoline and oxygen in an automobile engine. Your brain is a major energy consumer. It is only 2% of the total body mass, but consumes 25% of the body's energy. How that energy gets used is determined by insulin secretion, which converts glucose to release energy. If you don't eat often, insulin secretion goes up and down like a roller coaster. If you have a "grazing diet," and eat every two hours, insulin secretion doesn't go very high or very low.

Impulses travel between muscle and mind. Energy consumption, fatigue, pain, or pleasure experienced by any emotion corresponds to this back and forth nerve impulse travel.

You get traffic congestion if impulses are too rapid and narrowed into fewer lanes. In a state of caring love, the nerve traffic is distributed into multiple channels, which leads to the release of tension and the onset of pleasure. Tomkin models this nerve impulse traffic.

Tomkin's Model of Nerve Traffic

Nerve traffic has three distinct patterns according to Tomkin.

1. **Sudden increase** of nerve traffic and tension, as in the cases of startled reaction, fear, and impulse of interest.

2. **Sudden decrease** of nerve traffic with a release of tension felt in the cases of laughter, joy, and love.

Tomkin's Model of Emotional Traffic

3. Nerve traffic is **high and sustained** in the cases of anger and distress.

Intrapersonal Energy Quadrants

You always have some kind of emotion. "You cannot *not* feel." The energy cost of each emotion decides whether or not you waste energy in misplaced effort.

We divide the emotions into four quadrants: high positive (pleasure, love, "flow"), low positive (sleep, rest, meditation), high negative (fear, anger), and low negative (guilt, sadness, and repression).

Energy Quadrants of Emotions

High + Pleasure Love Flow	*High -* Fear Anger
Low + Sleep, Rest Meditation	*Low -* Guilt, Sadness Repression

Scan your mind-body at any given time to see what each emotion is costing you in energy, and how much of it is misplaced. We'll explain further in the tool section.

Interpersonal Vectors of Emotional Energy

You gain or lose energy depending on how you interact in the horizontal axis and vertical axis of intimacy. Vertically, you deal with your higher self and your mind-body network.

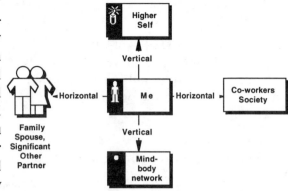

network. Horizontally, you deal with your spouse, partner, immediate family, or society at large. You can inventory directions of your own emotions. This graphic summarizes the concept.

6. EVOLUTION OF HUMAN EMOTIONS

Triune Brain

In the process of evolution, our brain came through three stages:

1. **The vital brain or reptilian brain** (like snakes): This part of the brain controls vital functions, such as heart rate, blood pressure, respiration, and temperature control. The vital brain is in the medulla and pons part of the brain stem.

This is the "cold blooded" part of the brain that does not have feelings. In fact, the reptilians kill their own species. That is why we use the expression "cold blooded murder"

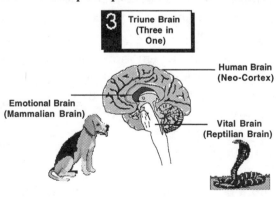

to denote merciless killing.

2. **The emotional brain** is in the limbic system. It is the mammalian brain because breast-feeding animals show affection and care towards their offspring.

The emotional brain gears up to move towards love, or away from fear. Fear in humans has shades of anger, guilt, and sadness as well. Biologically, humans have the same capacity for unconditional love as other mammals. But, as we evolved, we started suppressing this emotion to such an extent that caring love is in danger of becoming extinct in our lives.

3. **The human brain, neocortex,** or intellectual brain is a two-edged sword. It allows us to process information, think of the past, plan the future, use computers and solve problems by "data processing." But we also ruminate on the past and become anxious about the future. This suppresses our emotional brain, and we live a life of information processing, judging others, identifying and solving problems.

The cortical brain has two distinct levels of feelings: mindfelt feelings based on judgment, and heartfelt feelings inherited from our mammalian ancestors.

The true solace for humans is to recover and retrain the emotional part of the brain. This comes from learning how to experience caring love.

CONDITIONED RESPONSE OF EMOTION

The Russian physiologist, Pavlov, discovered conditioned emotional response. This conditioning occurs at three stages:

Before Training: The dog responds to the ringing of the bell by nonspecific orienting reaction.

During Training: The dog is fed while ringing the bell. The dog associates the ringing of the bell with meat feeding. The dog learns to associate and salivate with the ringing of the bell.

After Training: The dog salivates just at the sound of the bell, even if the meat is not given.

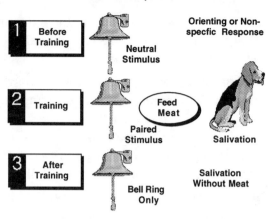

Conditioned Response

1. Before Training — Neutral Stimulus — Orienting or Non-specfic Response
2. Training — Paired Stimulus — Feed Meat — Salivation
3. After Training — Bell Ring Only — Salivation Without Meat

Conditioning any emotional response has a chemical basis. As a child, we all associated contact with people as a feeling of affiliation and love. This condition was associated with the release of endorphin-like chemicals which made us feel happy and euphoric.

During our teens, we changed. New contacts with people might be competitive, or at least, interruption in our personal agenda. This perceived "interruption" released stress hormones, such as adrenaline and noradrenaline. Thus, we began feeling grouchy and disturbed when we met new people. Along with the chemical changes in the body, the conditioning causes changes in the autonomic nervous system, muscles of the body, and heart. This is **state dependent learning** because the state of anger or state of caring love gets associated with a particular situation.

The beauty of state dependent learning is that if we can learn any particular behavior, we can unlearn or superimpose the learning with a new learning. We use caring love as a tool to develop this new learning. The following is the sequence of events in this new learning:

Childhood: Contact with people we learn as a caring love state with a release of endorphins.

Adulthood: Contact with people we learn as a vigilant or hostile episode, with release of noradrenaline.

Heartfelt Resonant Image Training: You relearn the childhood reflex of caring love by focusing on your heart area and asking the question, "Can I experience caring love towards this person, animal, or object?" The heart always says yes, and when it does, you are releasing endorphins and creating the childlike new association. Thus, you rediscover caring love for the second time in your life.

The key point of learning the new biology of emotions is to develop skill for synchronizing your heartfelt and mindfelt feelings. This removes the conflict between your brain and heart and releases endorphins (chemicals of caring love) in place of catecholamines (chemicals of anger and frustration). One of our young patients suggested this graphic to illustrate the point.

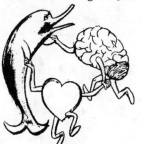

When the heart and brain dance in sync, the dolphins (endorphins) jump high.

15
How Anger Kills *You*

The number one killer in the world is anger. On a death certificate, it gets translated as heart disease or cancer.

How Anger Kills You

In this chapter, we will answer two basic questions:

1. How does anger kill?
2. Will it kill *me*?

WHAT IS ANGER?

We can show it visually using the iceberg model of human behavior.

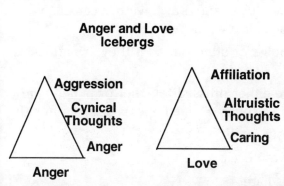

Anger and Love Icebergs

Aggression

Cynical Thoughts

Anger

Anger

Affiliation

Altruistic Thoughts

Caring

Love

Iceberg of Hostility

As we've shown earlier, human behavior is like an iceberg. The tip of the iceberg symbolizes actions. The middle, thoughts, and the base, feelings. The tip of the *anger* iceberg is aggression, the middle part is cynical thoughts, and the base is anger.

AGGRESSION: When you attack someone or yourself with anger, it is aggression. You assault others verbally or physically. If you choose not to express your aggression, you attack your own body by suppressing anger. Aggression is easily visible as verbal or physical attack. Less visible is aggression expressed through subtle body language.

CYNICAL THOUGHTS: Cynical thoughts come from the basic motive of "what's in it for me?" and "you're disturbing my personal agenda." Sometimes we refer to these thoughts as cynical mistrust. For example, in the supermarket express lane, which allows only nine items or less, the cynic counts items the person ahead has, because the cynic doesn't trust that person.

ANGER: The base of the iceberg is anger with its biochemical component. The chemistry of anger is felt as muscle contractions in the "pumps and pipes" of the body. Collectively, these sensations are anger.

EXPRESSION OF ANGER AND LOVE

Anger is expressed by holding your breath, rapid or irregular breathing, and tense muscles all over your body, and most noticeably, in an "angry face:"

• Your eyebrows lower and draw together, causing vertical lines between them. In a word, you frown.

• Your eyes bulge or stare out as if they are attacking someone.

• Your lips are either pressed together or pulled apart, exposing the teeth in a square shaped opening of your mouth.

• You grind your teeth.

• You squint your eyes.

• Your nostrils flare.

• You clench your fists.

• You talk louder than usual.

Love and pleasure are expressed by momentary breath holding followed by regular breathing.

• Your laugh lines or crow's feet wrinkle around your eyes, creating "smiling eyes" from "smiling mind."

• The corners of your lips turn up. In a clear smile, the upper lips pull up, causing wrinkling around the nose and exposing the upper teeth.

Expressed anger is mostly created by adrenaline and noradrenaline (catecholamine–like chemicals). Expressed love is mostly created by endorphins (opioids), phenylethylamine (in romantic love), and oxytocin (cuddling love).

It takes at least seventy–five muscles to frown with anger, but only fifteen muscles to smile with love.

Big and Small Anger

You may think you very rarely "explode," and so you can escape the killer trap of anger.

Research shows this is not true. It is the small hassles that make a big difference in the basic question: "Anger kills, but will it kill *me*?"

Anger releases adrenaline and its brother, noradrenaline.

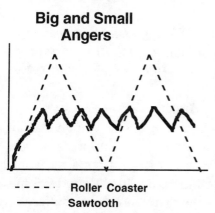

Big and Small Angers

– – – – Roller Coaster
——— Sawtooth

We call this family of these anger chemicals catecholamines. Love releases endorphin and its cousins, enkephalin and dynorphin. This family of love chemicals is known as opioids. All are released throughout the body in a split second. For example, if somebody steps on your toe, you instantly get angry. Chemicals are the cause. If you see a beautiful flower, at a glance, you fall in love with it , thanks to pleasure chemicals instantly released.

There are such moments; totaling hundreds in a minute; thousands in an hour and millions in a day. The graph shows pleasure and pain produce the biological effects of healing and illness in frequent, saw–tooth–like, small increments, rather than in a few extreme roller coaster highs and lows.

The anger which is present in you at all times is triggered by trivial happenings, or **free–floating hostility.** It floats free because there is no specific stimulus for such anger. The importance of trivial free–floating hostility is well–summarized by anger researcher, Redford Williams, in his book, *Anger Kills:*

"Anger kills. We're speaking here not about the anger

---

that drives people to shoot, stab, or otherwise wreak havoc on their fellow humans. We mean instead the everyday sort of anger, annoyance, and irritation that courses through the minds and bodies of many perfectly normal people.

If your immediate impulse when faced with everyday delays or frustrations – elevators that don't immediately arrive at your floor, slow–moving supermarket lines, dawdling drivers, rude teenagers, broken vending machines – is to blame somebody;

If this blaming quickly sparks your ire toward the offender;

If your ire often manifests itself in aggressive action; then, for you, getting angry is like taking a small dose of some slow–acting poison – arsenic, for example – every day of your life."

Covert or Overt Expression of Anger

If you express your anger by acting it out, you give away the original and keep a carbon copy. If you suppress it, you save the original and give out a carbon copy. No matter what, the harmful chemistry of anger takes place in your body. Some do not overtly express their anger. They are silent sufferers. Yet their body language shows anger; their thoughts are cynical, and the biochemical changes of anger simmerbeneath the surface. All cultures read the basic emotions of joy, fear, anger, guilt, and sadness in others. We act and interact with each other's emotions as if we constantly hold a mirror to each other.

You'll see this in type A and type C behavior. (Incidentally, we prefer the term type A and type C *behavior* rather than *personality types*. The same person will display type A, B, or C behaviors at different times.)

Type A behavior takes the form of overt and open anger, and verbal or physical aggression. Type C behavior is stoic, silent suffering of suppressed and repressed anger. Type B behavior falls in the middle, with a balanced expression of anger at the present moment, and a recovery to a normal state at the

---

next moment (like a child or lower animal). Type A behavior is associated with high blood pressure and heart attacks; type C with cancer, autoimmune disorders, and depression.

Type A Behavior and Hostility

Two San Francisco cardiologists, Meyer Friedman and Ray Rosenman, published research of type A behavior in 1959. By the 1970s, type A behavior was widely accepted in the scientific community as at risk for heart attack. Type A behavior has three parts: time pressure or hurry sickness, excessive competitiveness, and hostility. Time pressure shows up as talking, walking, eating fast, and thinking multiple thoughts at a time.

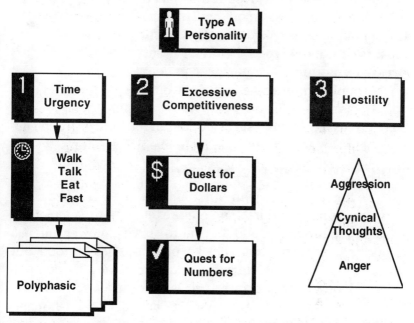

Excessive competitiveness appears as a quest for dollars and for achievement in life. Hostility looks like our iceberg, with a base of anger, a middle portion of cynical mistrust, and a tip of aggressive acts. **The most toxic part of type A behavior is hostility,** as clarified by Duke University research.

Type C Behavior and Hostility

Type C behavior was first described by San Francisco researcher Deborah Temoshok. The type C cascades progressively from level to level: from resistance, to resentment, to rejection, to repression, and finally to alexithymia. With your hostility, you first resist, then resent and reject, while still suppressing your emotions. You continue to suppress your anger, and when suppression becomes subconscious (repression), you finally lose your ability to experience or express emotions. This emotional numbness is called alexithymia. **The most toxic part of type C behavior is suppressed emotions.** Many cancer patients have trouble expressing emotions. Women with breast cancer felt angrier in the year before their illnesses were discovered. Expressing emotions in the form of group support helps breast cancer patients to live twice as long.

Type C Cascade

Resistance

Resentment

Rejection

Repression

Alexithymia

WHERE DID ANGER COME FROM?

We humans share with other animals the basic needs for survival. We hunger, thirst, and require temperature regulation. We also require anger, and arousal to survive. Lower animals either hunt or are hunted. They kill other species for food, but love their own species. Humans are different. We kill other animals for food, and kill our own species out of anger. In the movie, "The Jungle Book," Mowgli says, "We animals kill for hunger; you humans kill for anger."

In this information age, biological survival of the fittest becomes survival of the smartest. Humans not only get angry with other humans as other animals occasionally do, but we remember grudges in the future, and ruminate on past grudges in the present. This leads to litigation and war.

Today, war among nations is less likely. The biggest war is within ourselves: ruminating on past errors anxiously worrying about the future. In the rat race to become the smartest information processor and problem solver in life, we compete with each other. With subtle hostility, we figure how to accomplish personal agendas in the least amount of time and in the most productive way. This "what is in it for me" attitude preoccupies our minds with self–talk of "I, me, mine, myself." An interesting research from Larry Sherwitz at the University of San Francisco shows this preoccupation with the self carries a high risk of heart attack.

Were You Angry As a Baby?

All babies are born with the potential to love and be loved. Why then, do humans become angry most of the time? We can learn from a scientific study comparing how Japanese and American children are raised.

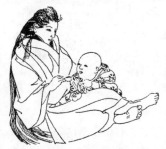

In the American system, we want the child to become "independent" as early as possible. The child sleeps in its own crib in a separate room. The mother pays attention to the baby's cry only at feeding time or if the diaper is wet. The child is given "conditional love" only when the mother feels it is appropriate for the culture. The idea is to make the baby independent and avoid "spoiling."

In many Eastern countries, the baby sleeps with the mother. There is immediate attention to the baby's cry with touch and "unconditional love." This study by Caudill of the National Institute of Mental Health showed that Japanese children age two to six are more affiliative and *interdependent*. American children are more *independent*. The hostility score tests showed that Japanese children are less hostile than American children. The Japanese culture calls caring love *"amae."* The standard psychological tests to evaluate hostility (Ho scale of MMPI) show that because of *amae* from childhood onwards, Japanese people have less hostility, atherosclerosis, and coronary artery disease than Americans.

The unconditional trusting trait of Japanese people is called *amae*. Type A behavior expert, Friedman, in his book, *Treating Type A and Your Heart,* states lack of unconditional love and affection during childhood leads to type A hostility in adulthood.

Children up until age six or seven are like the lower warm-blooded animals, either in a playful mood (bubbling with endorphin–like chemicals) or in a state of restful alertness in a meditative alpha–theta state. In this state, the only emotion they know is unconditional love. If they get angry, it's momentary. They forget quickly, as do lower animals.

The spoiled child is conditioned to a "self–fulfilling prophecy," and becomes hostile when its self–righteousness is not realized. In a way, we all are spoiled children. We keep tracking life with this selfish judgment, and when we do not get our way, we get angry. But it's not all bad news. If we can learn to get angry, we can learn to love again as well. The ability to love like a child is wired in our nervous systems and we can reclaim it.

How We Learn Anger

Anger is a conditioned reflex. It is Pavlov's dog, all over again. We develop an adrenaline-releasing, anger-provoking conditioned reflex every time other human beings who interfere in the personal agenda of our busy lives. You become conscious of your own personal agenda as you grow up. You feel the presence of another person around you as a subtle nuisance. Each time you experience this you release anger chemicals. Several thousand repetitions later, you've created a cause and effect for every time you meet someone. Ask yourself, "Do I feel a subtle disturbance in my mind, as if this person is intruding in my personal agenda?" If your answer is yes, you are experiencing subtle anger towards that person.

COST OF ANGER

The cost of anger is summarized in the graphics: biological damages by anger.

Biological Cost of Anger

1. **Anger and stress:** Anger causes an immediate fight or flight (acute stress) reaction and sustained vigilance (chronic stress). The fight-or-flight reaction comes from adrenaline and noradrenalines.

2. **The vigilance reaction** is due to testosterone and cortisol–like hormones. Together, they affect the nervous system by weakening the calming branch (parasympathetic) of autonomic nerves. This leads to stress arousal and all the disorders of stress that follow. The calming branch of the nervous system is the feminine part, or yin part of the balancing force. Anger opposes this force. That is why anger is symbolic of the "macho" or masculine power.

3. **The anger takes away pleasure and love** in life. This leads to a low brain serotonin level as a cause and effect chain event. Risky behaviors, such as overeating, smoking, and alcohol consumption, are attempts to recover this pleasure by raising brain serotonin levels. Depression and isolation continue. This is death in installments or suicide.

4. **The suppression of the immune system** is shown as a decrease of immune globins and decreased T–cell and NK cell activities. At an atomic level, stress hormones attack the nucleus of the cell and change the structure of DNA, resulting in immune disorders. The suppressed immune system can cause infections, allergies, cancer, or autoimmune disorders.

Actually, immune suppression by an episode of anger lasts five to six hours. This is why you notice the after effects of an anger episode for the rest of the day. Change in the calming branch of the nervous system makes the mind–body very sensitive to trivial challenges, such as mental arithmetic or the mere presence of another person in one's vicinity.

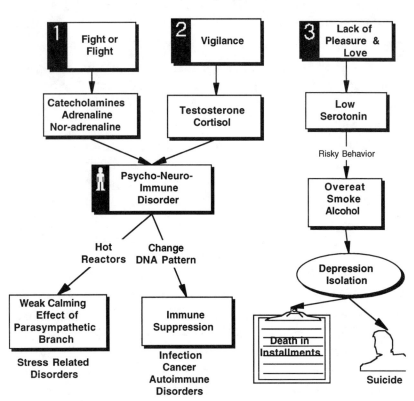

Biological Damages by Anger

This is called **"hot reactors"** by researcher Robert Eliot. Hot reactors react to minor challenges in life with high blood pressure and rapid heartbeat.

Intrapersonal Costs of Anger

HOSTILITY: Hostile people are lonely. They go to cocktail parties, but cannot come out of their hostile shell to mix with others in a caring way. A hostile person ruminates in his own thoughts and is preoccupied with himself. As mentioned earlier, Larry Sherewitz at the University of California, San Francisco shows the more a person thinks of the first person pronouns (I, me, mine, myself), the the greater the risk for a heart attack. Your preoccupation with self makes you more hostile, because you do not include others in your agenda.

DEPRESSION can coexist with type A behavior because both have the common biological marker of reduced brain serotonin. A 1990 report in the *American Journal of Cardiology* involved 342 people with depression showed they had a higher risk of cardiac arrest. Depression is linked with a first heart attack. A National Health Examination follow up study involving 2,832 men and women found that depression is associated with a 50% increase in fatal heart disease.

SELF–HATRED is low self–esteem. Low self–esteem underlies type A behavior. The individual tries to do more and more in less and less time to prove he/she is worthy. This hurry sickness and competitiveness leads to more hostile feelings towards others.

One example of a vicious cycle of self–hatred is to negatively visualize an afflicted organ in the body. If you have heart disease, and dwell on your blocked arteries, sending negative command patterns to the arteries, you make them worse. This self–directed anger can be reprogrammed with positive imagery work and using love as a tool.

PRE-MENSTRUAL SYNDROME (PMS) is a condition in which the brain serotonin level decreases as the progesterone level goes up near the next menstrual period. During PMS, self–hatred rises.

SEASONAL AFFECTIVE DISORDER (SAD) is another condition in which brain serotonin level drops. The cause: low exposure to sunlight in winter. Overeating and binge eating are instances of trying to induce the "high" of increased brain serotonin levels. Irritability and anger in overeaters relates to roller coaster–like insulin secretion, which leads to roller coaster brain serotonin levels. Overeaters hate themselves in that state, yet feel imprisoned by the addictive habit. Overeaters substitute the sweet taste for a sweet experience in life.

Isolation and Lack of Social Support

A **lonely heart** is more vulnerable to an attack. A 1960's, Alameda County, California study followed 7,000 adults for nine years. It showed people with less social support by marriage, friends, relatives, church, etc. are two to three times more likely to die from any cause than people who have social support (Berkman). A Swedish study by Orth Gomer (a ten year follow–up of 150 middle–aged men) showed that social support is an important predicter of coronary artery disease. The Reed study of Honolulu Heart Program looked at 4,653 men of Japanese descent and their social networks. This study found that lack of social support is a major risk factor for coronary artery disease. In 1979, at the Three Mile Island nuclear accident in Pennsylvania, those reporting lower social support had higher levels of stress hormones in the urine. All of these studies show social support is crucial for surviving, thriving, and healing.

Hating Your Spouse

People closest to you are like the sweet spot in a tennis racket. When strings are broken in the "sweet spot," they become "bitter." Because your spouse, significant other, partner, or roommate is close to you, your anger interacts with them the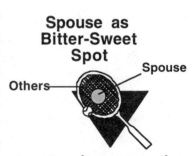

Spouse as Bitter-Sweet Spot

Others

Spouse

most. Minor irritations and resentments release stress hormones all day long. As this anger in the presence of the other person repeats, your body chemistry develops a conditioned reflex of anger with that person regardless of what that person does right or wrong. The basic problem here is that your own "anger chemicals" put you on a treadmill. You can create the reverse chemistry by applying HRI and caring love towards that person. One study of ten thousand men with heart disease found a 50% reduction in anginal chest pains as a result of supportive loving from their wives.

Social Cost of Anger and the Power of Love

Love and caring release pleasure chemicals (endorphins). This is true in animals, also. If the endorphin receptors in an animal are blocked by a drug called nalorphine, the animal becomes hostile. If the animal's endorphin is repeatedly blocked while in the presence of others, the animal learns to associate hostility with every contact with others. In another experiment, an animal given morphine, (an endorphin–like drug) starts loving, caring, and playing with other animals.

In this busy information age, when you come in contact with people, you are so preoccupied with the "report visit," you do not develop a "rapport visit" with that person. Thus your endorphins remain suppressed. In due course, you learn to associate any human contact with hostility. The reason is, you're not keeping your endorphin system tuned up with love. This is the logic of the flip–flop, duck–rabbit, report visit and rapport visit to kindle the internal pharmacy of love.

Hostility kills in three different ways:
1. By reducing social support and and causing isolation.
2. By increasing biological reactivity.
3. By encouraging risky behavior such as smoking, drugs, alcohol, and overeating.

A Western Electric study of 20-year mortality in 1,877 men shows death from all causes more than doubled as the hostility score increased. The following two graphs schematically reconstructs a 25-year follow up of doctors and lawyers starting from medical school and law school.

ANGER KILLS DOCTORS

Doctors, nurses, psychologists, and other health care professionals have a high incidence of stress-induced problems such as divorce, substance abuse, suicide, and heart attacks. These are not due to compassion fatigue or overcare, **but to lack of compassion or caring love in the modern mechanistic and robotic approach to health care.**

How Doctors Became Wounded Healers.

The current system of medicine is the result of a scientific revolution started in the 17th century. Rene Descartes, a philosopher, introduced the mind–body dualism into medical science. In his scholastic work Principles of Philosophy (1644), Descartes proclaimed the universe is a big machine that works on the principle of matter and

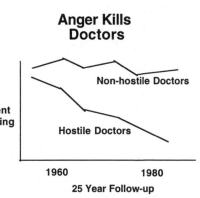

Anger Kills Doctors

Percent Surviving

Non-hostile Doctors

Hostile Doctors

1960   1980
25 Year Follow-up

motion. Spirit, in the form of God, prevails outside of the universe and does not have direct influence over the universe.

Humans have the ability to break everything into components. Thus they can understand the principles of matter and motion by the process of reasoning. **Descartes reiterated that the mind is the *disembodied thoughts* and the body is the thoughtless *machine*.** The domain of the soul and spirit went to the clergy. The domain of the mind went to the psychologist and psychiatrist. The domain of the physical body went to the physicians, hence the name. The 19th century physiologists and medical scientists continued the Cartesian tradition.

In the 20th century, technological advances created diagnostic and therapeutic gadgets that focused more on organ systems than the whole body, totally neglecting the soul. Illness was a pathophysiological event, with a counteracting cure possible by treatment. Here, on the edge of the 21st century, organ specialists like cardiologists, neurologists, urologists, etc. focus on various diseases with funnel vision and microscopic amplification. In reality, there are no diseases, only people with diseases. **A disease is not an event, but a process or pattern in a person.**

A plethora of computer-based information processing has revolutionized the practice of medicine by creating a robotic atmosphere. Doctors are busy making a "report visit" rather than a "rapport visit" with the patient. These are two polarities in medical practice.

The feelings of love, compassion, appreciation, and caring – the model traits of the noble profession – are in one hand, and the information processing automatic, robotic model is in the other. The mind dislikes polarities because the ego seeks clarity. The ego prefers to dwell in one pole at a time. Because of social, legal, scientific pressures, and time constraints, a physician spends most of his or her time with the patient creating a good "report visit." This suppresses the emotions of the physician, leading to compassion fatigue. The current system does not allow the health care worker to interact emotionally with the client.

As one physician put it, "the breasts of compassion are not sucked dry, but became dry by not being sucked at all." The solution for doctor's anger is to learn the skill of the duck–rabbit flip–flop during each client contact, so that the doctor heals himself with endorphins of a "rapport visit" overlapping the adrenalines of a "report visit."

Lawyers Lose Balance by Anger

Lawyers are expected to be angry at the other party because a law suit is an aftermath of a client's anger. This message gets transmitted to a lawyer's body parts, including his heart. It is ironic that in attempts to balance the two sides, the lawyer's own mind–body gets out of balance.

In our stress clinic, we train lawyers to learn the skill of HRI and implement the message Jesus gave, "love thy enemy."

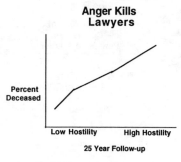

Anger Kills Lawyers

Percent Deceased

Low Hostility   High Hostility

25 Year Follow-up

HOW ANGER CAUSES HEART ATTACKS

Anger attacks the heart in the following way:

1. There is a brain–heart dissonance . The brain says get angry and the heart says love. This tug of war between brain and heart strangulates the mind–body and leads to **stress arousal.**

2. **Over–breathing** occurs, which leads to alkaline blood and buffer loss. Calcium, potassium, and magnesium go into the cell and cause neuromuscular irritability all over the body. massive amounts of catecholamimes are released.

This leads to changes in heart-related **pipes and pumps** Two major pipelines are affected: **coronary arteries and peripheral arteries.**

The coronary arteries are either kinked or clogged. Kinking or spasms occurs due to a sudden command from the brain via exciting branch of the nervous system. Clogging of these arteries occur by acute clot formation or by a slow deposit of atherosclerotic plaques. This clotting is called **coronary thrombosis**.

Three different factors contribute to coronary thrombosis: injury to the artery wall; rupture of atherosclerotic plaques; and stickiness of platelets. These are due to free radicals and

**How Anger
Attacks The Heart?**

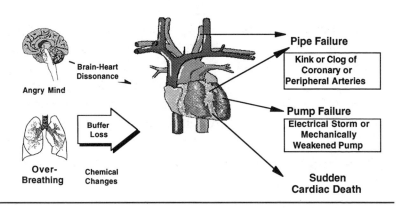

catecholamines in the blood.

Chronic deposits atherosclerotic plaques in the arteries is due to free radicals oxidizing the LDL, "bad cholesterol" and the white blood cells (macrophages) eating these oxidized cholesterol. Finally, the cholesterol-filled macrophages invade the wall of coronary arteries and deposit the plaques. This process, inflaming the tissues, originated from the spark of angry atoms, called free radicals.

In the peripheral blood vessels, anger causes pulse pressure rise with each beat of the heart. This in turn damages the artery walls.

The anger message from the brain affects the mechanical and electrical activity of the heart. The heart muscle becomes less effective with each beat, or there is an electrical storm of irregular heart beat. This electrical storm is called **ventricular fibrillation** and may lead to sudden cardiac death.

SOLUTIONS FOR DEADLY ANGER

There are three ways we try to control anger.

 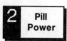

1. **Will** leads to overcontrol of type A, or loss of control of type C behavior. The more you try to control anger with will power, the more is your frustration and loss of control. Now, you are angry at your own anger. Logical reasoning is ineffective in anger control because the anger chemistry remains unchanged.

2. **Pill power** is the external pharmacy of tranquilizers. Pills are effective in changing the chemistry of brain cells. Most of them reduce the mind-to-muscle traffic; some relax the muscles and reduce the muscle-to-mind traffic. They are particularly helpful to calm down the "kindling phenomenon" of an irritable brain center. However, pills are habit forming and have other side effects.

3. **Skill power** is the choice. Skill is the ability to do something well.

Anger – an emotion – has to be replaced by another emotion. To do this, two parts of the iceberg – thoughts and body actions – must team up to replace the angry atom of the moment.

It's like a hand gun. Body arousal is the bullet, and the trigger is a thought. The most crucial intervention is to take the hand off the trigger. But, even if your hand is on the trigger, if the gun is not loaded, it will not fire. Similarly, if your body arousal of muscle contraction is not geared towards anger, the trigger will not cause any havoc.

Trigger control comes by instantly focusing on your heart and doing your HRI. Now, you are in a "loving your enemy" mode because you are heart centered. This momentary shift in your vantage point from your head to anatomical heart will instantly take the hand away from the trigger. You cannot be angry and in a state of love at the same time. You cannot blow hot and cold air simultaneously. This is how HRI works to replace anger. In summary, anger control has two steps:

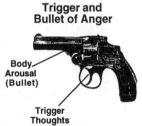

Trigger and Bullet of Anger

Body Arousal (Bullet)

Trigger Thoughts

Step 1. **Replace trigger thoughts with altruistic thoughts** instantly by doing HRI.

Step 2. **Calm down body arousal:** The body arousal is controlled by muscle–to–mind and mind–to–muscle tools (explained in the reactivity control chapter). Muscle-to-mind tools are easy to use because you have more control over your muscles than the mind.

Handy Muscle-to-Mind Tools:

1. Breath out three times, proloning your exhalation. This shifts you to the calming branch of the nervous system.

2. Motion controls emotion. Simply move around, take a walk, or rotate your arms like a windmill.

3. Chew a carrot, or eat a piece of fruit to dissipate your "biting" instinct.

4. Dissolve your negative imagery on the situation, or person, by eyeball desensitization. Move your eyeballs with a tic to the left, a toc to the right, while bringing the imagery of the anger scene to your mind. This erases the angry images in your brain.

Handy Mind-to-Muscle Tools:

1. Adapt a beginner's mind to the situation with a fresh, nonjudgmental look.

2. Open your mind's focus by simultaneously being aware of different body parts, rather than being head-centered.

3. Meditate with your eyes closed, focus on breath and mantra.

4. Speak into a tape recorder; write out your anger; or do self-disclosure to your partner.

5. Transcend with spiritual rituals.

Of the three approaches, skill power to control anger is the most effective, because it is a lifetime relearning.

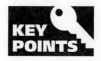

1 Anger is the result of your body arousal and trigger thoughts.

2. You control your body arousal by stress control methods of muscle-to-mind and mind-to-mucle tools.

3. You reframe trigger thoughts and replace anger with caring love by the HRI tool.

16

Mother Teresa Effect–
Love as a Tool

Mother Teresa Effect– Caring Love as a Tool

In this chapter we will help you answer two questions:

Can Caring Love Save Me?

If so, How Can I Learn it?

We start by providing scientific evidence to support the Mother Teresa Effect. Then we'll show you how to use love as a tool.

MOTHER TERESA EFFECT

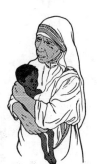

Mother Teresa is an 85-year old nun and winner of the 1979 Nobel Peace Prize. She dedicated her life to **caring love** of the sick and poor in Calcutta, India. Her altruistic care has become a symbol of unconditional love.

The Mother Teresa Effect is the physiological changes that occur in the mind-body during moments of caring love.

Caring love is affectionate, non-judgmental, affiliative feeling towards another person, animal, or plant. In English, the word "love" is a generic term, which includes all shades of meaning to the opposite of hate. Commonly, love refers to superficial waves of romantic, conjugal, or erotic love.

In Sanskrit, there are different words for different kinds of love. Love between a mother and her child is called *mamatha or vatslya*; love for God is *bhakti;* love for a friend is *mytri or preeti. Love* with concern is called *karuna;* love with pity is called *daya*; romantic love is called *prema*; and erotic love is called *kama.*

The underlying strata of all of this (love) is being connected by a caring and sharing. In our clinical work, we have found that the best words to express this form of love is **"caring love."**

We can measure and monitor biological or physiological

---

changes of caring love in the hard wire, liquid media, and vibrational whisper of mind-body connections.

Mindfelt
Feelings

1	Hard wire
2	Liquid Media
3	Direct Vibrations

Heartfelt Feelings

The overall effect is pleasure in the mind, healing chemistry, balance of *yin-yang* opposites in the body, and unconditional affiliation with others. We basically have two feelings: love and non-love. Heartfelt feeling is always love. Mindfelt feelings can be non-love as well. Non-love ranges from apathy to fear, worry, anxiety, anger, guilt, and sadness. We're able to measure love and non-love on the physiology of the *anatomical* heart.

HARD WIRE CONNECTIONS

These connections between heart and brain follow three distinct paths:

1. Sympathetic nerves (yang branch)
2. Parasympathetic nerves (yin branch)
3. Baroreceptor system

The sympathetic branch speeds up the heart and increases blood pressure. The parasympathetic branch calms it down and reduces blood pressure. This is how anger gives you palpitations and high blood pressure. The change in blood pressure is sensed by the baroreceptors found in big blood vessels, like the aorta. The baroreceptor provides the main feedback from heart to brain.

Heart Rate Variability

Heart rate is how many times the heart beats in a minute. Normal rate is about 70 per minute. Each beat has a variable distance from the next beat. In other words, the time between beats one and two can differ from the interval between beats two and three, four and five, and so on.

This beat to beat time variation is called heart rate variability. This variability can be small and erratic, or large and balanced. Imbalance in heart rate variability is a sensitive index of mind-body malfunction. In fact, low and erratic heart rate variability is a predictor of sudden cardiac death in people recovering from a heart attack. Erratic heart rate variability puts extra wear and tear on blood vessels and the heart.

Positive emotions, caring love, appreciation, and compassion allow a smooth, harmonious, even heart rate variability.

Negative emotions, anger, frustration, worry, anxiety, fear, guilt, and sadness cause erratic and non-harmonious heart rate variability.

LIQUID MEDIA EFFECT

There are three groups of messenger molecules, or liquid ingredients to your "body soup." All your body cells swim in this soup. The soup's taste depends on what ingredient is dominant at any given moment. These ingredients are:

1. **Neurotransmitters.** During positive emotions–such as caring love–we release endorphins, serotonin, and phenylethylamine. During negative emotions of non-love–such as anger and fear–we set loose adrenaline and noradrenaline.

2. **Hormones.** During caring love, we turn out oxytocin (cuddling chemical). During anger and fear, in addition to adrenaline-like hormones, we pump out cortisol.

3. **Immune transmitters.** With caring love, the immunoglobins increase, particularly the secretory immunoglobin (IgA) secreted in saliva. With anger and frustration, IgA is suppressed.

Some scientific proof of these effects:

Harvard Research on the Immune System: Harvard Medical School's David McClelland is the leading authority on human motivation. He studied students watching a documentary film of Mother Teresa administering love to the sick. He measured their immunoglobin (S-IgA) before and after the film. S-IgA is a first line of defense against infections in the respiratory, gastrointestinal, and urinary tracts. A normal level of S-IgA in saliva protects against the common cold, sinusitis, and pneumonia. Stress reduces S-IgA level in saliva.

IgA rose significantly in those who watched Mother Teresa and whether or not they agreed with her philosophy. McClelland found similar effects when students thought of being appreciated and loved by someone, or about appreciating someone else.

Increased S-IgA returned to base line after about an hour. If subjects were asked to "replay" the positive feelings of love and appreciation, the high IgA level persisted. **Consciously maintaining or "recharging" your love chemicals keeps your immune system primed.** It even stops the common cold! McClelland's study scientifically validates the **healing power of love.**

People with a natural loving and caring tendency have increased levels of the neurotransmitter dopamine; increased natural killer cells; higher S-IgA secretion rates; decreased stress hormone levels, and fewer illnesses.

HeartMath Research: HeartMath Institute at Boulder Creek, California, reproduced the Harvard research. Moreover, these scientists correlated heart rate variability findings with immune system changes. They found caring love and appreciation

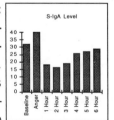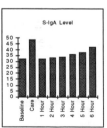

(L) Anger and frustration decrease immune response up to 6 hours. (R) Caring love increases immune power up to 6 hours.

increases IgA levels in saliva, lasting 4-6 hours. Five minutes of "replaying" an anger experience in the mind *suppressed* IgA for the rest of the day. They used Mother Teresa movie-watching, comparing it to self-generated emotions of replaying past experiences of caring love and anger. Self-generated emotions had a more profound effect on the immune system.

Animal Model of Love, Peace, and Play

Bowling Green University scientist, Jack Panksepp, did experiments with rats, chicks, and pups using the endorphin blocking drug, nalorphine, and came to the following conclusions:

1. If the animals' natural endorphins are blocked by nalorphine, they stop playful behavior and instead, get angry and fight with each other.

2. Give animals morphine, codeine, or heroin to stimulate opioid receptors, and they show playful, loving, and cuddling behavior.

The National Institute of Mental Health research found that anger and aggression are stimulated by catecholamines, such as adrenaline and noradrenaline.

Brain opioids stimulate social comfort, love, bonding, peace, joy, and play. **Brain catecholamines generate anger and aggression.**

VIBRATIONS OF LOVE

The main power center for vibrations of love is the heart. Heart and brain both generate electricity. But the electrical power of the heart is 40 to 60 times stronger than that of the brain. The heart generates 205 watts of electrical power with its own automatic rhythm and transmits it to every cell in the body.

Imagine your mind-body as two brothers. The heart is the bigger, wiser one. Your brain is the little brother. The two meet. Big brother heart shakes hands with the brain in a state of caring love. The trouble-making little brother brain twists the arms

---

of big brother heart in a state of anger and frustration. The aftereffects of these "handshaking" or "arm twisting" episodes are visible in each cell of the body. HeartMath Institute scientists have studied the changes in DNA cells.

DNA is the smallest code of message in your cells. These molecules act as antennas receiving vibratory pulse from the heart. Caring love produces coherent frequencies in the heart, which, transmitted to the DNA, harmonize the DNA's winding and unwinding.

Biology of Altruism

Altruism is unselfish concern for others. In Sanskrit, it is called *seva*, which means *you are also included in my agenda*. Altruism creates healing chemistry in the body. In childhood, we all had a natural tendency to bond and love. We secreted endorphin-like chemicals whenever we met people. Growing older, we treated each human contact with suspicion and competition. In our money-oriented society, we evaluated each new person from the perspective of economic gain or loss. Such judgmental mindfelt feelings released more adrenaline and noradrenaline than endorphins. This led to habitual competitiveness and outright cynicism instead of trust and altruism.

Rockefeller and Fetzer Stories: In his book, *How to Stop Worrying and Start Living,* Dale Carnegie tells the story of John D. Rockefeller. He made his first million at age thirty-three, and was a workaholic. His mindfelt feelings were fear, anger, guilt, sadness and "phony love" in the "business as usual" way of dealing with people. At age fifty-three, the richest man in the world was hit with an ulcer and heart problems. His condition was so severe, he was prescribed a diet of human milk. He suffered near death and the misery of ill health for about a year, in spite of well-wishers and compassionate caretakers.

Then he suddenly decided to donate his wealth, establishing the Rockefeller Foundation and making many charitable gifts to people around the world. What happened? He recovered completely, and he lived to be ninety-eight. The moral is, mindfelt feelings and caring from others did not help John D. Rockefeller. **Only his caring love and altruism restored his health**. *When he became the sender of caring love, he recovered and lived another forty five years.*

Kenneth Pelletier, in his book, *Sound Mind, Sound Body,* studied fifty-three rich and famous people who had balanced lifestyles. Pelletier quotes John E. Fetzer's case. He had a near fatal heart attack in 1980 at age 79. He focused his attention on energy management of the mind-body and became a visionary philanthropist, creating the Fetzer Institute for the study of mind, body, and spirit. This altruistic self-transcendence let John Fetzer live to be ninety. Pelletier's research shows altruism is the single common denominator among people who are both rich AND healthy.

Mother Teresa herself had heart problems due to biological aging. But, in 1995, at the age of 85, she is doing well serving the needy and sick in Calcutta. *She produces the Mother Teresa Effect on herself and keeps healing herself.*

Sender and Receiver of Love

Caring love has two ends: sender and receiver. The sender initiates and actively participates. The receiver reflects caring love. For example, a birthday girl's caring love is most intense as she appreciates the people who brought her gifts. Not while she is the center of attention while cutting cake and having happy birthday sung to her. In our biofeedback laboratory, we find physiological balance is greater when one **sends** caring love than when one receives it.

This **other directed care** is what Hans Selye called **altruistic egotism.** It corresponds to the "autotelic flow" experience of Mihaly Czsikentmihaly, and yogic union, in which viewer, scene, and the process of seeing become one and the same, with the viewer initiating the process.

Love of Social Support

Those who are naturally loving and caring have increased levels of neurotransmitter dopamine; increased natural killer cells; higher S-IgA secretion rates; decreased stress hormone levels; and fewer illnesses.

Stanford Research led by David Spiegel has shown social connectedness doubles survival years for breast cancer patients. In this case, it was active participation in caring love of other patients, producing the Mother Teresa Effect.

A University of California at Berkeley study by Reynolds and Kaplan shows women with the least amount of social contact had twice the incidence of cancer over 17 years.

A University of San Francisco study of 7,500 people told us that single men between age 45 and 54 had twice the rate of mortality of a control population with married men in it.

A University of California study by Siegel of 345 pet owners indicated that owning pets decreased doctor visits.

LOVE AS A TOOL

The Mother Teresa Effect is a behavioral tool (we call it **"love as a tool"**). This tool activates your *internal* healing pharmacy. It energizes you by removing the misplaced effort of stress. To use love as a tool, we follow a ritual called Heartfelt Resonant Imaging (HRI). The technique is rather simple. You just focus your awareness on your heart and ask yourself, "Can I experience caring love towards this person, animal, or plant?"

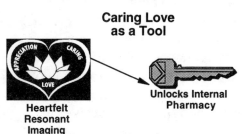

We will elaborate on HRI later. For now, let us look at some of the basic principles on which love as a tool works.

What happens in using love as a tool, is it produces biochemical changes in the body as you experience the state of caring love. These biochemical changes involve electrical changes in the heart. We measure the changes as heart rate variability. This is like checking the chemistry of your car battery by measuring the voltage with a voltameter. The chemistry of caring love is influenced by the following:

1. Thought vs. images.
2. Focusing on the anatomical heart.
3. Mindfelt vs. heartfelt feelings.
4. Sender vs. receiver of love.

THOUGHTS AND IMAGES

Just a thought of caring love does not produce biochemical changes. You need to focus your awareness on your anatomical heart and stay focused for at least the time it takes to breathe in order to observe the effect. Thoughts are just electrical sparks. It is when you stay with the thoughts long enough that the messenger molecules connect the body and mind and create an image. The image releases the chemicals.

FOCUSING ON ANATOMICAL HEART

You have to learn how to focus on your anatomical heart. First, think of the left side of your chest. Then become aware of the heart underneath. We use computer feedback of heart waves to prove you remain focused on your heart. You can focus your awareness to your head and return back to your heart. This flip-flop between heart and head gives you the contrast of two feeling states: mindfelt and heartfelt feelings.

HEARTFELT VS MINDFELT FEELINGS

The heart does not have rational thinking and it does not know how to hate or resent. Buddha used the word, *ajatashatru,* to refer to the heart, which means that the heart has no ability to create hatred. Your heart is not only your friend, it cannot hate anybody. In our worldwide Stress Cybernetix seminars, we typically ask three to four hundred people in the audience to close their eyes, focus awareness on the heart, and ask the question, "Can I experience caring love towards the person that I dislike or hate the most?" The answer is always yes. When you stay focused on your heart, it is rather impossible not to

---

enter into a state of love. In other words, if you learn the art of focusing on your anatomical heart, you have relearned the art of using caring love as a tool.

"Love thy enemy," said Jesus. Jesus did not say "do not have an enemy." You can have mindfelt feelings of dislike or hatred toward someone, but your heart still loves that person. You can prove this by closing your eyes, focusing your awareness on your heart, and asking your heart if you love that person. The heart says "yes." President Nixon once said, "Let anybody hate you. You lose when you start hating that person." The idea is to not stew in the juices of hatred, even if your rational mind judges the other person as wrong.

SENDER AND RECEIVER OF LOVE

The most effective way to activate your love chemistry is to initiate caring love, rather than passively receive it. You want to be the one shaking somebody's hand or hugging someone rather than expecting the others to do this to you. **When you send love, you are in the driver's seat. You maintain control and choice.** HRI as explained below allows you to be in the driver's seat all the time.

HEARTFELT RESONANT IMAGING (HRI)

Heartfelt feelings are based on unconditional love, without any element of judgment. When we say, "hearty congratulations," "sweetheart," "cordially," etc., we refer to heartfelt feelings. New research shows heartfelt feelings have to do with anatomical heart-centered orienting of energy patterns. This is the "intuitive field of heart." The mother's caring love for her infant is an anatomical heart-centered energy field. This is not a theory. It can be reproduced in the heart rate variability as shown earlier.

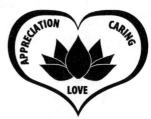

In summary, two things happen when you are in a state of caring love:

1. You experience unconditional love.
2. **Your energy system is centered around your anatomical heart.**

In HRI, you do the second thing as a first step and allow step one to take place. In other words, you focus your awareness on your anatomical heart and ask yourself what is your dominant feeling at the moment.

Removing the Tug of War

In our busy life, we constantly have the tug of war between head and heart. This conflict is the single most important cause of stress in modern life. We deal with the "report visit" (mindfelt feelings or mind talk) and "rapport visit" (heartfelt feelings or mindfulness) unknowingly all through the day. We all experience heartfelt feelings for 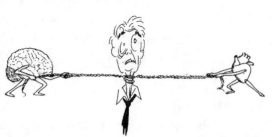 people, animals, and plants for a few moments in spite of our busy life. With HRI, we deliberately increase the number of moments we spend in rapport visits, and take advantage of the biological value.

Conditioned Reflex

With HRI, you replace one conditioned reflex with another. The conditioned reflex of anger tries to release adrenaline-like chemicals at the moment of contact with people. You simply replace that reflex with the reflex of caring love. This cannot be done as a statement, declaration, or pep talk. It has to be developed as a biological reflex. If you diligently "practice" over 24 hours, you will be able to develop the new reflex. If you stay with it everyday for a week, you will master the new reflex. You will enjoy the unconditional caring love state for the second time in your life—the first being when you were a child.

The HRI steps are simple:

1. Focus awareness on your anatomical heart.
2. Ask yourself, "Can I experience caring love towards this person, animal, or plant?"

The following exercises facilitate the learning of HRI:

1. Where are you right now? In the head or in the heart?
2. Can you center yourself in the heart now?
3. Can you center yourself in the head again?
4. Can you toggle between your head and heart several times?
5. Can you stay anchored to your heart?
6. Can you observe your breathing in your belly as you stay anchored in your heart?
7. Repeat these drills until you are able to shift your centering from head to heart and head to belly effortlessly.

Benefits of HRI

1. HRI balances your yin-yang cycles.
2. Your heart heals, as shown by heart rate variability.
3. Your immune system becomes stronger.
4. You resolve conflicts in your mind and feel better.
5. You feel less stressed and more energized.
6. You develop biologically effective altruism. This is healing by your internal pharmacy. You upgrade your emotions from apathy to empathy and from anger to caring love.

When to Use HRI

Three common situations in which to practice and use HRI:

1. At every opportunity to meet another person.
2. Every time you imagine a living thing (person, animal, or plant).
3. At the time of every phone call.

Duck-Rabbit Flip-Flop

If you look at the picture on the right, it looks like a rabbit vertically and a duck horizontally. You can flip-flop and toggle your mind from one to the other. Similarly, with every person you interact with, you can switch from the "report visit" of information exchange and "business as usual" to the "rapport visit" or caring love for your own biological sake of healing.

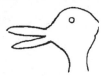

**Duck-Rabbit
Flip-Flop**

"Felt Sense" Differences in Mind and Body

The felt sense is how you orient yourself in your mind or body. For example, the body part of the felt sense of anger is frowning or clenching of the jaw. The mind part of the felt sense of anger is the feeling of distress or restless mind state. Which is easier to orient? Obviously, the muscle action of frowning and jaw clenching. If you first do frowning and jaw-clenching, it is easier for you to recall and "replay" an episode of anger from your recent past. In the case of caring love, the felt sense is focused on the anatomical heart area. In HRI, you take advantage of this anatomical fact, get oriented to your anatomical heart first, and then ask your mind what kind of feeling the mind is registering.

In summary, the felt sense of caring love is easier to get oriented in the muscles of your heart area before you "feel" it in the mind. It is easier to change an emotion from muscle-to-mind than from mind-to-muscle.

Putting the Cart Before the Horse

Normally, when you are in a state of caring love, the energy in your mind-body is heart centered. Conversely, if you focus your energy to your heart area, you enter into a state of caring love. This is like putting the cart before the horse and turning the horse around.

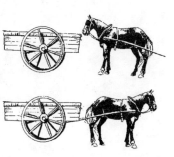

---

1. The Mother Teresa Effect refers to the biological benefits of caring love in the form of enhanced immune system, balanced heart rate, and healthy winding of DNA.

2. The biological state of caring love can be produced by choice simply by focusing on your anatomical heart and orienting toward your emotion.

3. You can flip-flop between the achievement-oriented, information-processing, problem-solving life on one moment and the affiliation oriented, caring love life the next moment.

17

Reactivity Levels of the Heart

Reactivity Levels of the Heart

WHAT IS REACTIVITY?

Reactivity refers to the result or sequence of an action. The action in your mind–body is muscle contractions, thoughts, and emotions. Reactivity is best understood through analogies: the domino effect, a treadmill; an echo; and chemical reactivity.

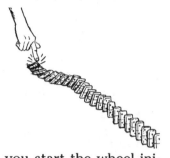

In the domino effect, the initiating force transmits to the second, third, and fourth dominoes in a progression.

On a treadmill or a treadwheel, you start the wheel initially at your own speed, and you are in control. As you push the wheel faster and faster, you reach a point where you lose control, and the machine controls you.

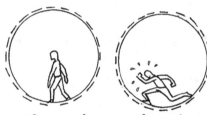

In an echo, sound continues after you have created it.

In a chemical reaction, as in the case of sodium and chloride joined as salt (sodium chloride), the compound continues to exist, rather than its components.

The heart is a pump attached to pipes. According to Newton's third law of motion, every action or force has an equal and opposite reaction. The heart is a major actor and reactor. We can look at action–reaction in the body using the heart as the central vantage point.

1. The Heart as a Pulsating Pump and Pipes:

The heart has its own pulsating rhythm, and reacts to other rhythms in the body. The pipes into which the heart pumps blood directly influences its pumping action. The reactivity of the heart pump and pipes shows up as an increase or decrease in heart rate variation from beat to beat (heart rate variability); increase or decrease in pipe pressure (blood pressure); and change in quality and quantity of blood itself. The change in heart rate and blood pressure during stress arousal is the hot reactor state.

Feedback from the Pumps and Pipes of the Body: Other pumps and pipes send feedback messages to the heart. These systems include the muscles, urinary bladder, reproductive organs, gut pipes, etc. Of these, the major muscles take an active part in regulating the heart. The pumps and pipes of the mind–body are summarized in the graphics at the end of this chapter.

2. The Brain as Pump Regulator:

The brain is a command center sending messages to the heart to speed up or slow down, and beat more forcefully or less.

Mind–Heart Reaction: All these actions and reactions are observed by the mind as a bystander. Sometimes the bystander intervenes in the 'pumps and pipes' affairs. Often the mind becomes perturbed with the reactivity of the body. This leads to a restless mind and insomnia.

3. The Lungs as Balancer of Heart–Brain Regulation:

The lungs are a major pump and pipe system that changes the heart pump. Hyperventilation or over breathing is the lungs trying to catch up with the needs of other pumps in the body.

4. Stress Chemical Reaction as Messengers:

The chemicals released during stress and strain on pumps and pipes interact with the heart and change its activity.

HOT REACTING HEART PUMP

Cardiologist Robert Eliot coined the term "hot reactors" for people who respond with rapid heart beat and increased blood pressure when stressed. Hot reactors react at the pump (heart) level, pipe level (blood vessels constrict), or both. This

---

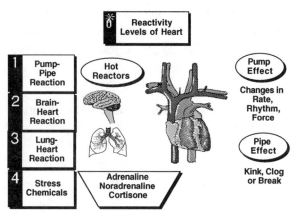

Reactivity Levels of Heart		
1 Pump-Pipe Reaction	Hot Reactors	Pump Effect — Changes in Rate, Rhythm, Force
2 Brain-Heart Reaction		
3 Lung-Heart Reaction		Pipe Effect — Kink, Clog or Break
4 Stress Chemicals	Adrenaline Noradrenaline Cortisone	

pump and pipe reaction show the classic action-reaction effect. The pump exerts pressure on the pipes, and they constrict. That puts an extra load on the pump. Both suffer.

In a hot reaction, nerve impulses and stress chemicals travel to the heart and blood vessels. At the pump level, the hot reaction causes rapid heart beat and erratic beat-to-beat variation. The rapid beat can be measured and monitored by counting your pulse rate. Heart rate variability (covered in the next chapter) requires sophisticated electronics to be seen. The pipe reaction is measured by taking blood pressure. Hot reactors have a higher risk of hypertension and coronary artery disease.

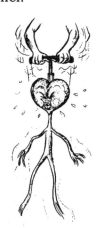

Are You a Hot Reactor?

Eliot's Hot Reactor Test:

1.   Measure your resting blood pressure.

2.   Give yourself a mental challenge, such as a video game or a simple arithmetic problem of subtracting sevens continuously starting from the number 1000. Do this for three minutes.

3.   Record your blood pressure at the end of three minutes. You calculate your *mean* blood pressure from the systolic and diastolic pressure recorded on the instrument. For example:

Your blood pressure is 140/90.

Take 140 (systolic) and subtract 90 (diastolic) from it. You get 50. Divide the result by 3, which gives you 17. Now add this 17 to the diastolic pressure of 90. The final number is 90 plus 17, or 107. Your pulse pressure is 107.

Calculate pulse pressure by adding one third of the difference between systolic and diastolic pressure to the diastolic pressure. If you have a resting pulse pressure over 107, you probably have hypertension. You can interpret your reading as follows:

Below 107 – Cool Reactor.

107 to 117 – Lukewarm (Mild)

117 to 127 – Moderate

Above 127 – Severe (Hot)

You should take the readings immediately after the stress challenge. Take several readings over two weeks and compare them. You can use an electronic blood pressure unit. These days, doctors use **ambulatory blood pressure** monitoring to measure the hot reactor's blood pressure in real life situations. A **Holter monitor with a heart rate variability indicator** measures the balance of the parasympathetic (calming branch) and sympathetic (exciting branch) system.

Global Hot Reactions

The heart acts as the body's master oscillator or global reactor. Body reactivity can be easily remembered as "pumps and pipes."

THE BRAIN AND HEART REACTION

The brain and heart react to each other through:

1. Hard–wire connections.

2. Liquid–media messenger molecules.

3. Direct vibrational waves.

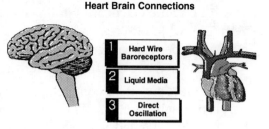

Heart Brain Connections

1 Hard Wire Baroreceptors

2 Liquid Media

3 Direct Oscillation

HARD WIRE CONNECTIONS

The direct hard wire connection goes from brain to heart and heart to brain. **The brain to heart connections** are either sympathetic or parasympathetic pathways. The sympathetic stimulates the heart and speeds it up. The parasympathetic slows and calms it down.

The **heart to brain connection** is the Baroreceptor system. It sends messages from the heart and aorta to the brain. These baroreceptor strings act as "reins" from the heart controlling the brain.

LIQUID MEDIA CONNECTIONS

Hormones, neurotransmitters, and immunotransmitters make up the "biochemical soup" in which the body cells swim. At any given time, contents of this soup determine heart rate variability, brain waves, or emotions. If you wash out these chemicals as you do in blood dialysis for kidney patients, heart rate variability changes, as does the person's mood.

You release hormones such as adrenaline, noradrenaline, and cortisol according your emotional response. The neurotransmitters, endorphins and serotonin, affect the pleasure and pain centers and cell-to-cell junctions of the nervous system called synapses. Immunotransmitters, such as interferon and interleukins, connect the mind–body by the psycho–neuro–immune network.

DIRECT VIBRATIONAL "WHISPER" WAVES

The heart marches to its own rhythmic beat. Heart waves show up on an electrocardiogram. The brain also has its own rhythm by which it creates brain waves. These waves appear on an electroencephalogram. As we said earlier, the heart has 40 to 60 times more electrical power than the brain.

The most sensitive connection between emotions and the heart is through the lungs. When you hyperventilate, your blood chemistry is changed with each breath, and this affects the heart. Also, the respiratory center in the brain communicates

---

with the centers regulating blood pressure and heart rate. Thus, breathing, emotion, heart rate, and blood pressure are all interdependent.

Breathing and the Heart

Breathing is the bridge between the mind and body. The alarm reaction in the breath holding reflex, is common to all animals. Vigilance and competition of modern life has caused us to develop this conditioned response of faulty breathing. We hold our breath and take shallow breaths. This over breathing is hyperventilation. That leads to mechanical and chemical disturbances in the body. In the heart, hyperventilation can cause chronic atherosclerosis, pump failure, acute spasms of coronary arteries, and heart attack or cardiac arrhythmia leading to sudden death. Effortless diaphragmatic or deep breathing can be learned by retraining the mind–to–muscle behavior patterns. As you breathe in, the heart speeds up. It slows down when you expel air. This is sinus arrhythmia, and it results from parasympathetic or *yin* control. In a stressful state and after a heart attack, the sinus arrhythmia decreases and becomes erratic. Breathing and its effects on the heart are explained in greater detail in the next chapter.

Chemical Stress Reaction

Chemicals released during acute and chronic stress are like a bowl of soup in which body cells swim. These chemicals cause the heart to react. Our graphics illustrate acute and chronic stress reactions and how they affect the entire mind–body.

Acute Stress Reaction

In acute stress reaction, first described by Cannon as a fight or flight response, there is a release of adrenaline and noradrenaline. There is a quick startle–the heart beats fast and hard in response to the direct commands from the brain. Adrenaline–like hormones directly stimulate the heart.

The typical acute anger reaction of type A behavior is helped along by the adrenaline and noradrenaline type of hormones. The behavior comes out as rage, fear, and frustration.

Type A behavior reacts with anger, aggression, and cynical mistrust to acute stress. In a normal reaction, acute stress response is followed by a "calm after the storm" type of overshooting and return to baseline.

Chronic Stress Reaction

Chronic stress reaction is a conservation and withdrawal response. It was first described by Selye as the General Adaptation Syndrome. The body releases pituitary hormones and adrenal cortical hormones, such as cortisone. The heart's irritability increases in response . The vigilance reaction leads to type C behavior of defeat, despair, helpless, hopeless states, and isolation from society. The heart carries an extra load. The immune system is suppressed. Physiological reserves go through an acute alarm, a resistance to combat, and exhaustion by consumption.

Comparision of Acute and Chronic Stress

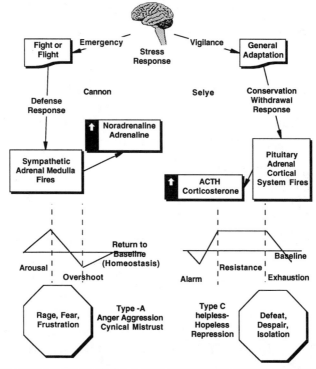

REACTIVITY OF BODY'S PUMPS AND PIPES

The basic reaction is stress chemicals which make calcium, potassium, and magnesium flood the cells, affecting the pumps and pipes of the body. At the atomic level, free radicals attack and distort the cells.

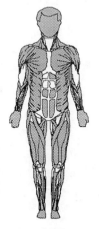

Blood Pipes in Brain Constrict:
1. *Restless Mind During the Day.*
2. *Restless Sleep at Night.*

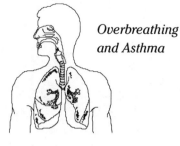

Overbreathing and Asthma

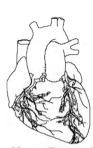

Muscle Pumps :
TMJ, Back Pain,
Tension Headache
Chronic Fatigue
Fibromyalgia,

Heart Pump: *Irregular Heartbeats* Yin-Yang *Heart Rate Imbalance (Emotions* Interact *with Heart) Pump Failure of Heart.*

Heart Pipes: *Coronary Blockage, Angina, Heart Attack, High Blood Pressure, Migraine, Cold Feet and Hands.*

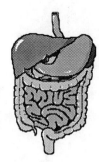

Gut Pipes:
Spasm of Esophagus
Ulcer, Irritable Bowels,
Colitis, Constipation.

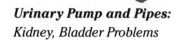

Urinary Pump and Pipes:
Kidney, Bladder Problems

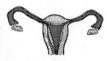

Reproductive Pump and Pipes:
Menstrual Cramps
Infertility, Sexual Problem

---

1. There is a continuous process of action and reaction going on at a chemical level in the body.

2. This chemical reaction manifests in different pumps and pipes of the body.

3. The heart is the master commander of the reactivity of the body.

4. You can memorize the pumps and pipes reactivity as given in the diagram. Every day you can relate your anger level and stress level to the pumps and pipes of the body.

5. Reactivity can be changed by interrupting the treadmill. This means slowing down your muscles before you slow down your mind.

Heart Disease and Cancer

18

Breathing and the Heart

Breathing and the Heart

Breathing is the bridge between your mind and body. It plays a key role in stress and relaxation response. Breath patterns reflect undercurrents in your body chemistry, thoughts, feelings, and even the programming of your subconscious mind.

Breathing has two basic chemical functions: 1) bring in energy - oxygen, and take out metabolic waste products - carbon dioxide; 2) to regulate the acid base balance of your body.

Normal and Abnormal Breathing

Normal breathing is effortless, without your conscious control. Most of the movement is in your abdomen's diaphragm. Your abdomen or belly bulges out as you breath in (inspiration) and collapses as you breath out (expiration). What is abnormal is either holding your breath, or hyperventilating. Breath holding is often a response to sudden sympathetic arousal-anxiety, or fear. It is followed by sighing and panting. Hyperventilating is rapid, shallow breathing, like a dog panting.

Breathing and Stress

When you are stressed, your sympathetic nervous system gets stimulated. Your breathing becomes more rapid and centered in the chest (thoracic area). This leads to excessive blowing out of carbon dioxide. Your blood turns alkaline and your kidneys receive a message to dump bicarbonate buffer from your body. If you try to relax, your breathing slows down and your blood becomes more acidic. Because your buffer reserve is depleted, your body cannot balance itself and the stress cycle continues. This vicious cycle creates a physiological **addiction to stress**.

Motion Controls Emotion. Breathing movements of the abdomen, chest, and shoulder muscles send messages to your brain, keeping it stimulated. Both holding your breath and shallow breathing intensify emotions. When you breathe into the

---

upper chest, you activate your sympathetic system, stimulating the stress arousal response. When you breathe into the abdomen, you activate the vagus nerve, stimulating the parasympathetic system and activating the relaxation response.

Startle (Alarm) Reaction: When you are startled, the typical reaction is a sharp intake of air or holding your breath, followed by shallow breathing in the chest area only.

Anger or Fear causes breath holding or rapid, shallow breathing.

Anxiety and Panic

The anxiety is accompanied by: breath holding, shallow thoracic breathing, increased breath rate, and irregularity. The decrease in carbon dioxide constricts blood vessels in the brain, thus reducing the oxygen supply, which results in behavioral changes and difficulty concentrating. The anxious person talks after taking a breath in a high voice. The depressed person talks after exhaling in a low voice. With panic, you hyperventilate, feel anxiety and a loss of control.

BREATHING AND THE HEART

The diagram summarizes the interdependent connections of various body functions and breathing.

1. **Hyperventilation:** When you over breathe, several changes occur in your body's physiology. For one, your lungs blow out excessive carbon dioxide and your blood pH becomes alkaline. Changing your blood's pH changes body chemistry in your heart and brain.

Your body has a fixed range of chemical balance, or *homeostasis*. One of the major components of your body chemistry is the acidity and alkalinity (pH) of body fluids. This is influenced by foods you eat as well as the motion and emotion in your body. Breathing is the pivotal factor for controlling motion and emotion.

2. **Bohr Effect:** Alkaline blood affects oxygen exchange in

---

Breathing and Heart

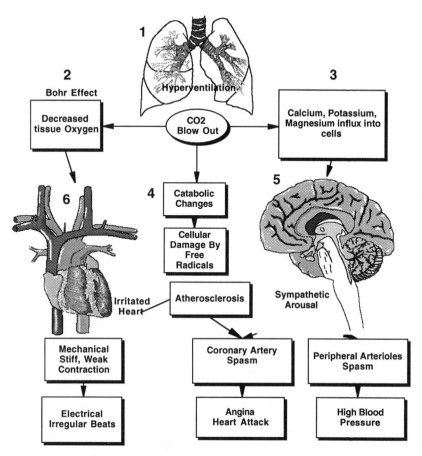

1 Hyperventilation

2 Bohr Effect

Decreased tissue Oxygen

CO2 Blow Out

3 Calcium, Potassium, Magnesium influx into cells

4 Catabolic Changes

Cellular Damage By Free Radicals

5 Sympathetic Arousal

6

Irritated Heart

Atherosclerosis

Mechanical Stiff, Weak Contraction

Coronary Artery Spasm

Peripheral Arterioles Spasm

Electrical Irregular Beats

Angina Heart Attack

High Blood Pressure

tissues. The bonding affinity of oxygen with hemoglobin in the red blood cells is stronger in alkaline blood. Not enough oxygen gets released to tissues. This is the Bohr effect. A low oxygen supply means less energy and less healing for the tissues. Low oxygen in the brain causes restless mind and memory loss.

3. **Mineral Changes:** Alkaline blood puts calcium, potassium, and magnesium into the cell. This mineral imbalance leads to irritability of nerves and muscles.

4. **Metabolic Changes:** You release adrenaline and noradrenaline during hyperventilation. That increases blood glucose,

fatty acids, and LDL cholesterol so you have extra energy to cope. Insulin secretion increases too, adding deposits of cholesterol in the blood vessels. The blood's ability to coagulate increases. Over time, "bad cholesterol" causes arteriosclerosis, coronary artery spasms, and peripheral arteriole spasms that lead to high blood pressure. Metabolic changes at the atomic level come from membrane damage or nuclear damage by the free radicals.

5. **Changes in the Brain:** Mineral changes and low oxygenation affect the brain and nervous system. This arouses the sympathetic nervous system. Peripheral arterioles begin to experience spasms, resulting in high blood pressure.

Hyperventilation increases neuromuscular excitability, causing pain, muscle tension, twitching, tremors, and fatigue. You can also include psychological factors such as tension, anxiety, phobia, panic, insomnia, nightmares, worry, fear, depression, anger, and feelings of loss of control. This hyperexcitability comes from calcium and potassium moving into the cells from the blood stream. The result is twitching or muscle contractions. Light is brighter, sound is louder, and you startle more easily.

6. **Changes in the Heart:** Adrenaline–like hormone and mineral changes in the blood strike the heart as well as the nervous system. The heart's mechanical pumping becomes weak, leading to stiff, ineffective emptying of the heart. And, because its electrical system is affected, heart beats become irregular.

Breathing and Sudden Cardiac Death

Hyperventilation can kill you. Actually, it is cardiac arrhythmia or a heart attack. Sudden spasm of the coronary artery cuts off oxygen to the heart muscles, causing cardiac arrhythmia. You may experience angina pains due to a coronary spasm - with or without preexisting narrowing of these arteries. In one study, eight out of nine patients who had variant angina, showed coronary artery spasm on angiography x–ray studies within five minutes of hyperventilating.

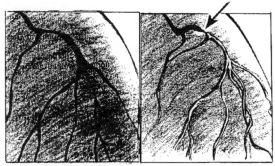

The dramatic effect of almost complete blockage of coronary arteries during forced hyperventilation is shown in the graphics on the left.

Before Hyperventilation Angiogram **After Hyperventilation Angiogram**

Sudden shocking can cause fatal hyperventilation. The first death as a result of the 1985 TWA flight hijack, was Benjamin Zimmerman. He died on the ground, in his home after receiving a phone call that his son, a flight engineer, was in the hijacked aircraft. Researchers found that 86% of NASA workers with sudden cardiac death had ruptured heart muscles (contraction band lesions) due to a sudden surge of catecholamines. Most of these patients had no coronary artery disease.

Diaphragmatic Breathing

The diaphragm muscle separates the belly from the chest cavity. The diaphragm normally does 80% of the breathing. You see diaphragmatic breathing in the pushing out of your abdomen with each breath taken in.

The benefits of diaphragmatic breathing include: less stress arousal, less fatigue, better circulation, enhanced lymph flow and immunity, a stronger and more stable heart, more positive emotions, and improved healing.

How to Practice Diaphragmatic Breathing: The simplest way to learn diaphragmatic breathing is to put one hand on your belly and one on your chest. As you breathe in, make sure that your belly bulges out like a balloon. Repeat this exercise for five to ten minutes until you are able to get a feel for belly breathing without your hands on your belly. While lying down, put a book on your belly and make the book go up with each breath in the cycle. After about five minutes, take the book away,

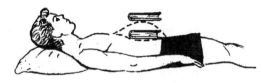 and repeat the belly movements by recalling the book experience. Do this for about a week, and you'll have a pretty good feel for what diaphragmatic breathing really is.

BAD BREATHING HABITS

BREATH HOLDING:

It is the natural fight or flight response. This stimulates your sympathetic nervous system, increasing stress. If you just let go and breathe out, you immediately feel better. The easy pun to remember is "When you inhale, you are in hell." Just getting into the exhale cycle helps you feel more relaxed.

THORACIC BREATHING:

This is with the chest wall muscles, which are less efficient than those of the diaphragm. Shallow breathing with chest wall movements blows out carbon dioxide and makes your blood more alkaline. This increases the rate of nerve impulses and muscle tension. It also requires more breaths to maintain an adequate supply of oxygen. It is another misplaced effort.

HYPERVENTILATION

This is rapid breathing which sets up a chain reaction. It starts with excessive exhalation of CO_2. Usually, it includes thoracic breathing. You sigh frequently in order to catch up with the loss of breath. Reduced carbon dioxide makes your blood more alkaline. That makes you hyperexcitable, anxious, and stressed. Calcium, magnesium, and potassium are driven into the cells, which irritates your heart, brain, and peripheral tissues. Blood pressure goes up and your heart has to work against an additional load, causing it more stress.

Causes of Hyperventilation

Two types of factors can start you hyperventilating:

Body factors Metabolic, physical, and chemical disorders

---

of bodily organs stress the system. A fever is a metabolic example. Chemical factors include foods and drugs. Physical factors may be exercise or lack of it.

Mind factors - stress due to activation of the sympathetic nervous system.

Hyperventilation Cycle

You can trace the cycle from initiating mind–body stressors to the final common pathway of hyperventilation. Once started, hyperventilation leads to chemical changes in the body (carbon dioxide blow out, alkalosis, calcium, potassium influx into cells) and unpleasant body sensations. You experience rapid heart beat, emotional sweating, and tense muscles. These sensations make you anxious, which provokes further stress and hyperventilation. You can interrupt

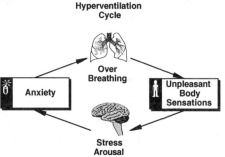

Hyperventilation Cycle

Over Breathing — Anxiety — Unpleasant Body Sensations — Stress Arousal

this cycle by conscious diaphragmatic breathing, which will correct the chemical changes and break the cycle.

Catabolic Effects of Hyperventilation

Your body's metabolism can be regenerative (anabolic) or degenerative (catabolic). The catabolic changes of hyperventilation include a halt in synthesis and increased breakdown of protein, fat, and carbohydrates. These changes lead to:

1. Elevated blood levels of glucose, free fatty acids, and LDL cholesterol, increased liver enzymes and red blood cells for mobilizing energy.
2. Damage to bone, mucus membranes, skin, immune system, and nervous system.
3. Decreased sexual hormones.
4. Retention of salt and water. Increased output of blood from the heart.
5. High blood pressure.

Symptoms & Signs of Hyperventilation

You see hyperventilation's effects in the "pumps" and "pipes" of the body.

Respiratory: Asthma, cough, sighing, shortness of breath.

Cardiovascular: Palpitation, angina, irregular heart beat, heart attack, high blood pressure.

Neurological: Dizziness, fainting, migraine, numbness.

Gastrointestinal: Lump in the throat, dry mouth and throat, indigestion, constipation, diarrhea.

Muscular: Shoulder pain, tense muscles, twitches, tremors, pain, fatigue.

Psychological: Tension, anxiety, phobia, panic, insomnia, nightmares, worry, fear, depression, anger, feeling of loss of control.

How to Measure Hyperventilation

Hyperventilation is a subtle physical, chemical, and behavioral change in response to stress you can measure by:

1. **Self–Observations:** Put one hand on your abdomen and one on your chest. Watch which hand moves more. Over breathing is usually thoracic. Your chest moves more than your abdomen. Count your respiration – if it is more than 12–15 per minute, you are over breathing. Look at the proportion of inspiration to expiration. A normal ratio is 1:1. When you breathe in more than you breathe out, it is hyperventilating. Notice what hyperventilation does to your neck and shoulder muscles. If you hyperventilate, you will feel aches and pains. Observe your sleep pattern – if you wake up with a restless mind and sweating, it is most likely you are hyperventilating during the day.

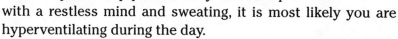

2. **Biofeedback:** We place elastic around your chest and abdomen that measures the rate and the degree of movement. Another biofeedback measure (called EMG) directly monitors

---

muscle tension in abdominal, shoulder and neck muscles with each respiration.

3. **Capnometer:** We use a special machine that measures the amount of CO_2 (end tidal carbon dioxide) in exhaled air. The normal capnometer value is 38 to 42 torr units. A value less than 38 indicates hyperventilation. In severe hyperventilation, it is less than 20.

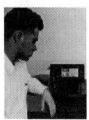

Treating Hyperventilation

Treatment is generally the same as managing stress arousal. The approach is either muscle–to–mind or mind–to–muscle.

Muscle–to–Mind Approaches

1. Deliberately switch to diaphragmatic breathing.

2. Increase physical activity by walking around to manage your acute hyperventilation. This exercise increases the carbon dioxide production and balances the body's chemistry.

3. Do yoga and stretching exercises to increase the length of muscle fibers and decrease muscle–to–mind traffic of nerve signals.

Mind–to–Muscle Approaches

1. Remove conflicts in the mind by heartfelt resonant imaging (HRI).

2. Desensitize your haunting negative imageries and major worries by eyeball desensitization; meditation and imagery; the open focus exercise, etc. These are explained under restless mind control.

3. Balance your rest and activity in life as outlined in the chapter on rest and activity.

1. Hyperventilation is rapid thoracic breathing which leads to alkaline blood and chemical changes.

2. Chemical changes lead to a restless mind, insomnia, and reactivity of the pumps and pipes of the body.

3. You control thoracic breathing by using muscle-to-mind and mind-to-muscle tools.

19

Heart Rate Variability and Emotions

Heart Rate Variability and Emotions

Once, a doctor's stethoscope was the major magic diagnostic instrument. Today, thanks to high tech computers, we can measure, monitor, and modify each beat of the heart. You can also modify your body chemistry and emotional state by modifying your heart rate.

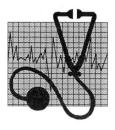

The Heart as a Powerhouse

Your heart is your body's main source of electrical power.

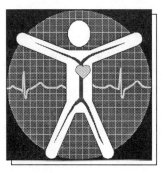

It produces an electrical output of 2.5 watts, which is 40 to 60 times stronger than the brain's. The heart's electrical power is transmitted to each organ and every cell in the body. The smallest cell part of the cell, such as DNA, dances to electrical virbrations as the heart commands. The heart and blood vessels have the largest body surface, covering an area over half the size of a football field.

Electrocardiogram (ECG or EKG)

The heart generates an electrical wave with each beat. The EKG complex includes several wave segments called P,Q,R,S, and T. The P wave represents contraction of the atrium or the upper chambers of the heart. The QRS complex represents contraction of the ventricles, or lower chambers of the heart. The T wave represents repolarization or electrical recovery of the ventricles. Strong emotional states, such as anger, frustration, and fear, immediately change the shape of these waves. Anger stimulates the emergency branch of the nervous system (sympathetic branch) and releases adrenaline-like hormones.

When you're angry, the T wave flattens, indicating insufficient recovery of the heart muscle with each beat.

Holter Monitor

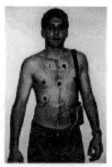

The Holter monitor is a battery-powered recording device connected to the heart by electrodes placed on your chest. As you wear this device, it measures each heart beat for 24 hours. Then a computer analyzes the tape. This Holter study gives the character of each heart wave, beat by beat. It also calculates your heart rate and heart rate variability.

Heart Rate Variability (HRV)

This refers to the number of times your heart beats per minute. The normal adult rate is about 70 beats per minute. This is an average because time intervals between heart beats are always changing. **Heart rate variability is a measure of these beat-to-beat time interval variations as the heart speeds up or slows down.** Mathematically, heart rate variability is the fluctuation of the heart rate around a mean heart rate. Let us take a person who has a mean heart rate of 60 beats per minute. This would mean that his heart beats one time every second. In reality, the heart never beats that regularly. There are always minor changes in the time interval from one beat to the next. If the interval between beat one and two is one second, beat two and three could be 0.75 seconds, beat three and four could be 1.5 seconds apart, and so on. In this case, heart rate variability is irregular. It could be regular if the variation follows an even pattern; it is irregular if the variation does not follow an even pattern.

A normal EKG shows variability with each breath. There is a rhythm of variation with each breath. We call it **sinus arrhythmia.** This sinus arrhythmia itself can be low, less than 50 milliseconds from beat to beat on average, or big, more than 50 milliseconds.

Cardiac Arrhythmia or irregular heart beats is commonly diagnosed in the doctor's office. This refers to irregular beats originating in the ventricles, or

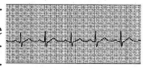

above the ventricles. This is diagnosed by a common electro-cardiogram or EKG. The patient may feel these beats as palpitations. This example shows such premature ventricular beats.

HEART RATE VARIABILITY

Cardiac Arrhythmia

The HRV we refer to is not these irregular beats; rather, it is the variation in sinus rhythm itself as it changes from beat to beat. Recording HRV requires more sensitive computer equipment to calculate the distance from one beat to the next. When we measure peak-to-peak distance of two QRS waves from one beat to the next, we call it a time domain analysis. If the wave pattern itself is measured in each beat, with its accompanying harmonic derivatives, it is a frequency domain analysis. The newer high tech computers can analyze these wave patterns. Modern fast computers have made these fine tuned analyses practical in your doctor's office.

What Controls Heart Rate Variability?

Heart rate variability (HRV) depends on three connections between the brain and the heart:

1. **Hard-wire connections** between sympathetic and para-sympathetic nerves.

2. **Liquid media** connections by messenger molecules.

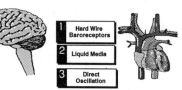

Heart Brain Connections

3. **Direct vibrational waves.** The hard wire connection has three parts: sympathetic and parasympathetic branches which act as opposites, bringing messages from the brain to speed up or slow down the heart; and the barorecep-tor system which takes messages from the heart to the brain. So it is a two-way communication system.

Yin-Yang Balance and HRV

Your body has two opposing systems: female and male, yin and yang (Chinese), or prakriti and purusha (Sanskrit).

Yin System: The yin system in the hard wire section is made up of parasympathetic nerves which slow down the heart and let it recover. The liquid media of yin includes endorphin-like chemicals which also make you feel good. The yin vibrations are smooth, regular, and change rhythmically with each breath.

Yang System: The yang system in the hard wire is made up of sympathetic nerves which speed up the heart and cause wear and tear. The liquid media of yang includes adrenaline-like chemicals which also make you feel agitated and angry. The yang vibrations are erratic and irregular. When yin-yang is out of balance, your heart becomes brittle and vulnerable to serious irregularity or heart attack.

Brittle Heart and Sudden Death

In a normal person, the HRV is rhythmic, with a value of more than 50 milliseconds on average between beats.

A Multicenter Postinfarction Research Group study found that low heart rate variability, less than 50 milliseconds, has a 5.3 times higher chance of sudden death. This is due to dampening of the parasympathetic pathway.

A new study by Algra looked at 6,693 consecutive Holter records of people who died suddenly. Low heart rate variability was associated with double the risk of sudden death. Heart rate variability itself is an independent risk factor for sudden irregular heart beat and death. **Sudden death in low HRV people is due to a "brittle heart" not being able to withstand stress and strain.**

Coronary Artery Disease

Coronary artery disease, congestive heart failure, and hypertension change heart rate variability. Change is due to suppression of parasympathetic vagal tone and stimulation of sympathetic tone. In heart attack patients, the damage done to the heart affects HRV sensitivity. Diabetes and certain neurological diseases affect heart rate variability as a result of damage to the nerve pathway.

Drug Effects

Heart rate variability is affected by drugs that stimulate or depress the sympathetic and parasympathetic pathways or brain centers. Atropine blocks the vagal nerves and decreases HRV. Beta-blockers block the sympathetic nerve receptors and increase HRV. That is why beta-blockers are given to increase HRV after a heart attack. Calcium blockers, ace inhibitors, uppers, and central nervous system downers affect HRV as well.

Emotional Opposites

Caring love, appreciation, joy, and peace go with high and regular heart rate variability, below:

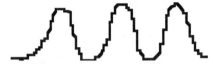

Frustration, anger, fear, and guilts accompany low and irregular heart rate variability, below:

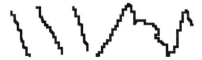

State Dependent Learning

Heart rate variability graphs in a biofeedback computer monitor the state of caring love and contrast it with frustration and anger. This allows you to differentiate between mindfelt feelings and heartfelt feelings. By repeatedly focusing on the anatomical heart and recalling feelings of caring love, you release endorphins into the blood and dicover the sense of peace and joy within yourself. This conditioned learning is just like Pavlov training his dogs to salivate at the ring of a bell.

Putting the Cart Before the Horse

When you are in a state of caring love, such as feeding a

baby or "whole heartedly" helping someone, your heart rate variability is smooth and rhythmic. This sequence is reversed in training with biofeedback of heart rate variability. First, you focus on your anatomical heart – this makes your heart rate variability smooth and rhythmic.

Second, in this heart-anchored state, you orient yourself to your caring love feelings and develop a conditioned response to enter into this state.

1. Heart rate variability (HRV), is a new scientific discovery. HRV refers to change in the distance between one heart beat and the next one.

2. New research by Holter monitoring thousands of people has shown that erratic and low HRV may herald sudden death.

3. Anger and frustration causes erratic and low HRV. Caring love causes smooth, and rhythmic HRV.

4. Focusing on your anatomical heart causes smooth, and rhythmic HRV. This phenomenon is used in developing the tool called HRI (Heartfelt Resonant Imaging).

20

Restless Mind Control

Restless Mind Control

Restless mind and insomnia are interdependent with a common biochemical basis. A restless mind is the result of a restless body. A restless body contains agitated chemistry and tense muscles. A restless mind has a corresponding imbalance in three systems:

1. **Hard wire of neuromuscular connections**: (Tense muscles and increased nerve traffic).
2. **Liquid media of messenger molecules** (Stress hormones, neurotransmitters, and immune transmitters).
3. **Vibrational waves of the heart and brain** (heart rate and rhythm; brain waves pattern).

The mind and body are two ends of the same bridge with a traffic terminal at either end.

This is a recirculating traffic system: what goes up comes down. You have up–going traffic from the muscle to the brain (sensory nerve pathway) and down–going traffic from the brain to the muscle (motor nerve pathway). The muscle–to–mind pathway carries muscle tension or agitation that interferes with mental calmness. The mind–to–muscle pathway delivers the restless, racing mind that often triggers nervous muscle movements and tension.

You can control restless mind traffic at either terminal, but it is easier to control it at the muscle terminal. Once you reduce the muscle–to–mind traffic, it is easy to control your mind (just like it's easier to control an automobile at a reduced speed). Reducing muscle and mind traffic makes your mind more sensitive to subtle differences. Imagine holding a hammer in one hand and a feather in the other. If a fly lands on the feather, you will notice it more than if it lands on the hammer. The goal of relaxing muscle tension is to reach this subtle level of perception.

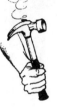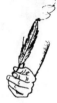

You reduce traffic at the muscle end by lengthening muscle fibers. Yoga postures, stretching, or contraction and muscle relaxation of your muscles will do the job. When muscle fibers lengthen, the relaxed muscles send fewer signals to the brain, reducing traffic congestion at the mind level. To reduce traffic at the mind, you distribute sensations or thoughts into multiple, parallel channels. This process is called opening the focus or simply open focus.

Breathing connects two terminals. When you synchronize your mind in a rhythmic fashion (repeating a mantra and connecting it with the rhythm of breathing), you simultaneously reduce the traffic congestion at both terminals (mind and muscle). This is because you calm the mind and muscle at the same time.

Your restless mind control tool consists of several exercises, both muscle–to–mind and mind–to–muscle.

INTRODUCTION TO MUSCLE–TO–MIND EXERCISES

The part of your body over which you have direct control is your skeletal muscles. That is why they are called voluntary muscles. These muscles control the arousal level of the brain and autonomic nervous system, which in turn changes the hormonal and immune functions. **The first step in self–regulation starts with control of skeletal muscles.**

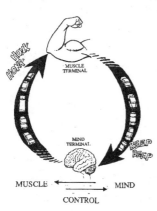

Two sets of voluntary muscle make important contributions to the *mind–to–muscle* connection and the restless mind. These are the *muscles involved in sight*, both outer vision and inner vision (visualization), and the *muscles involved in speech,* both outer speech to others and inner speech (self–talk).

The restless mind is a series of thought waves mixed with emotions. There are two distinct control signals for this "thought wave machine."

Heart Disease and Cancer

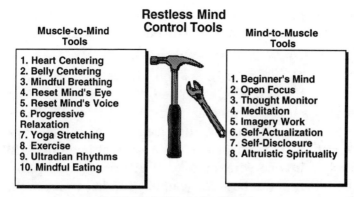

Restless Mind Control Tools

Muscle-to-Mind Tools

1. Heart Centering
2. Belly Centering
3. Mindful Breathing
4. Reset Mind's Eye
5. Reset Mind's Voice
6. Progressive Relaxation
7. Yoga Stretching
8. Exercise
9. Ultradian Rhythms
10. Mindful Eating

Mind-to-Muscle Tools

1. Beginner's Mind
2. Open Focus
3. Thought Monitor
4. Meditation
5. Imagery Work
6. Self-Actualization
7. Self-Disclosure
8. Altruistic Spirituality

Meditation Begins When Restless Mind Ends

Let's call these two signals the *"mind's voice"* and the *"mind's eye."*

The mind's voice is your talking mind. When you engage in restless mind–talk, there is hidden tension and muscle movement in your jaw, lips, tongue, throat, and vocal cords that parallel your thoughts. Your mind's voice uses non–vocalized impulses to your real mouth and vocal cord to keep on talking to itself. We've recorded this with electromyography machines used in biofeedback training.

The mind's eye is your visualizing mind. Your mind's eye uses your real eyes as a buddy. Whenever you think, you visualize images. When your mind's eye is restless, you usually visualize negative images. They provoke negative emotions, such as fear, anger, guilt, and sadness. Because of the muscle–to–mind connection, you have indirect control over the seemingly uncontrollable: restless mind–talk of your mind's voice; and negative imageries of your mind's eye. You take control through specific voluntary muscles.

We will show you how to control your mind chatter by controlling the real muscles of your mouth and vocal cord; and then how to control the flickering of your mental eye by controlling your real eyeball muscles. We will show you a few drills to develop muscle relaxation skills. The goal is to identify the control signal for contracting each muscle. Your control signal is the feeling of tension in each muscle. You want to become aware of the tension that goes with each restless mind activity.

Muscle–to–Mind Exercise Instructions

1. **Heart Centering:** Focus your awareness on your anatomical heart area, and ask yourself, "Can I experience caring love towards this person, animal, plant, or object?" Differentiate between mindfelt and heartfelt feelings, and the sender and receiver of love. **Use this Heartfelt Resonant Imaging (HRI)™ as a tool to invoke your biology of altruism (endorphin release).** The tug of war between your head and heart is the single most important cause of a restless mind.

2. **Belly Centering:** Simply shift your awareness to your belly button and breathe. Centering is basic to all muscle–to–mind exercises for quieting the restless mind.

3. **Mindful Breathing:** Find, follow, and link the breath to your restless mind. Focus on the exhaling sigh and slightly prolong it. Breathe with awareness focused on the abdominal area. Develop a rhythm of diaphragmatic breathing by imagining the metaphor of a pyramid with the base in the pelvis and the apex at the throat, filling from bottom to top with each breath.

4. **Reset Mind's Eyes:** Imagine a pendulum swinging in front of your open or closed eyes and move the eyeballs "tick" to the right, and "tock" to the left with the swing of the pendulum. This resets the mental eye because the imageries in your mind do not get the corresponding feedback from your real eyes. In other words, this eyeball desensitizing erases the negative emotional charges of haunting thoughts. **This exercise is very effective for calming down at night if a restless mind keeps you from getting back to sleep.**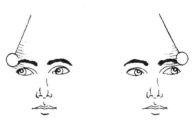

5. **Reset Mind's Voice:** You calm the the talking muscles by imitating the kissing movement of "eee" and "ooo." Move

the tongue in all directions. Count down from ten to one and simultaneously reduce the volume of the imaginary voice in your vocal cord. Clench your jaw tightly; feel the control signal (of tension), then relax or "let go" and open your jaw.

The jaw muscle is the first to tense due to our primitive "biting instinct." Your mind's voice tends to make your jaw muscles bite down hard on problematic, ruminating thoughts.

6. **Progressive Muscle Relaxation:** Contract and relax muscle groups starting from the head and proceeding to the toes, paying attention to the different sensations in the muscles as you contract and relax them. Think of the slogan, **"find and follow."** This is another way of saying "Pay attention to the control signal." Once a muscle contracts, relax again. It lengthens more than it was before. You can do a muscle relaxation exercise quickly, progressively focusing on the main muscles of tension. You can also do it over a longer time period. Include more muscle groups or repeat those that continue to have unwanted tension. Use this list to assist you:

- Forehead – raise eyebrows and frown.
- Eyes – close tightly; move eyeballs up, down, left, right, and all around.
- Jaw and lower face – clench jaw.
- Head – touch left and right shoulders, then put chin to chest.
- Shoulders – lift and shrug.
- Arms – squeeze upper and lower on each side.
- Abdomen – tighten belly.
- Legs – squeeze thigh and calf on each side.

7. **Yoga Stretching**: Motion controls emotion. When your mind is restless, just stand up and walk around in the room. Changing your posture stretches the contracted muscle and reduces the up–going traffic to the brain. You can use different muscle stretching routines throughout the day to relax your

---

mind–body. The parent system of stretching routines is various yoga postures.

What is Yoga? The literal meaning of yoga is union. By union, we mean uniting parts of systems and subsystems. From a practical standpoint, this union is of the mind, body, emotions, spirit, and the universe–at–large. It is a union of two sides of human existence: *yin–yang*, female–male, and parasympathetic–sympathetic. That is why yoga balances your life. Yoga reconnects the mind–body's two oscillating cycles (mind–to–muscle and muscle–to–mind) in the same process, in the, here and now.

Body-minded Yoga: Commonly, yoga refers to yoga postures. Traditionally, however, that branch of yoga is known as **hatha yoga.** We like to use yoga in a "body-mindful" way. Stretch and strengthen muscles by moving very slowly, with particular moment–to–moment awareness of the body part being stretched and the control signals of the stretched muscles. In body–minded yoga, you get centered by paying attention to your breathing. Direct the breath and mind to the part of the body being stretched. This opens the focus of your "head strong" mind to the "body strong" mind. Yoga is stretching your mind to the entire extent of the body. This is the fundamental principle of self–study, or *svadhyaya,* as Patanjali, the father of the yoga system, put it in his *Yoga Sutra* treatise.

Your awareness of the body parts in question brings that part into order and regulation. This is just like the way a class in school comes back to order when the teacher returns. Our awareness to a certain part of the body revitalizes that part.

Being rather than Doing Yoga: The common error people make in stretching or yoga exercises is they pay attention to the outcome and extent of the stretch. This is *doing yoga;* trying to achieve something. But, what is most important is "*being with it*" in the process of stretching, moment by moment. This orients you to the body and heals that part by directing the vital energy, *prana, or chi t*o it.

Yoga Itself is Meditation: In the classical teaching of Patanjali, yoga postures prepare one to enter into the meditative state. The body–minded diffusion of thinking energy gets you into a passive state ready for meditation. But, in reality, if you do each posture mindfully, paying attention to the present moment, then that itself is meditation. Yoga postures can also help you prepare for sitting meditation.

Mathematics of Yoga Stretching: Ultimately, how much of stress impulse goes to your brain depends on how many of your muscle fibers are shortened and how many are lengthened. You have approximately 1,030 muscles in your body. Hypothetically, if you imagine there are 1,000 feet of fibers in each muscle, you have a total of 1,030,000 feet of muscle fibers.

So, if you stretch any of these muscles, regardless which, you add to the total fiber length. And **the longer the muscle fibers, the less impulse traffic to the brain** and the less restless the mind. This is the rationale for athletic and yoga stretching.

8. **Physical Activity: Race the Body with the Mind**: If your mind is still restless, take a brisk walk or rotate your arms like a windmill, or simply sit and stand to dissipate the pent–up adrenaline and other hormones. If you are inside your room and feel stressed, a quick and simple way to release tension is to swing your arms like a windmill.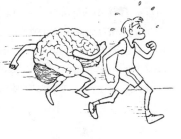
The principles of rest and activity are outlined in the Rest and Activity chapter.

9. **Respect the Rhythms of Life: Sleep, Daydream, etc.**: The earth moves on its axis and around the sun. This gives your body the symphony of a round–the–clock **circadian rhythm** (day–night or "circle the day") that regulates such factors as hunger, temperature, mood, and alertness. One third of us are night people, who like to go to bed late and get up late.

Another third are morning people, who like to go to bed early and get up early. The remaining third can go either way. The morning larks are energetic in the morning and the nightowls at night. Learn your own biological rhythm and set your productive and meditative time accordingly.

Due to periodic and natural fluctuations in the earth's magnetic field, our mind–body operates in a cycle of 90-minutes activity and 20 minutes rest.This is the **ultradian rhythm.** Natural cues tell you to give your body a 20 minute break. You want to stretch, yawn, snack or urinate. Your mind wanders, your performance levels drop sharply. Use these natural cues. Take a one to five minute break every 90 minutes. Some suggested break time activities include: closing your eyes, doodling, urinating, meditating, diaphragmatic breathing, daydreaming or fantasizing, eating healthy snacks, and stretching.

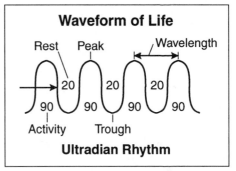

10. **Mindful Eating:** Eat six meals per day to keep your insulin and blood sugar level even. This also keeps your restless mind under control. Eat starch based, low fat, fruit and vegetables. Add a fruit and vegetable snack between breakfast and lunch, lunch and dinner, and bedtime. Vegetable snacks satisfy the chewing instinct and eliminate the "biting instinct"that goes with a restless mind.

INTRODUCTION TO MIND–TO–MUSCLE EXERCISES

Mind–to–Muscle Exercise Instructions

1. **Beginner's Mind:** Look at a person, animal, plant, or object as if for the first time, in a non–judgmental way. Here's an exercise to help you. First, look at a tree and analyze it. Make judgments about its features, such as its leaves. Are they green enough? Now get centered by focusing on your belly–button.

Look at the tree as if you are looking at it for the first time. Simply look at it mindfully and notice the difference in your perception.

2. **Open Focus™**: Open Focus™ refers to opening up your sensory awareness from a "tunnel vision" to a "funnel vision." Often, you may have a one–track mind which inhibits entry of all the other information at the same time This restraint leaves you tense because the restraining order in your brain consumes a lot of energy.

Your mind has parallel processing powers. It is a multi–tasking, multi–channeled computer. When you shut down a channel of information, then all of these sensory energies get narrowed down into one channel, which produces congestion and tension.

When you open all your channels, your mind automatically relaxes because the pressure is distributed into multiple channels. You can open all your channels by **simultaneously and equally** allowing your mind to be available to experience. The most effective drill for this skill, called open focus, was developed by Les Fehmi.

Fehmi shows that the easiest way to open focus your mind is to think of space in and around your body. Basically, you conceptualize yourself and your surroundings as interconnected space. This imagined interconnected space in and around your body automatically disembodies your mind from your head to your body, and relaxes you completely.

To do the drill, ask questions: With your eyes closed, can you imagine that your left eye is full of space? ...that your right eye is full of space? ...there's space between your eyes? ...space above, below, behind, and in front of your eyes?

Ask these questions of your whole body, your immediate surroundings, and finally, the entire intergalactic space and the universe. Distribute your senses *simultaneously* and *equally* to what you see, hear, smell, taste, and touch at the moment. This parallel distribution of impulses reduces traffic. Imagine your left eye is space, your right eye is space, your head is space, and your whole body is space. This space awareness relaxes your muscles.

3. **Thought Monitor:** Observe your thoughts as a spectator. There are three kinds of baby–sitters: one overcontrols the baby, the second neglects and falls asleep, and the third just observes the baby. Baby–sit your thoughts as a spectator and observer.

4. **Meditation:** Observe your breathing in your belly. Mentally, say "so" as you breathe in and "ham" as you breathe out. If your mind wanders, bring it back to your breath and the "so–ham" sound. Deepen meditation by rolling your eyeballs up as if to watch the sun rise to midday.

5. **Imagery Work:** Close your eyes and breathe out three times, slightly prolonging expiration with a "haam." Now, you are in the alpha–theta state. Create mental pictures (such as a seashore) for relaxation, healing, problem solving, or creativity. An effective way to calm your mind is to imagine you are in a pleasant setting, such as a beach. A beach is ideal for most people because it involves many senses: the sight of surging waves, the sound of surf, the feel of warm sun and sand, the smell of seaweed, etc. That opens up inhibited channels of your mind.

6. **Self–Actualization:** Observe your mind–body muscles in relation to your thoughts and feelings. Figure out your perceptual type, mindfelt and heartfelt feeling level, physiological signature, money style, gender differences, and explanatory style. Speak this out to a tape recorder or write it down for your self–actualization.

7. **Self–Disclosure:** (Three T's) Time, Touch, and Talk with a partner. Express and explain how your body changes with each emotion. Dovetail your feelings with your partner's feelings. Do the three T session every day. Write out difficult feelings and read them to your partner. (Self-actualization and self-disclosure are discussed in detail in Chapter 24.)

8. **Altruistic Spirituality**: Spirituality is the recognition and acceptance of a Higher Power over and above your own intelligence and will. An entity with which you can have an intimate relationship. **The essential concept is the transcending of your own personal self.** "Modern" individuals often feel a sense of "existential anxiety." There is a vague sense of tension, of boredom, and a quiet desperation. They wonder if they are all that they can be. Many cannot escape from self–imposed confines of existential anxiety. It is here that a sense of spirituality provides solace.

Spirituality suggests a higher self, a higher power, God, Nature, Universal Energy. It often involves a quest for happiness, or inner peace. Spirituality is that part of us which connects us with the positive forces of the universe. The great 20th century philosopher, Aldous Huxley refers to human purpose as "perennial philosophy." According to perennial philosophy, we all came from a spiritual source – a dimension more than our mind and body. Huxley quotes an anthology of passages from great religions and spiritual systems in the world. He concludes that truth is one and paths are many.

The central core of all spiritual beliefs is that every form of dedication and purpose in human life is ultimately spiritual – be it literature, art, music, religion, etc. The purpose of science itself is to understand Nature. The spiritual quest can be undertaken by a religious person, atheist, agnostic, or anyone.

The only thing that separates from this spiritual connection is our belief we are separate. Our soul yearns to unite with a spiritual source. The moment we realize our interconnectedness with each other and our interdependent existence, we begin our journey towards the higher power that ties us together. This pursuit is called self–actualization by Abraham Maslow. Maslow named it "peak experience" or sense of unity with the cosmos, or oneness with higher self. Hindus call it yoga or union with God.

The dualistic concept of "spirit" or higher self as different from "matter" has created two opposite camps: sacred (spiritual) and secular (scientific). Science has focused on measurement of Nature, with the yardsticks of scientific experiments and data collection. However, this view of Nature is limited. Humans have an inner urge to leave this self–imposed restraint of looking at the scientific horizon as the ultimate destination.

Altruism is living with the feeling "you are also included in my agenda." This is called *seva* in Sanskrit. This feeling can be cultivated in a biological sense by heart centered living. The heart knows only how to love. Heart centered living connects you to others and your own higher self. In his treatise, *Yoga Sutra*, Patanjali said, *Tapaha swadhyaya ishwarparanidhanmiti kriya yogaha,* which means that the ultimate solution for a restless mind is to surrender to the ultimate power.

1. Restless mind is due to restless body.

2. Restless body has agitated chemistry and tense muscles.

3. You can control restless mind in two ways: muscle-to-mind, or mind-to-muscle pathways.

4. Muscle-to-mind pathway is always easy because we have more control to change the muscle contraction.

5. This chapter lists muscle-to-mind and mind-to-muscle tools used in the rest of the book.

21

Insomnia Control

Sleep as a Slayer, Sleep as a Saver

Insomnia –
Sleep as Slayer or Saver?

Sleep is a litmus test of health. You often hear someone say, "don't lose sleep over it" or "get a good night's sleep." But sleep (or lack of it) is a slayer. Protein synthesis and cell division occur during sleep. Throughout the day, you have cells die and be repaired. Healing repair happens during sleep because that's when you release healing growth hormones and endorphins.

What is Insomnia?

Insomnia is qualitative or quantitative sleep loss, or both. There are two types:

1. **Sleep onset insomnia** (difficulty falling asleep - taking more than thirty minutes to fall asleep),

2. **Sleep maintenance insomnia** (difficulty staying asleep, with sleep interruption of longer than thirty minutes or waking up too soon and being unable to return to sleep). The result is fatigue, impaired performance, and mood disturbances.

What Causes Insomnia

First, you may be **predisposed.** That is, you tend to be obsessive, worrisome, hypervigilant, and anxiety prone. It may be an inherited trait, and women are twice as prone to insomnia. Physical or mental stress and illness can **precipitate** the problem. Ffinally, maladaptive habits and irrational thoughts about insomnia **perpetuate** sleep loss. **This is a state of learned helplessness**, or mind–body conditioned response. We call it psychophysiological insomnia. It can be unlearned using the state-dependent learning principles.

Cybernetic Model of Insomnia

Insomnia is when the wakefulness center in the brain overpowering the sleep center. It sets up a vicious cycle.

1. **Stress arousal:** You go to bed with rapid breathing, rapid

Cybernetic Model of Insomnia

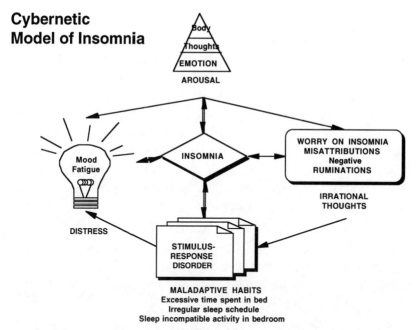

heart, higher temperature, increased muscle tension, etc. which causes (or is caused by) thoughts (intrusive worries), and emotions (anxiety, anger, guilt, or sadness).

2. **Irrational thoughts:** That spurs worries about sleep loss; ruminations on daytime problems; more muscle tension, and restlessness. Trying hard to sleep creates anxiety. You overestimate your sleep loss and become even more anxious. How can you possibly fall asleep under those conditions!

3. **Maladaptive habits:** Other factors that don't help: Excessive time in bed, irregular sleep time, and arousal producing activities - watching TV, reading, arguing with partner, etc. Being awake to these stimuli provokes more wakefulness, and the vicious cycle continues.

4. **Distress** Insomnia leaves you fatigued, irritable. You have social and relationship problems. Your job performance drops. This creates guilt and helplessness in the downhill spiral of loss of control. So you attribute insomnia to external factors, rather than seeing the vicious cycle you are in.

Stress Addiction — "Sour Sleep"

As discussed earier, stress addiction follows a pattern: 1) stress leads to hyperventilating, 2) you blow out carbon dioxide, 3) your system becomes alkaline, 4) buffer reserve suffers, 5) calcium, potassium, and magnesium flow into cells, 6) the neuromuscular system becomes excited, 7) causing more stress, 8) insomnia, and 9) the cycle starts all over again. Typically, buffer loss reduces the flexibility of your acid–base equilibrium system, and the slow breathing of sleep for three to four hours leads to acidosis. So you wake up between 1:00 and 3:00 AM with a restless mind and emotional sweating . We call this "sour sleep" because acidity in the blood triggers it.

The solution for sour sleep is to cut day time arousal. Take a break every two hours. Breath diaphragmatically, and meditate. The more diaphragmatic breaths you take during the day, the better your buffer reserve is at night.

Behavioral Treatment of Insomnia

1. **Sleep Hygiene:** Maintain a healthy lifestyle to minimize sleep–disturbing physical and chemical activities.

(i) *Food and Drugs:* Avoid nicotine, caffeine, and alcohol. Caffeine in the afternoon reduces the quality of sleep at night. Alcohol may induce sleep, but later interrupts deep sleep. Avoid stimulant drugs in the afternoon. A complex carbohydrate meal aids sleep. Protein enhances alertness. Tryptophan in the form of milk helps sleep. Fruits at bedtime help to balance the acid–base problem by increasing the alkaline tide at night, strengthening the buffer system.

(ii) *Exercise:* Exercise in the early afternoon or in the morning promotes sleep. But exercise late in the evening keeps some people awake at night.

(iii) *Worries:* Meditation, self–disclosure, and cognitive restructuring help reduce mind restlessness.

(iv) *Environmental:* control stimulants, such as noise, light, and improper temperature.

(v)   Maintain a regular wake up time and bed time to keep your body clock synchronized with your physiology.

2. Stimulus Control: Stimulus control training re-associates the bed and bedroom with sleep and relaxation. Then you don't have to try hard to sleep.

Two stimuli: bed time, and where you sleep, help or hinder sleep, depending on how you use them. You can control these stimuli. One way is to leave the bed if you are awake for more than ten minutes. In this way, the bed and bedroom remain associated only with sleep, and not awakefulness. This is the Bootzin technique.

The Bootzin technique:

(i)   Go to bed only when you are feeling sleepy.

(ii) If you are awake for more than 10 to 15 minutes, leave the bedroom and come back only when you feel sleepy.

(iii) Use the bedroom for sleep and sex only.

(iv) Maintain a regular wake up time in the morning, regardless of when you get to sleep.

3. **Sleep Restriction:** The idea is to limit the amount of time you spend in bed to actual sleep. Let us start with a hypothetical sleep duration of three hours. In the first three or four days, restrict time in bed to three hours. If you sleep the full time, increase it by half hour increments. Should you not be able to sleep, go back to the previous stage and start over . This reconditions the sleep center and develops a sense of self–mastery.

4. **Response Control:** We have found the following response control method is very effective in combating insomnia.

(i) *Sit up:* First, sit up if you cannot fall asleep. We feel most helpless lying down.

(ii) *Do not turn lights on too long* (preferably use a flash light), otherwise light-sensitive melatonin and wakefulness- producing chemicals are activated.

(iii) *Go to the bathroom.* Emptying the bladder stimulates the parasympathetic, yin branch of the nervous system and reduces arousal. Also, walking to the bathroom builds up the carbon dioxide level, thus reducing hyperventilation–induced acid imbalance.

(iv) *Progressive Relaxation:* Sit in bed, keep your eyes closed, and do muscle–to–mind progressive relaxation. Simply contract and relax different muscle groups: frown , relax and let go. Similarly, close your eyes tight, let go, clench your jaw, shrug your shoulders, tense your right arm, left arm, legs, abdomen, etc.

(v) *Eyeball Desensitization:* This is very effective. When you wake up at night with a restless mind, your mental eye is constantly creating images. Along with this, your real eyes flicker to catch up with your mental eyes. You can prove this. Ask your partner to close his/her eyes and imagine a pendulum swinging with a "tick" to the left and "tock" to the right. Observe the eyeballs moving left and right with the imagined pendulum movement. The mental eyes make the real eye movement and vice versa. Your restless mind can be quieted by deliberately moving your real eyes with a "tick" to the left and "tock" to the right. You can use the tick–tock of the clock to time it. Continue till your eyes are tired and your restless mind calms down.

(vi) *Diaphragmatic Breathing:* Put one hand on your belly and one on your abdomen and check your breathing. Shift to belly breathing.

(vii) *Drift into a Mind-to-Muscle Meditative Trance:* Observe your breathing, and say "so" as you breathe in and "ham" as you breathe out. The slow brain waves help reduce your restless mind and metabolism. Soon you will fall asleep. Even if you do not fall asleep, your metabolism in the meditative state is 16% lower than in the awakened state. In normal sleep, metabolism reduces by only 8%. So, you get better returns in metabolic energy savings from the meditative state.

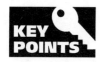

1. Stress arousal and maladaptive habits are two common perpetuating factors of all cases of insomnia.

2. Hyperventilation during the day causes buffer loss and insomnia during the night.

3. Stimulus control and response control are two components of insomnia management.

4. Stimulus control disassociates the bedroom from the fear of insomnia. This is reestablishing the conditioned response of sleep in relation to the bedroom.

5. Response control is sitting up when you cannot sleep, and using   muscle-to-mind tools of progressive relaxation, eyeball desensitization and diaphragmatic breathing and then drift into the meditative state. Once the restless mind is controlled, lie down, and sleep will follow.

22

Biofeedback – Reactivity Monitor [1]

---

1. *Thomas Browne, PhD helped edit this chapter.*

Clinical Biofeedback – Reactivity Monitor

Bio means life, and *feedback* means return of information. You constantly receive and respond to information from your bodily functions. For example, when you run fast, your heart rate increases to an uncomfortable level, and you slow down. At rest, you are usually not aware of your own heart beating. But, you can use a stethoscope and listen to your heart beat. You can connect the stethoscope to an amplifier and several people can listen to your heart beat. In this example, the stethoscope is a biofeedback instrument.

Clinical biofeedback instruments amplify and transform the internal body processes into audio and video signals, so that a person can sense the changes in subtle physiology. Since 1970, the biomedical technology and availability of fast computers have made clinical biofeedback a commonly used means for measuring, monitoring, and modifying human behavior.

COMMON CLINICAL BIOFEEDBACK MODALITIES

EMG (Electromyography Feedback)

The EMG measures and monitors your muscle tension with the help of surface sensors (electrodes) placed on your muscles. The muscle tension is depicted on the computer screen as graphs, or heard as sound with an audio amplifier. With EMG feedback, you can learn to relax particular muscle groups, or learn generalized relaxation of your mind-body. EMG feedback is often used for tension headache, back pain, TMJ disorders, and general relaxation training.

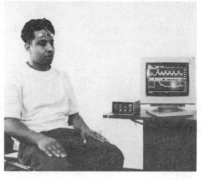

Temperature Feedback

A temperature sensor (thermistor) is placed on your finger and the feedback is shown on a computer screen or heard as sound. Hand temperature represents the degree of constriction of blood vessels. Stress makes your hands and feet cool down by the narrowing of blood vessels and restriction of blood supply. Relaxation warms your hands and feet. Temperature feedback is used for migraine, hypertension, anxiety, Raynaud's disease, and relaxation training.

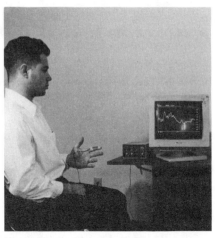

Emotional Sweating Feedback

When you are nervous, you start sweating in your hands, feet, forehead, etc. The electrical conductance of your skin in your hands is monitored with electrodes. Sweating increases the conductance of electricity, and this signal is amplified. Emotional sweating is the basis of the lie detector test. When you lie, the autonomic nervous system sends messages to your sweat glands and you undergo emotional sweating. Emotional sweating feedback is used for anxiety, desensitization of fears and phobias, conflict resolution, and relaxation training.

Pulse Rate and Pulse Pressure Feedback

A sensor attached to your finger measures and monitors your pulse rate and pulse pressure. These values reflect heart rate and blood pressure. Heart rate variability is monitored by the same device. Heart rate changes from one beat to the other, and also with respiration. Heart rate variability monitoring is the most sensitive biofeedback for the heart function as well as the yin-yang balance monitoring of your whole body. Pulse feedback is used for hypertension, anxiety, anger control, and cardiac arrhythmias.

Respiration Feedback

Sensors are wrapped around your chest and abdomen to monitor the expansion of your body with each breath. This modality is used to train diaphragmatic breathing by encouraging belly movement. Respiration feedback is used for asthma, anxiety, panic, heart conditions, and relaxation training.

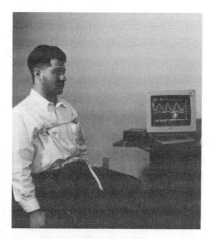

Brain Wave Feedback (EEG) – Electronic Meditation.

Electrode sensors are placed on your scalp and the electrical changes from your brain are monitored on the computer. In the normal awakened state, the EEG waves are beta waves (12-25 Hz), whereas in the meditative state, the waves slow down to alpha (8-12 Hz) and theta (4-8Hz). The alpha-theta brain wave feedback is often referred to as electronic meditation. You can learn to enter and exit the alpha-theta meditative state with your eyes open or closed by brain wave feedback. We have used this method to teach meditation at our Stress Cybernetix Clinic in Concord, California.

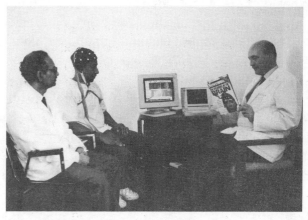

Window into Your Mind-Body

Each biofeedback method is a window to look into your physiology. Some windows make certain aspects more visible. But they all look into the same body and give their own pictures of internal body processes.

Stimulus and Response Patterns

Every aspect of the functioning of your mind-body can be interpreted from the action end (stimulus) or reaction end (response). Once the body process is in progress, the response of one stimulus acts as a stimulus for the next reaction, and so forth. Each one of us has individualized and stereotyped behavior patterns based on stimulus or response.

Stimulus Stereotype

Habitual insomnia is a good example of a stimulus stereotype. The insomniac gets aroused by the familiar cues of his own bedroom. Whenever the person lies down in the same bed, his/her nervous system gets aroused (thoughts of insomnia and worry take over) and he/she cannot sleep. If our subject goes to another room, he/she is able to fall asleep, because the stereotyped cue of the bedroom is eliminated. In fact, to treat this kind of insomnia, the person is encouraged to step out of the bedroom if sleep doesn't come easily after 10 to 15 minutes.

Once a patient is diagnosed to have a heart condition (e.g. coronary artery disease), the stimulus of stressful thoughts creates stressful imageries. This makes the condition worse. The solution is to overlay the imageries of blocked coronary arteries immediately with positive imageries of unblocked arteries. If the emotional sweating biofeedback monitor is attached, it will show that sweating goes up with the imagery of one's own blocked arteries. If the new, healed, and unblocked artery imagery is overlaid, emotional sweating immediately decreases. This method of decreasing stress response focusing on stimulus stereotype is called desensitization. Fears and phobias (of public speaking, snakes, heights, flying, etc.) can be effectively desensitized in this way.

Response Stereotype

Every person has his or her own physiological signature or finger prints. For example, some people get sweaty hands and feet, others get palpitations, shoulder pains, or jaw clenching as the first and prominent symptoms of stress arousal. Biofeedback helps to figure out such stereotypical response patterns. The dominant response pattern is used to train the person in relaxation drills. Heart rate monitoring with pulse pressure and breathing monitoring are the most commonly used responses to train the heart patient.

Heart Rate Variability (HRV) for Anger Control

Breakthrough scientific research has shown that monitor-

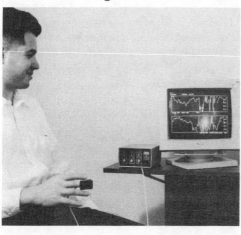

ing HRV is an effective biofeedback way to train people to control anger. When you are angry, the HRV becomes erratic and low. When you are in a state of caring love, the HRV becomes smooth, rhythmic, and accentuated. Focusing your awareness on your anatomical heart switches your head centered thinking to your heart and balances the HRV into a new rhythm.

Conflict Resolution

The most common reason for excess stress in our society is mental conflict: mindfelt judgments antagonize heartfelt feelings. These conflicts can be effectively resolved using a heart rate variability monitor. You can learn to switch between head centered and heart centered feelings while observing the heart rate variability on the computer screen.

Escape from Whirlpool Effect

People afflicted with catastrophic illness, such as heart disease or cancer, feel as if a rapid current has pushed them into an inescapable whirlpool. They feel that their physiology of stress, insomnia, helplessness, and depression cannot be changed, and their condition is permanent and pervasive in all aspects of life. This is the result of a particular messenger molecule circulating in their immune system. This whirlpool effect can be effectively reversed by biofeedback training. The biofeedback training to control one's own physiology resets the immune system. Taking the whirlpool analogy further, biofeedback is the helping hand to pull you out of a whirlpool.

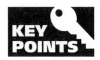

1. Clinical biofeedback is like a mirror reflecting your mind-body. Biofeedback measures and modifies your body functions so that you can learn to modify them.

2. Biofeedback helps you to identify your stimulus and response patterns and change your reactivity accordingly.

3. The latest discovery in biofeedback is heart rate variability monitoring to resolve conflicts in your mind and control anger and frustration.

4. Biofeedback training helps to overcome the whirlpool effect of learned helplessness. This is how biofeedback awakens your suppressed immune system.

23

Meditation and Imagery

Meditation and Imagery

In modern times, man or woman looks at meditation with two basic questions:

Is there scientific proof that meditation will help me? If so, how can I learn meditation and make it a part of my daily life?

Three scientific milestones have validated the role of meditation in our life here at the dawn of the 21st century. These three breakthrough researches are:

1. In 1975, Herbert Benson from Harvard transformed the sacred ritual of meditation into a secular method of *relaxation response* that anybody could learn without a teacher present. This discovery was done in the wake of Maharishi's introduction of Transcendental Meditation™ to Western countries.

2. Dean Ornish's Coronary Artery Disease Reversal (1991) and Carl Simonton's Cancer Healing (1978) programs scientifically proved that meditation is a major component in restoring mind–body balance.

3. Eugene Peniston discovered that alpha–theta brain wave training (electronic meditation, late 1980's) can reprogram the brain to heal from serious addictions, such as alcohol.

In this chapter, we will study meditation under the following basic headings:

- What is meditation?
- Why meditate?
- Why do people fail to meditate?
- How do you meditate?
- How do you fit meditation into your busy life?

WHAT IS MEDITATION?

Meditation is a state of mind. Sleep is another state of mind. To understand the different states of mind, scientists use brain waves.

Brain Waves and Levels of Consciousness

Brain Wave	Frequency	Subjective Experience	Sleep Cycle
Beta	14 - 35 Hz	Awake and Alert	25
Alpha	8 - 13 Hz	Meditation	12
Theta	4 - 7 Hz	Twilight State	9
Delta	0 - 3 Hz	Deep Sleep	4

Beta State: This is the normal awake and alert state with a brain wave range of 14–35Hz.

Alpha State: When you close your eyes, or when you open focus your mind into multiple channels, you enter alpha state (8–13Hz).

Theta State: This is the twilight state, being on the threshold of sleep, but not yet asleep. You enter into this state normally as you enter sleep (hypnagogic) and as you exit sleep (hypnopompic). Passive problem solving and creativity occur in this state (4–7hz).

Delta State: This is deep sleep without dreams (0–3Hz).

Meditative State includes alpha and theta state. The meditative state is also known as the transcendental state (*turiya* in Sanskrit). During sleep, the drop in energy consumption (metabolic rate and oxygen consumption) varies from 2–10 % of the awakened state. During the meditative state, this drop goes as much as 16%. Sleep is not a substitute for meditation. The meditative state is an interface or relay station between your conscious mind and subconscious mind.

Why Meditate?

Meditation is a state of the mind–body in which the muscles are relaxed and the mind is restful and alert. Stress is a state in which the muscles are tense due to misplaced effort and the

Why Meditate?

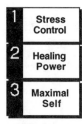

1	Stress Control	Fear and Anger Control
2	Healing Power	Survive from Heart Disease, Cancer, etc.
3	Maximal Self	Creative Thriving in 21st Century

mind is restless with fear, anger, and loss of control. Meditation is an antidote to stress arousal. Meditation reduces the metabolism and eliminates misplaced effort. Meditation reduces the traffic in the hard wire of the nervous system by controlling the restless mind and relaxing the muscles. It switches from the exciting branch of the sympathetic system to the calming branch of the parasympathetic system.

Meditation changes the liquid media of the body by reducing the stress chemicals (catacholamine) in circulation. Meditation resets the brain waves and synchronizes the waves of the brain with the waves of the heart. This, in turn, makes the waves of your mind–body dance in sync with the waves of Nature and Universal Mind.

Meditation allows your body to heal itself. Dean Ornish's reversing heart disease and Carl Simonton's cancer healing use meditation as an effective tool to heal. The meditative state is an interface between the conscious mind and subconscious mind. Meditation makes it easy to exchange the symbolic messages between the mind and body. In the meditative state, self–destructive negative images can be superimposed with positive healing images.

The meditative state brings out your inner child, and makes you more creative and more effective at problem solving. Meditation helps you to maximize your intellectual power and capacity for unconditional love. The maximal self has two components: achievement and affiliation. Meditation optimizes both. In the 21st century lifestyle, human efficiency is measured with the yardstick of problem solving and information processing. Meditation helps to enhance the immediate problem solving (presence of mind) and long term solutions (creativity).

Why Do People Fail in Meditation?

We have found four major reasons why people fail in their attempt to meditate.

1. **Lack of Time:** People often complain, "I do not have enough time to sit for meditation." We have solved this problem by showing people how to meditate in one moment, one minute, and five minute increments.

2. **Restless Mind:** The restless mind during meditation is handled by resetting the mind's eye, resetting mind–talk, reducing the volume of the mental voice, and relaxing the muscles.

3. **Cannot Concentrate:** People often complain that they cannot meditate because they cannot concentrate on their breath or a mantra. Meditation is not an exercise or challenge of your ability to concentrate. You use the tools, breathing awareness, and mantra as anchor devices. When your mind wanders, you focus on the area of the breath and mantra, just like focusing a camera on an object. This is not a pinpoint, laser sharp concentration process. Instead, it is a state of passive awareness.

4. **Doubting the Method:** People often feel guilty that they may have chosen a less effective method to meditate, and keep shopping for a better one. All methods lead to one final destination: a meditative state. It is like learning to ride a bicycle, if you sit on a bike and keep pedaling, no matter what method you chose, you pick up the same balance. Once learned, you will never forget how to ride a bike. Similarly, once you learn to enter the meditative state, you own it for the rest of your life.

How Do You Meditate?

The method of entering a meditative state is surprisingly simple. Many of the gurus and preachers have made meditation into a pious and difficult–to–learn ritual. Lower animals, such as dogs, cats, or lions, are mostly in alpha–theta meditative states. Children below age seven enter into a meditative state quite often even with their eyes open. We teach the following simple method of meditation to hundreds of our heart clinic patients. We have verified the method by brain wave monitoring. We call our method CyberZen™. (And after learning this method, you will be able to direct your own "internal navigation," no matter what external meditation techniques are used.)

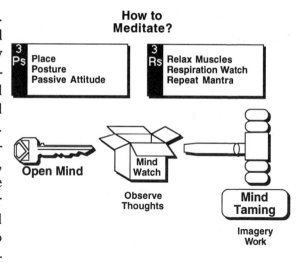

How to Meditate?

3 Ps | Place / Posture / Passive Attitude

3 Rs | Relax Muscles / Respiration Watch / Repeat Mantra

Open Mind — Mind Watch — Observe Thoughts — Mind Taming — Imagery Work

The essential principles of meditation can be summarized into 3 P's: Place, Posture, and Passive State; and 3 R's: Relax Muscles, Respiration Watch, and Repeat Mantra.

Place: You can meditate in any place during the day. For morning and evening meditation, you can select a specific location in your home. Sitting up in your own bed or favorite chair on a regular basis develops a cue-dependent conditioned meditative response.

Posture: The ideal posture for meditation is with your eyes closed (this removes 85% of distractions from the outside), and sitting up with your head, neck, and back in a straight line. Your head should be free without a head rest to avoid falling asleep. Doing yoga postures before starting meditation is helpful to de–focus from your head to body and achieve a passive attitude.

Passive Attitude: A passive attitude is a "let go" state. It refers to opening up the channels in your mind in such a way that the mind–body is simultaneously and equally available to experience the present moment. If there is a noise, such as someone talking, incorporate this sound into meditation without any resentment. This is called open focus. You achieve this passive state by de–focusing from your narrow–focused head. The muscle–to–mind way to open focus is to alternately contract and relax different parts of your body, visit different parts of your body mentally, or visualize each part of your body as an empty space, while paying attention to each part. The mind–to–muscle way of open focusing is to observe your breathing and link your breath to a mantra or sound.

Two examples will make the passive state clear. One, when your urinary bladder is full, if you try hard to urinate, the urine does not flow. Instead, if you just relax and let go, the flow starts. Second, the monkey in the picture is unable to take his hand out of the bottle, unless he lets go of his grip on the banana.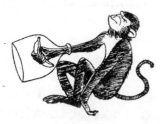

Relax Muscles: Relaxing muscle tension reduces up–going nerve traffic to your brain and relaxes your mind. Contract each muscle group, observe the tension, and relax. A suggested sequence from head to toe is as follows: frown your forehead, close your eyes tight, clench your jaw, shrug your shoulders, tense your right arm, left arm, right leg, and left leg. We recommend two levels of body work during meditation: body watching (body scan) and body taming (resetting muscles of the body, mind's eyes, mind–talk, and mental voice).

Respiration Watch: Find your breath in your belly and follow it. When you breathe in, your belly bulges out like a balloon. When you breathe out, your belly collapses. If your mind wanders, bring it back to your breath.

Repeat Mantra: *Mantra* is a mono syllable sound that keeps you occupied so that you do not get carried away by your mind's automatic self–talk. The simple mantra we recommend is to say "soo" as you breathe in and "ham" as you breathe out. This link between mantra and breath synchronizes your mind–body and puts you into a meditative state.

What Do You Do During Meditation?

The meditative state is the key to entering the dynamics of your mind. You can watch or monitor your mind, called mind–watching, or modify your mind, called mind–taming. You can also watch and modify your muscles during meditation. Inside meditation you do two kinds of work: Body work (body watching, and body taming) and mind work (mind watching and mind taming). First, let us look at what to do with your body or muscles.

Body watching (body scan) refers to focusing your awareness on different parts of your body. A suggested sequence is: forehead, eyes, jaw, neck, arms, legs, abdomen, and chest. **Body taming** refers to resetting the muscles of your body. You contract muscles in each area of your body and relax them. Like a pendulum pushed from midline overshooting to the other side, your contracted muscles relax to a state better than base line. In the popular European method of autogenics training, you visualize heaviness and warmth of different parts of your body.

When your mind is restless, it keeps on talking to itself (self–talk) and creating various mental pictures. With each mental picture, there is corresponding eyeball movement. When you have haunting thoughts, these eyeball movements covertly follow the mental pictures. You reset these mental pictures by deliberately moving the eyeballs all the way to the left and then to the right. It is like a pendulum swinging "tic" to the left and "toc" to the right. Keep doing this eyeball movement until your haunting imagery fades away. Similarly, you reset your mind–talk by moving your lips and tongue. One easy way to move your lips is to do "eee" and "ooo" movements of your lips alternately. You move your tongue inside your mouth forwards and backwards to reset it. You reduce your mental voice by counting down from ten to one as you reduce the tension in your vocal cord.

You can do these body watching and body taming exercises in any combinations and permutations to reduce the muscle–to–mind nerve traffic during meditation.

Mind–watching allows you to observe your thoughts and emotions non–judgmentally. Become a spectator of your own thoughts and observe the patterns of your thoughts without analyzing them. Mind watching helps you to understand your mind–body communication, which leads to unconditional acceptance of the self.

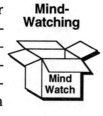

Mind-Watching

Mind–taming refers to modifying the pattern of thoughts for healing, personal growth, creativity, and problem solving. In mind–taming, you are creating imageries in your mind to modify your thoughts and emotions in this subtle, restful alert state. The meditative state is most

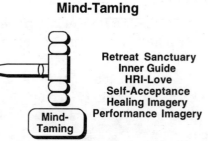

Mind-Taming

Retreat Sanctuary
Inner Guide
HRI-Love
Self-Acceptance
Healing Imagery
Performance Imagery

conducive to mind–body communication because your analytical left brain is temporarily put out of circuit. Examples of mind taming exercises are:

1. **Retreat Sanctuary:** Imagine a beach scene or meadow and take a retreat from your restless mind. Use all of your senses to see, hear, touch, taste, and smell the beach scene.

2. **Inner Guide:** You can conceptualize an inner guide as a divine figure, light, or symbol to come and guide you with your problems in life.

3. **Heartfelt Resonant Imaging (HRI):** Can you focus on your anatomical heart and experience caring love to yourself, your body parts, your family, and the society at large? Can you bring the imagery of people you dislike and "love your enemy" for the sake of healing your heart? Forgiveness is changing your perspective of judgment towards the other person. In fact, you forgive yourself for your wrong perspective. This requires the biological state of altruism. You arrive at the altruistic caring love state by focusing on your heart area during meditation. If your mind tries to judge and starts disliking the other person,

again refocus to your anatomical heart area and enter into a caring love mode. Each time you become heart centered, you are releasing endorphins and equipping yourself with the "chemistry" to forgive.

4. **Self–Acceptance:** In the meditative state, visualize the abundance of your health, wealth, and relationships. Mentally smile at each of your possessions and validate them. This meditative acceptance of abundance leaves you with contentment and fulfillment when you come out of meditation.

5. **Healing Imageries:** In the meditative alpha–theta state, your mind–body communication is directly on–line. First, you greet your affected organ with love and then you visualize the organ being healed. For example, you can visualize your coronary artery being opened up, the cancer being engulfed by your white cells, your muscle injury being repaired, and so on. Focus your awareness on your heart zone and send heartfelt caring love to the organ.

6. **Performance Imageries:** In a meditative state, imagine yourself successfully performing the action in an interview, examination, public speech, etc. This message gets transferred into the waking state later.

Meditation Balances Your Mind and Body and Heals You.

You don't have time *not to* meditate. We prescribe meditation in our clinic in one office visit of 15 minutes. Meditation comes in one moment, one minute, or five minute increments. Once you know how to meditate in small increments, longer meditation is a simple multiplication of these increments.

Now that you have read the details of how to meditate, let us show you how you can just do it.

Mindful Meditative Centering

(One moment, Please).

Simply drift your awareness to your belly center or heart area **AND CONTINUE TO BREATHE FROM YOUR BELLY.**

Use belly button centering for a balanced assessment of

Just Do it
Meditation Prescription

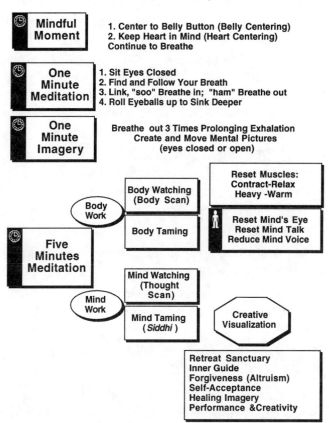

Mindful Moment
1. Center to Belly Button (Belly Centering)
2. Keep Heart in Mind (Heart Centering)
Continue to Breathe

One Minute Meditation
1. Sit Eyes Closed
2. Find and Follow Your Breath
3. Link, "soo" Breathe in; "ham" Breathe out
4. Roll Eyeballs up to Sink Deeper

One Minute Imagery
Breathe out 3 Times Prolonging Exhalation
Create and Move Mental Pictures
(eyes closed or open)

Five Minutes Meditation

Body Work
- Body Watching (Body Scan) → Reset Muscles: Contract-Relax Heavy -Warm
- Body Taming → Reset Mind's Eye, Reset Mind Talk, Reduce Mind Voice

Mind Work
- Mind Watching (Thought Scan)
- Mind Taming (*Siddhi*) → Creative Visualization → Retreat Sanctuary, Inner Guide, Forgiveness (Altruism), Self-Acceptance, Healing Imagery, Performance &Creativity

the moment, and heart area centering for accessing caring love feelings. This helps you shift away from your usual head–centered, intellectual state.

Mindfulness Explained

Your mind has two operating systems: mind–talk and mindfulness. Mind talk is the ongoing self–talk. The contents of this self–talk come from your past experiences stored in your memory and current perceptions from your sensory organs.

The default mode of your mind is mind–talk. There are two problems with mind–talk: one, self–talk is often judgmental with the hidden motive of "what's in it for me;" second, you

---

are diverted from enjoying the experience of the present moment. Mindfulness is shifting your operating system from this self–talk to the bare perception of the present moment. All systems of meditation in the world use mindfulness as the basic stepping stone. Mindfulness is also called beginner's mind because you are experiencing the present moment for the first time. The word beginner's mind applies to the fact that when you first experience an event or meet a person, you accept that experience unconditionally without any judgment.

Belly centering allows you to be mindful of your whole experience of the moment. Heart centering allows you to be mindful of the present moment from the vantage point of heartfelt feelings.

ONE MINUTE MEDITATION

1. Close your eyes (You can do this with eyes open as well, but closed eyes work better).

2. Focus your awareness on your breath as follows: Find and follow your breath in your belly and slightly prolong your exhalation.

3. Use a mental sound or mantra as follows: Mentally say "soo" as you breathe in and "ham" as your breathe out.

4. Deepen your meditation as follows: Roll your eyeballs up as if watching a sunrise and following the sun to midday over your head.

As your mind wanders, bring it back to the breath and mantra and repeat.

ONE MINUTE IMAGERY

1. Close your eyes (You can do this with eyes open as well, but closed works better.)

2. Follow and link your breath as in the one minute meditation, but make sure that you prolong your breathe–out by three times.

3. Focus your awareness to your heart area and ask your

---

heart "Can I experience caring love towards me, my heart, etc.?" Can I visualize the opening up of my heart like a lotus blossoming, and my coronary arteries opening wider and wider?" (Visualize any afflicted organ and see it healed).

Once experienced, you can do the imagery concurrently focusing on the heart zone and prolonging the breathe–out slightly with each breath.

FIVE MINUTE MEDITATION

Basically, all you are doing is adding muscle–to–mind and mind–to–muscle tools to make the meditation deeper and longer. A typical sequence would be:

Body work: Body scan, contraction and relaxation of body parts, eyeball movements, lip and tongue relaxation, counting ten to zero to relax vocal cords.

Mind work: Observing the thoughts, and then doing various imageries for healing and personal growth.

Detailed Meditation Script

For all practical purposes, you simply close your eyes, observe your breathing, and say mentally "so" as you breathe in and "ham" as you breathe out. This is the heart of meditation. The following script gives you additional details for adding muscle–to–mind and mind–to–muscle tools to your meditation. You can speak the following script to a tape recorder and replay it with closed eyes.

Posture and Passive Attitude

1. I am sitting up with **my head and neck straight** and comfortable, with or without back support.

2. I **close my eyes** and withdraw from the outside world. **I feel this clearing my mind**.

3. I **am allowing all the sensations from the outside** world to be a part of my meditation. I do not try to control them, but observe them as a **spectator** and let go.

4. I **allow all the sensations from my body** to be part of

my meditation by observing them passively in a non–involved way.

5. I **allow all the thoughts** in my mind to surface to my awareness as I observe, acknowledge, and let go.

Body Work (Body Scan)

I "visit" my forehead, eyes, jaw, tongue, neck, shoulders, arms, legs, and abdomen. (This body scanning can be done before or after contracting and relaxing different body parts).

Body Taming (Resetting Muscles)

1. I **contract and relax muscle groups** by observing **control signals** of tension from head to toe, one by one.

- I **frown my forehead**, feel tension, and let go.
- I **squeeze my eyes**, feel tension, and let go.
- I **move my eyeballs**, side to side, up, down, and let go.
- I **clench my jaw,** feel tension, and let go.
- I **touch my chin** to my chest, feel tension, and let go. I touch **my left ear to my left shoulder**, feel tension, and let go. I touch my **right ear to my right shoulder,** feel the tension, and let go. I **shrug my shoulders**, feel the tension, and let go.
- I **tense my arms**, feel the tension, and let go.
- I **tense my legs**, feel the tension, and let go.
- I **tense my belly,** feel tension, and let go.
- I **observe my belly** as I breathe and let go.

2. I allow my body parts to feel **heavy and warm** for relaxation.

My forehead is heavy, warm, and relaxed.

Eyes – heavy – warm – relaxed.

Jaw – heavy – warm – relaxed.

Tongue– heavy – warm – relaxed.

Shoulders – heavy – warm – relaxed.

Neck– heavy – warm – relaxed.

Right arm– heavy – warm – relaxed.

Left arm – heavy – warm – relaxed.

Right leg – heavy – warm – relaxed.

Abdomen– heavy – warm – relaxed.

Resetting Mind's Eye

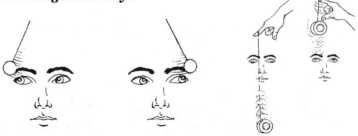

'Tic-toc' eyeball movement to reset mind's eye

Yo-yo imagery to quiten mind's eye

I move my eyeballs by watching an imaginary pendulum moving "tic" to the left and "toc" to the right. Also, I move the eyeballs up and down by watching an imaginery yo–yo bouncing up and down. I repeat these eye movements several times to erase the mental pictures and reset my mind's eyes.

Resetting Mind–talk

I reset my lips by saying "eee" and "ooo." I reduce the volume of my mental voice by counting down from ten to zero.

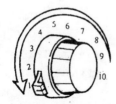

Reduce volume of mind's voice by radio knob count down from 10 to 0.

Meditation
(Breath and Mantra Meditation)

1. I **find and follow my breath** in my belly one after the other.

2. I **link my breath to a sound (mantra),** mentally repeating: "So" as I breathe in and "Ham" as I breathe out.

As my mind wanders, I **bring it back to my breath and mental sound** (*mantra*). I roll my eyeballs upwards as if following a sunrise to midday, and **go deeper into a meditative state.**

Mind Watching

I watch my thoughts one by one and acknowledge each one without judging or controlling them. I observe my thoughts

---

but come back to the breath and mantra again.

Mind Taming –Imageries

I direct my mind to different imageries. As the picture fades away, I enlarge it, move it back and forth, color it, or change its shape.

- I visualize the **seashore and a calm beach** as a sanctuary.

- I visualize my **inner guide** to help me solve my problems.

- I visualize **my heart area** and ask myself, "Can I experience **caring love** towards my spouse, children, parents, co–workers, etc.?" I **forgive people** by separating my heartfelt feelings from my mindfelt judgments and by separating events from people.

- I **accept the abundance** of my home, my present wealth, my car, my job, my family, and my health.

- I visualize my **coronary artery opening up** and my heart opening up like a blossoming lotus.

- I visualize **successful performance** in forthcoming public speaking, job interview etc.

Now, I observe my breathing and slowly open my eyes and feel wide awake and alert.

For personal verification on the "before and after" changes that occur, Experiential Verification exercises are shown in the Appendix.

Note: This is a secular form of meditation and imagery we teach in our Stress Cybernetix Institute, located at 2182 East St., Concord, California 94520. The phone number is (510)–685–4224. This method encompasses all other systems of meditation and does not conflict with any one system. It is practical and effective in producing the alpha–theta– brain wave state very quickly. This system was choreographed by Naras Bhat, MD and Thomas Browne, PhD.

How to Fit Meditation into Your Busy Life

The first thing to remember is that you should meditate several hundred moments every day. This is possible if you learn how to meditate in one moment and in one minute increments. Every 90 to 120 minutes, your mind–body goes through an ultradian healing rhythm of drifting into a daydream state. This is an ideal time to close your eyes and do a one minute meditation, one minute imagery, or a good five minute meditation. Every time you have an acute stress or anger episode, simply drift into a one moment or one minute meditation. This synchronizes your mind–body connections.

In the morning, as you get up, sit up in your bed and meditate for one to five minutes. Most people find it convenient to do 10 to 20-minute routine of yoga stretching and meditation in the morning before breakfast. As you sit for breakfast, you can meditate for a moment and be mindful of your food and eating. When you reach the office, as you get set for work, meditate for a moment or a minute. During the day, put in scattered moments or minutes of meditation as often as you can remember. An extended 20 minute session in the evening or before you go to bed is helpful as well. Just before you go to bed, meditate for one to five minutes.Because you can meditate in small increments, the excuse of "not having enough time" does not exist. In our clinic, we have the slogan, "you cannot not meditate."

For an enhanced experience, we recommend you meditate for 40 minutes to an hour at least once a week for the first month, then once a month after that. The longer sessions of meditation help you to sharpen your tool and understand your own mind–body dynamics better.

21 DAY ROUTINE

For the first 21 days of learning to meditate, we recommend at least one 20-minute session per day. This frequent repetition helps to establish the state-dependent learning of meditation. This is like learning how to ride a bicycle – once you get the balance, you will never forget it. After learning our method here, you will always have your own "internal navigation," no matter what other external techniques of meditation you may try.

IMAGERY

Imageries are symbolic experiences without the object directly stimulating any sensory organs at that moment. There are two kinds of imageries: **receptive and guided**. Receptive imagery refers to being aware of the spontaneous symbols evolving from your subconscious mind. Guided imagery refers to the creative directing of your power of imagination for personal growth and healing.

Imagery involves using all the senses to create or recreate an experience in your mind. Although imagery is frequently called visualization or "seeing with your mind's eye," sight is not the only significant sense. Hearing, taste, smell, touch, and kinesthetic, or sense of "feel," are also included in the imagery process. The imagery process is a mental creation and does not require an external stimulus to produce it.

Imagery is the mind thinking in pictures instead of words. Mental imagery, like intuition, is nonlogical thinking. The left brain thinks logically and verbally in spoken language. The right brain thinks intuitively. The mind communicates with the body in symbolic pre–verbal language. The language of imagery is the same as the language of both night dreams and daydreams. Imagery is one of the foundation steps of healing.

WHAT TO DO

Close your eyes to get the mind–body into the imagery session. Breathe three times with a slightly prolonged expiration saying "hah." This stimulates the vagus nerve and switches the nervous system from the aroused sympathetic to the relaxed parasympathetic mode. With your mind's eye, start imagining what you want to create. This is called "guided imagery." You are directing your mind in what to imagine. Also, pay attention to your receptive imagery, looking at whatever pops up in your mind.

For healing, you can look at what is there, then modify it to be what you want it to be. For example, if an imagery of a blocked heart comes to mind, you would want to repair it.

Imagine the artery being opened up with a pipe roto–rooter or cleaning apparatus.

Caution: Your mind will wander while focusing on the imagery. You can control the tendency to wander by changing the submodalities of the image. Increase or decrease the size, movement, texture, or sound of the object you are focusing on. Give it different qualities. Changing the imagery in this way keeps your mind's attention. If you don't vary the image, it slips away.

How often should you practice imagery? Do it throughout the day, whenever you remember. Research has shown that synchronizing the imagery with the 90/20 minute ultradian cycle helps the body shift into a relaxed, daydreaming mode. This takes advantage of the body's natural day dreaming cycle and expands it into a guided imagery.

Imagery Prerequisites

1. An **altered state of consciousness** is needed to switch the brain from the logical left side to the symbolic right side. Also, shifting into an altered state of consciousness relaxes the body–mind, and changes the brain waves from active, high frequency beta waves to slow, rhythmic alpha waves. This physiological state is called an open focus and a passive attitude (described in Tools 3 and 4). The simple act of breathing out slowly produces this altered state by switching to the parasympathetic mode of the autonomic nervous system.

2. Imagery should be in your own **subjective format** rather than using quotations or suggestions from others. You can refer to anatomy books, discuss it with your doctor, or be personally creative in synthesizing your own metaphor or image.

3. Your imagery will **change as your physiology changes** with time. Accept the new version of the imagery as it varies from session to session.

MIND–BODY BENEFITS

Einstein once said, "If you can imagine it, you can create it." Everything created by human beings is first created in imagery. Just as an architect creates a blueprint to guide the building of a house, imagery creates a blueprint of "software" commands for any desired body activity, whether for healing or performance. It can create the foundation for healing your body's chemistry. It can also create additional rehearsal time for perfecting performance.

HOW IT WORKS

Imagery works by creating a mental blueprint in an innate, symbolic language. This blueprint creates a set of commands to be executed by the mind–body, just like computer software conducts a routine. The mind–body perceives imagery no different than it perceives real happenings. To the mind–body, the imagery is a real experience. **When you guide your imagery, you are not altering the past experience, but adding new experience to overlay the past experience.** The mind creates its own imageries depending on the physiological status of the body–mind at that time.

The body and mind are two sides of the same coin. These two sides are connected to each other by the hard wire of the nervous system, liquid media of neurotransmitters, immune transmitters and hormones, and vibrational whisper of electromagnetic waves. Each imagery produces neuronal, biochemical, and electromagnetic changes in the body.

In the "hardwire connection," the nervous system is connected to different parts of the body in a symbolic way. By activating the imagery, the symbolic connection comes into play. Symbolic language is the final common pathway to the brain's execution of a command. **An engram is a neuromuscular transmission pattern that is recorded in the brain in a particular sequence. The repetition of the imagery reinforces the engram.** It creates a blueprint of experience that can be recalled and replayed in the future.

The "liquid media connection" of imagery refers to the chemical components of the physiological state experienced in both the physical and imagined realities. By creating the imagery, you recreate the chemistry of the experience. In that way, you can recall and replay that chemistry. This deliberate activation of your "internal pharmacy," through the use of imagery, can be used for self–healing.

The "vibrational whisper" connection of imagery refers to the fact that nature has its own frequency and everything either corresponds with or goes against the waves of nature. By creating a favorable imagery, you synchronize your mind's waves with nature's waves. You set up a resonation between your mind, body, and nature so that you are in harmony with the body's and nature's healing forces.

HOW TO DEVELOP A SKILL

There are two forms of imagery: passive, receptive imagery and active, guided imagery. Receptivity is the state of being an observer of the phenomena of life. When you are in a receptive state, thoughts and feelings surface. You can become receptive to the perception of the feeling in a mindful, open focused way. This kind of receptivity to what is in the mind's eye helps to shape the direction of the creative guided imagery.

For example, in any given day, during meditation, your heart may look like a pump with valves that open and close. The next day, when you meditate, your road map may change because your physiology has changed. That day it may look like a valentine's heart. The day after, it may look like a lotus. Archetypal symbols may pop up. It doesn't matter. What matters is how it looks to you on that day. You'll find that patterns in receptivity will repeat themselves. Your physiology always picks up on the same blueprint for symbols. Then you learn in your pattern of thinking, your road map, that "Every time I see good things, a blue light comes up. Whenever I see negative things, a yellow light is present." Whatever it may be, it is most important to learn the pattern. Once you learn the pattern, you can take advantage of the information for rehearsal and get into the appropriate physiological "state" in real activity.

When you create healing imageries, it is necessary to **understand your own road map** or blueprint of the physiology in connection to the problem. For example, suppose you are a non-medical person and you have a heart problem. You have a conception of the heart as a valentine's heart. Then you went and took a course on human anatomy. With that information, your concept in visualizing your heart changes entirely. Imageries change and can be realistic, archetypal, or personal symbols at any given point in time. The mind-body connection is symbolic, not linguistic. You need to tap into the symbolism.

To learn how to deliberately create an imagery, mindfully observe a beautiful object or a pleasant scene. Take a mind–body snapshot of it. Then close your eyes and replay it in your mind's eye. Repeat this procedure 10 to 15 times to imprint it in your memory. Then recall this impression at will. Just 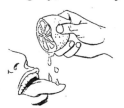 imagine yourself squeezing a piece of cut lemon onto your tongue and feel the magical response of imagery on your mind–body.

Imagery Tips

1. **Close your eyes.** Closed eyes tune you into the experiential mode.

2. **Breathe out three times** to stimulate the parasympathetic vagus nerve and induce an altered state. Do not breathe in deeply because you may get agitated and dizzy due to hyperventilation.

3. **Duration:** Each session of imagery **should last 1 to 5 minutes**. Do not stretch it too long, or else you can get stressed out by trying too hard. The short impulses act as quick oriented reflexes to heal. If you stay on the image for too long a time, the mind wanders and gets lost. To overcome this, change the quality of the image in size, color, movement, distance, etc.

These submodalities keep the image alive.

While your imagery work will last only a few minutes, the blueprint created by this imagery is doing the work in the subconscious mind all the time and producing the healing process.

4. **Frequency: Three regular sessions** should be timed for early morning after awakening, at twilight, and at bedtime. Every ninety minutes, your mind goes into a daydream cycle due to the earth's rotation on its own axis and around the sun. These naturally occurring ultradian healing breaks are ideal times for having imagery sessions. Also, you can have imagery sessions throughout the day, whenever you think of the problem, or when your body reminds you of the problem.

5. **How long to continue:** Research has shown that to develop a good conditioned response and to change the body processes, the imagery sessions should be continued **regularly for at least 21 days** at a stretch. After 21 days, you develop the habit of using the imagery and you will never give it up.

REAL LIFE APPLICATIONS

Two main areas of using imageries involve performance and healing. Research in sports psychology has shown that physical practice with equal or more time devoted for mental imagery (mental practice) enhances sports performance. Modern Olympic athletes devote considerable time to mental practice. Jack Nicklaus, perhaps the greatest golfer of all time, creates a "mental movie" before every shot. Tennis stars like Chris Evert and Jimmy Conners use imagery before the game. Golf, skiing, and tennis coaches frequently implement imagery in teaching. In stage fright, you can imagine giving a flawless performance in front of an audience. Repeated mental rehearsal like this desensitizes the fear and creates a storehouse of confidence building success patterns.

There are two famous models of the use of imagery in healing situations. The first is the Ornish program for reversal of coronary artery disease. In this program, arteries are visualized as being opened up. The second popular use of imagery

---

for healing comes from the work of Carl Simonton and Bernie Siegel in healing individuals with cancer. In this example, the immune system is imagined to create warrior macrophage cells which battle the cancer cells, engulfing and destroying them.

1. Meditation is a restful alert state of the mind–body. Today, meditation is used as a scientific tool prescribed by doctors rather than a sacred ritual.

2. You can meditate in one moment, one minute, or five minute increments. This is the solution for the common excuse of "I don't have time to meditate."

3. Mind–watching to observe yourself and mind–taming with healing and creative visualization are essential parts of meditation, and are easy to master.

24
Self–Disclosure

Self–Disclosure

What is Self–Disclosure?

The word "self–disclosure" refers to the exposure of the self to others. Self–disclosure is intimately **sharing your emotions with someone else.** Before you disclose the self, you first have to understand the self. Understanding the self is called self–actualization.

Report Visit vs Rapport Visit

In the modern information age lifestyle, when we interact with people, we typically relate to each other by sharing objective information. We call this way of communicating a "report visit." A report visit means that you share opinions, statements, and factual information with each other. For example, in a husband and wife relationship, most of the communication is filled with questions like, "Did you close the door?" or "Did you feed the dog?" In a work situation, the boss will ask you, "Have you finished typing that letter?" These are factual information exchanges. In our society, we rarely share our emotions with each other because we are preoccupied with solving problems and getting things done. This does not allow for intimacy and exchange of feelings. **Suppression of emotion is the fundamental cause of stress in modern life.**

Thoughts vs Feelings

Thoughts are often mistaken for feelings. **Thoughts** are automatic sparks in your mind which are often judgmental or have a hidden agenda of "what is in it for me?" **Feelings** are the mindful awareness of the state you are in, as experienced in body changes and accompanying thoughts. Every emotion has an accompanying body motion or muscle contraction. These muscle contractions function as markers of your emotions. Although there are accompanying chemical changes associated with each emotion, you need a physical "road map" to determine what is happening. It is easy to associate the tension or lack of tension of any body part as the identifying marker for each emotional surge. You can learn to observe the changes in your physiology as you experience a particular emotion. For example, a student may feel sweat on his hands whenever he is taking a final exam. A public speaker may sense his heart beating quickly just before he begins his speech.

Why Do Self–Disclosure?

Self–disclosure helps you develop **horizontal intimacy with others**, whereas self–actualization (understanding your patterns of behavior and the way feelings are expressed in your body) is the way you develop **vertical intimacy with yourself**. You have to have enough vertical support (understanding of yourself) to have horizontal support (caring sharing with others) and vice versa. To use a common analogy, a high, vertical structure, like the Eiffel Tower, needs horizontal support to stand straight. Likewise, you also need horizontal support for vertical extension. Otherwise, it is difficult to achieve your maximal self. Recall that the maximal self refers to the internal mind–body conditions which help you perform at your peak level. Disclosure of your emotions, first to yourself (self–actualization) and then to others (self–disclosure) helps you realize your maximal self.

Self–disclosure also allows you to **send and receive caring love**. Research has shown that when you send caring love, you benefit even more than when you receive it. Sending caring love enhances your immune system by releasing pleasure chemicals. It also increases the experience of pleasurable love in the emotional part of your brain. For example, the person initiating a hug enjoys it more and experiences more physiological benefit than the one being hugged. In other words, the initiator of the caring action gets more out of it.

The caring, nonsexual touch that we recommend as part of self–disclosure has additional mind–body benefits. When you touch another person, you are touched as well. Caring, nonsexual touch releases endorphins (hormones necessary to feel intimacy). Endorphins are released in mammals when they touch others of the same species. They are also released in humans who lovingly stroke animals, such as dogs. In this culture, we touch each other in relatively few ways, such as contact sports, social handshakes, and sexual contact. As a rule, we do not touch as other animals do, in an affectionate way. If you look at a cow, for example, it nuzzles and licks her calf or other cows. Often, we don't touch others because we fear this action will be interpreted as a sexual advance. In today's society, touching is considered to be infringing upon someone else's privacy or personal space. There are legal constraints surrounding touching. For example, in most work situations, touch between members of the opposite sex may be interpreted as sexual harassment and set up potential legal liability. Touch between members of the same sex may be construed as homosexuality. This is not true of all cultures. In many cultures, such as in India or Italy, it is common for men to walk with arms around each other. In western culture, this is tolerated in rare situations, such as at the height of athletic pride or extreme emotion. The touching we recommend is affectionate, non-sexual touch, like a mother to a baby.

Self–disclosure has many additional healing benefits for your mind–body:

1. It **boosts your immune system** by increasing the immunoglobin level, and enhancing T cell and B cell function.

2. It reduces **mind–body stress** caused by pent up emotions and associated muscle tension and restless mind. The effect of self–disclosure on your mind–body is analogous to removing your clothes from a dryer — when you open the dryer door, the agitation stops and the heat dissipates. Ultimately, you empty the load of wears from the dryer.

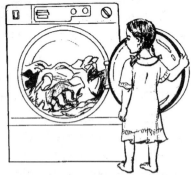

The agitation stops when you open up.

3. Self–disclosure **promotes a healthy heart**. When you suppress and repress your emotions, your heart rate variability, or the beat–to–beat variation of your heart rate, becomes very erratic. Research has shown that erratic heart rate variability is an indicator of sudden death due to a heart attack. This is because the yin and yang branches of your nervous system (the parasympathetic and sympathetic branches) go out of balance when you suppress your emotions.

4. Self–disclosure **promotes altruistic pleasure**.

Why We Don't Do Self–Disclosure

The main reason why we don't self–disclose is that we are conditioned to accept the problem solving, report style of communication as a norm in our modern lifestyle. We also hesitate to disclose our feelings because we are afraid we'll be misunderstood or misjudged by others in our society. Differences based on perceptual type, mindfelt and heartfelt feelings, physiological signature, gender differences, money style, and pessimistic or optimistic explanatory style can contribute to such misunderstanding.

The most common reasons people hesitate to do self–disclosure is the lack of common grounds between people and the fear of being misunderstood. Let us trace the path of communication from person A to person B step by step.

1. Person A has his experience in his body, thoughts, and feelings to share. He conveys this message as verbal statements (content) and emotional expressions (intent) directed to person B.

2. The message from person A gets encoded by the internal noise, or the peculiar message packaging system of person A.

3. The symbols of a message are transmitted to person B in the form of verbal and body language. Only 7% of the message is in the verbal language form. The remaining 93% is in body language. Body language includes 38% vocal qualities (pitch, resonance, articulation, tempo, and volume of voice)

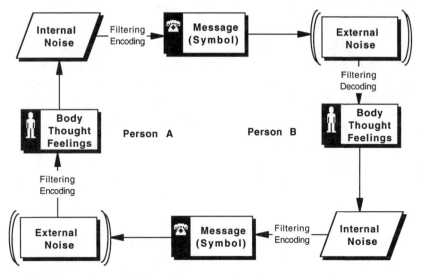

and 55% body movements (facial expression, posture, and gestures).

4. The message gets further distracted by external noise before reaching person B.

5. There is one more encoding and filtering process in person B before he interprets and acts on the message.

A similar encoding and filtering system interfaces when person B sends messages to person A.

These communication hurdles or filtering processes are based on individual differences of perceptual types, gender differences, money style, physiological reactions, and explanatory style of the individual. The common denominator for all human beings and animals is caring love. It is the non–possessive, nonsexual caring and altruistic feeling present in all mammals. To activate this state of caring love, one has to relearn the childlike altruism of accepting a playmate without any judgment.

Scientific Studies on Self–Disclosure

The following are some important research studies proving the healing value of self–disclosure.

Alameda County (California) Study: Researchers in Alameda County, California studied 7000 people for 9 years and found that death rate and illness correlated to four types of social support: marital status, extended family contacts, church memberships, and other associations. Individuals with the least social connections had twice the death rate.

Michigan Study: The James House study from Michigan looked at 2,754 adults and concluded that people with social support had three times less of a death rate over a 12 year follow up.

Berkeley Study: The Reynolds and Kaplan study from Berkeley followed up women for 17 years and found that lack of social support increased cancer related death by 2.2 times.

Duke University Study: Williams followed 1,368 people and found that the survival of heart attack victims after five years tripled by the support of a spouse or a partner.

Studies on Support Groups: The Spiegel study at Stanford found that the survival rate of terminally ill breast cancer patients doubled with supportive expressive group therapy. The Richardson study at the University of Southern California found similar results in lymphoma and leukemia patients. Fawzy at the University of California, Los Angeles found similar results in malignant melanoma patients. Dean Ornish's study of coronary artery disease showed that group support and self–disclosure heals coronary arteries.

Self–Actualization

Self–actualization is developing a road map to explore the contents and dynamics of your mind–body. The goal of self–actualization is to reach the maximal self in the material achievement of health and wealth, and in the human affiliation of connectedness to others.

The perennial questions brooding in the human mind are "Who am I?" and "What am I doing?" These questions are usually approached abstractly, both philosophically and religiously. Our approach is different. We answer this question from a physiological standpoint, embodying the concept of self–actualization. Our self–actualization definition refers to understanding your mind–body functions as they relate to your thoughts and emotions. "Who am I?" gets answered as "What happens in my mind–body when I experience various situations?" By repeatedly asking yourself this question under different circumstances, you come to realize who you are. You get to build a blueprint of what to expect from yourself. This is like having an owner's manual to understand your automobile.

What is Self–Actualization?

To create the blueprint of understanding in your mind–body, it is important to first understand the building blocks of human behavior. The actions of the mind–body are collectively called "behavior." Whatever you do is considered a behavior. That behavior can be understood with the three components of an iceberg. The tip of the iceberg is composed of the actions or muscle contractions; the middle part of the iceberg is composed of the thoughts (sparks of electromagnetic waves of the mind–body), and the base is composed of the emotions.

Bodily functions (the tip of the iceberg), such as breathing, posture, voice tone, muscle tension, sweating, coldness in the extremities, and heart rate, change according to two factors: the emotion that is predominant at any given moment and the level of intensity of that emotion. When you recognize these bodily changes and can associate them with each emotion, you have self–realized your emotions.

Thoughts are actually just sparks of electromagnetic waves in your mind–body. Thoughts are contents of your mind, just like written statements are contents of a book. Emotions add intent or purpose to these thoughts.

Emotions are the driving force of activity in the other two

areas of the human behavior iceberg. There are two basic emotions: pleasure or love, and fear or anxiety. Three additional negative emotions are derived out of fear: anger, guilt, and sadness. Humans have the innate capacity to have pleasure or love, but the negative emotions mask this inherent state. Michaelangelo once said, "The art is already hidden in the rock, you just have to chisel out the unwanted and the sculpture shows up." Similarly, once you "chisel out" your negative emotions, with self–disclosure, the underlying love surfaces.

With an understanding of this iceberg concept, you can develop vertical intimacy, or intimate knowledge of the parts of your own behavior. This intimacy has six components as you relate to yourself and others in this world. These components are as follows.

1. Perceptual Types.

2. Mindfelt vs. Heartfelt Feelings.

3. Money Style.

4. Gender Differences.

5. Explanatory Style.

6. Physiological Signature.

Before you proceed with self–disclosure, find out who you are in each of the above six areas.

What is Your Perceptual Type?

There are three perceptual types. Your type decides how you perceive the world. **Visual people** think in mental pictures and they express an opinion by saying, "I see your point..." **Auditory people** think in mental sounds and they express an opinion by saying, "It sounds like..." **Kinesthetic people** process information through feelings and express their opinion by saying, "My gut feeling is..."

Although you can register information in any of these styles at any given time, you have a dominant style of perception. That is the way you usually operate in the world. Once you understand your main perceptual type, it helps you understand other people's perceptual types. People are "wired" differently in their perceptual types. When you are interacting with another person and you have trouble communicating, it may be because each of you have different styles of perceiving.

To determine your perceptual type, ask a simple question, such as, "What did I eat for breakfast yesterday morning?" Or, ask someone to ask you questions demanding memory recall. As you start thinking, no-

3 PERCEPTUAL TYPES

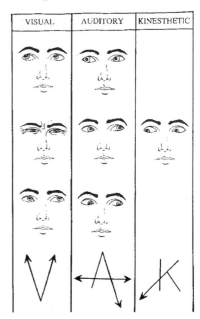

tice where you place your eyes. If you are a visual communicator, your eyeballs roll up; if auditory, they roll from side to side and to the left; if kinesthetic, they roll down. Although you have one predominant communication modality, at any given time, you may use another one.

Mindfelt and Heartfelt Contrasting Feelings

Part of self–actualization is to understand that you have two levels of feeling. One is your heartfelt feelings. This is your native way of feeling, the way a child feels, without any predetermined judgmental ruling in favor or against the object or person. The heartfelt feeling, or gut feeling towards any person or object, has its own propulsive power, but we frequently override it with a veto by the mindfelt feeling. The mindfelt feeling is an evaluation of the situation, object, or person, which is ruled by the basic motive of "What is in it for me?" You have both mindfelt and heartfelt levels of reaction, and these two may not always agree with each other. When they conflict, it creates internal stress. You have to resolve the stress either in favor of or against the heart.

In the Heartfelt Resonant Imaging Exercise (HRI), we train you how to focus your awareness on your heart, become aware of your heartfelt feeling towards any object, plant, animal, or person, and compare that to your mindfelt feeling.

Money Style

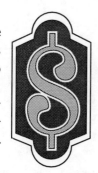

Because money is such an important issue in modern life, most people relate to their lives in terms of money. Money dictates the ability to perform in life and the success of performance, because everything is translated into a currency value. The following money styles, defined by Olivia Mellon, reflect imbalances in attitudes towards money:

- **Money monks**, who think money is evil.
- **Money amassers**, who scheme all the time about making more money, whether they need it or not.
- **Money avoiders**, who just do not want to think about the subject.
- **Money worriers**, who spend every waking moment totaling up figures in their heads, imagining total disaster.
- **Hoarders**, who believe the purpose of money is to save it.
- **Spenders**, who never have a penny in the bank.

A balanced attitude to money is to pay almost equal importance to the meaning of life – connectedness to people – without the price tag of money. This requires a heartfelt focus of caring love to people. We all had this attitude as a child, but the competition in society made us forget it. Relearning this attitude is done with the heartfelt resonant imaging (HRI) tool in a duck–rabbit, flip–flop manner, explained elsewhere.

Gender Differences

Men and women are not created equal in terms of their emotional and biological responsiveness.

Gender differences fall into the following domains:

1. **Right or Left Brain Dominance.**
2. **Contents of Thoughts.**
3. **Expectations of Intimacy.**

Right or Left Brain Dominance: Women are generally intuitive and emotional, and typically use their right brain dominant attitude to evaluate situations. Men are more left brain dominant and typically have an analytically oriented approach to life. When men and women deal with each other, this difference in ways of experiencing the world can create a potential conflict due to communication patterns based on these differences (called "**genderlect**"). This brain dominance theory of Roger Sperry from Stanford won the Nobel Prize. A recent study from Yale has confirmed that women use both sides of the brain to process sounds and words while men predominantly use the left brain. This new study is illustrated in the graphics below:

Contents of Thoughts: Research has shown that men and women think about different topics during the day. One study shows that, the majority of the time, men think either of sex, sports, or their career, while women, the majority of the time, think of their relationships. This indicates a gender difference in the filtering systems of men and women.

Gender Differences in
Thoughts

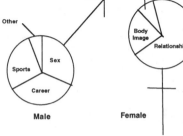

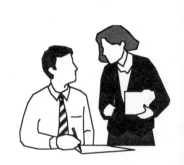

Heart Disease and Cancer

Expectations of Intimacy: The gender difference also refers to how men and women differ in their expectations of intimacy with each other. For example, men want to give the appearance of being "armored" and stoic. Women want to express intimacy and caring feeling.

Once you understand these gender–based differences, you realize that each of us has a different filter with which to experience a situation. The conflicts that normally arise during the day with members of the opposite sex (particularly partners or significant others) are often not because either person is difficult to get along with, but because both people, as different genders, have different attitudes in life. Knowing this reduces the conflicts and your level of stress.

Pessimistic and Optimistic Explanatory Styles

When faced with the problems and challenges of daily life, you develop habitual patterns of responding to these problems. These response patterns can be optimistic or pessimistic, depending on past experiences. If one person has a series of failures in life, for various reasons, they may develop a pessimistic attitude due to "**learned helplessness.**" With this attitude, people think that "Whatever I do, it is not going to work." The pessimistic explanatory style has three "P" components: **Permanence, Pervasiveness, and Personalization**. The pessimist thinks that "Everything is permanent; it will go on forever; it is going to be bad and I'm going to be unsuccessful." Pervasiveness means, "It involves everything I do. Regarding personalization, "It is just me that this all happens to; everything is conspiring to make me fail." When life accommodates this pessimism, it is called **learned pessimism**. If these people succeed in any particular task they try, this success immediately reprograms their whole system to do things differently.

This is called **learned optimism**. If you have fallen into the groove of learned pessimism, you need to do something that you do well in order to challenge this pessimism and reprogram your system towards success. For example, if you are doing poorly at math in school, you may develop the helpless, hopeless, pessimistic attitude that whatever you do, you'll fail. Instead, turn away from the math for a while and focus on another subject that you are good at. When you do something well, it gives you the power of a positive attitude and a positive immune response. Your mind–body learns that you can succeed. When you come back to the math, you'll do better because your immune system and mental programming is such that you are able to perform at your best.

Physiological Signature

Under stress, each individual has his or her own pattern of reactivity in the nervous system, chemical messenger system, and accompanying body organ response. This is what we call "physiological signature" (individual finger prints of mind–body response). For example, driving through rush hour traffic may make different people experience different body responses, such as a clenched jaw, sweaty palms, rapid heart, hyperventilation, uneasy stomach, or headache. You can learn to observe your own physiological signature to each situation in your daily life and develop an internal road map in such a way that you will be able to predict the outcome of a situation in advance.

How to Do Self–Disclosure

Self–disclosure requires certain rituals. It doesn't happen all of a sudden. You must learn from repeated trial and error. We have found that the **three T's of Time, Touch, and Talk** are an easy way to remember the self–disclosure ritual.

Time: Assign at least **15 to 20 minutes** in an undisturbed, dedicated fashion, for the sake of self–disclosure with your significant other, spouse, or partner of choice. For example, in a group therapy arrangement, two heart patients may join up as buddies to create a "self–disclosure club." You can have more than two in the club, but two is sufficient to create a self–disclosure pair. This reserved time can be broken down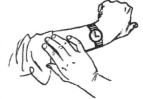

into smaller amounts of time initially, to get into the habit of sharing. The best time is at the end of the day.

Touch: Caring, affectionate touch while talking establishes greater intimacy. (By the way, intimacy can be defined as "in–to–me–see.") Sit within 18 inches of each other during a 3 T's self–disclosure session. This creates a comfortable reaching distance for touching and invites closeness.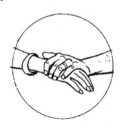

Talk: The first thing to consider in self–disclosure is to know what you are self–disclosing. In any communication between human beings, there is a body language and a verbal language. The body language conveys the intent and the verbal language conveys the content. The intent is the emotional background. Research has shown that only 7% or 8% of communication is by verbal language. Out of the remaining 92%, you use things like your posture, breathing, voice inflection, pitch, rhythm, and all body expressions and gestures to convey the message behind the message. That's why comprehension is so different when reading a book versus listening to a tape versus live interaction.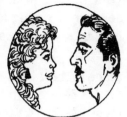

In attempting to communicate feelings, it is important to translate the feelings into body experiences and use these as the reference for the feelings. This helps the receiver to understand both the sender's content (words) and intent (body language). An example will clarify this. If you say that "every time I think of my high cholesterol, I get a palpitation in my heart area," you give a clearer understanding of what is going on within yourself than if you say, "I get 'scared' whenever I think of my high cholesterol." What does scared mean to you? However, when translated into body language (shoulder ache, palpitations, etc.), it is easier to understand. It creates an "exchangeable currency," or a common language. If you use an

---

abstract word, such as scared, it must be filtered through the receiver's own currency to understand it. This equating of currency is done by embodying emotions into a verbal "package" to be sent. That embodiment of emotions is nothing but self–realization, or knowing the self in the body.

Talk about your self–actualized feelings (rapport visit), rather than opinions and statements of news in the world (report visit). When we suggest that you talk about your self–actualized feelings, we are referring to sharing your feeling pattern of the day as you have experienced it in your mind–body.

The 3 T's Session is a good time to do a Heartfelt Resonant Imaging (HRI). While talking with the other person, focus on your own anatomical heart area and, from that feeling space, send your caring love towards the other person. The HRI enhances self–disclosure.

The process of receiving this shared communication takes place in three steps: 1) The receiver repeats a close paraphrase of the sender's message. This is called **mirroring back** the message; 2) The receiver gives a **validating acknowledgment** of the sender's message in the receiver's own language, and; 3) The receiver attempts to **empathically feel** the sender's message in his or her own body. The following information helps you understand these concepts better.

Mirroring: For visually oriented people, mirroring involves a visual duplication or use of visual imagery. For auditory people, it is an "echoing," or "parroting." For kinesthetic communicators, it is sharing the "gut feeling," "internal micons," or "movie strips." When you have successfully mirrored, you can paraphrase the content of the other person's emotions in your own words. Typical phrases of mirroring are, "I see that…, It appears to me…, I hear that…, It sounds like…, I feel…"

Validation: The content of the other person's emotion now has to be translated into the intent. The receiver of the message temporarily suspends judgment regarding the sender's message and makes a validating statement that the sender's experience is "worthy" of attention. Typical validating phrases are, "It makes sense to me…, I understand that…, I realize your point…"

Empathy: If you try to "relive" or make a carbon copy of the sender's feelings in your own body–mind, it is called empathy. When you try to duplicate the sender's message in your own body, you create a "feeling rehearsal," which gets expressed in your own body language. This deep level of communication heals both the sender and receiver.

Mirroring, validating, and empathizing give you a structure from which to talk and exchange feelings, which sets the stage for dovetailing.

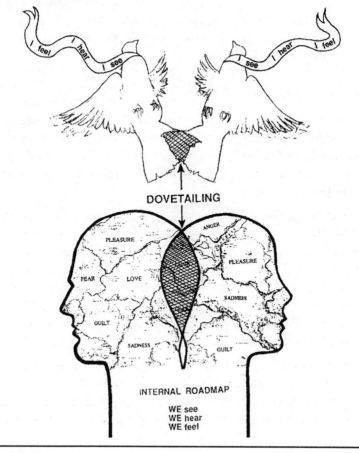

Dovetailing refers to the fact that the differences between people (gender differences, perceptual types, money styles, and pessimistic/optimistic explanatory styles) can be brought into a shared understanding. Each person has a way of looking at life. When you self–disclose to each other, you interlock each other's styles. This interlocking **allows the "your feeling" and "my feeling" to become "our feeling."** I feel, hear, see and you feel, hear, see becomes we feel, hear, see. It opens up your perception to their world and increases your joint intimacy because you **understand, accept, and acknowledge each other's differences in life**. This helps avoid conflicts. The primary reasons for dovetailing are for your personal growth in understanding the differences between two people and for the development of intimacy. With dovetailing, it is easier to get along with difficult people. By the way, the definition of a difficult person to get along with is — "the other person." There is no such thing as a difficult person, just your perception of the other person as being difficult, which you create based on your framework.

Steps in Dovetailing

The steps in dovetailing are:

1. Express your feelings in your own body language of
   a. I see.....
   b. I hear....
   c. I feel.....
   d. I want......

2. Now this message has to be translated or transposed into the map of the receiver and restated as:
   a. I find that you see.....
   b. I find that you hear......
   c. I find that you feel......
   d. I find that you want......

3. Now rephrase the sender–receiver complex as "MY/ OUR"

---

a. We found that you and I see.....
b. We found that you and I hear...
c. We found that you and I feel....
d. We discovered that we want...

At times, we don't have enough time or the right situation to self–disclose. One of the best ways to get around this problem is to record what you would disclose about yourself into a **tape recorder**. Later, you can replay it, along with a partner. Or you can write a letter indicating your feelings, then mail it or read it to the other person. Research on self–disclosure has shown the effects of journalizing feelings and sharing that **journal**. Medical students were put into two groups — one group kept a report visit type diary and the other group kept a diary of emotional feelings that occurred during the day. The emotional feeling group showed immune systems that were significantly enhanced compared to the other group. This indicates that disclosing your emotions, in some unknown way, enhances your immune system, thereby resetting your healing mechanisms.

Supportive Expressive Therapy

Supportive Expressive Therapy refers to the forming of a "buddy system" in which a person or group of people agree to be a support system for the person with a problem. This type of support is beneficial in lengthening the lives of people with life threatening diseases. This type of therapy allows you to get in touch with, and express your mind–body problems in the presence of, a helper who is available, in an informed and caring way. Specifically, if you are the afflicted person, you first identify in your own body the feelings and sensations you experience (self–actualization). Then, you open up and share this information with another (self–disclosure). It is important for the person with the problem to include close family members and children in the self–disclosure routine. Also, the person with the problem needs to learn to ask for specific help, then appreciate and acknowledge the help.

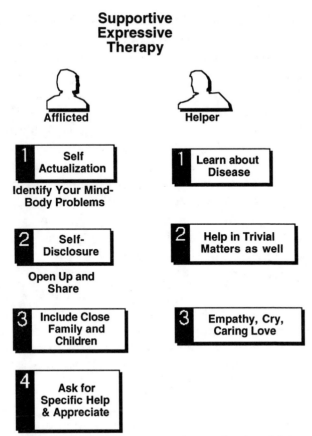

Supportive Expressive Therapy

Afflicted

Helper

1 Self Actualization

Identify Your Mind-Body Problems

1 Learn about Disease

2 Self-Disclosure

Open Up and Share

2 Help in Trivial Matters as well

3 Include Close Family and Children

3 Empathy, Cry, Caring Love

4 Ask for Specific Help & Appreciate

The helping person or group of people should first learn about the problem or disease. Becoming educated about the problem sheds understanding as to the symptoms experienced by the afflicted person. Then the helper should anticipate the afflicted person's need for assistance and offer to help in trivial matters as well as bigger ones. The helper should empathize with the afflicted person, even to the point of being able to cry along with them. Also, the helper should express caring love towards the afflicted person. This is best done with an HRI — Heartfelt Resonant Imaging. You do the HRI by accessing your own heartfelt feelings, concentrating on your physical heart area, then extending feelings of caring love towards the afflicted person. HRI can become part of the daily 3 T's Session.

Experimental Verification Exercises for Self–Disclosure

When you self–disclose, you feel a release phenomenon which you experience as better sleep, less restless mind chatter, reduced muscle tension, and improved bowel habits. Also, you may observe an immediate sense of connectedness with the person to whom you share your feelings. In addition, you may experience greater rapport with others, thereby improving communication. There is a need for self–disclosure every single day. One should be able to identify the pent–up feelings by the end of the day and share this information with another. By doing this daily, it will become routine to self–disclose.

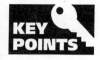

1. Self-disclosure has two parts: (i) Self-realization of your own mind-body characteristics in the area of perception, feelings, physiological signature, gender differences, money style and explanatory style. (ii) Disclosing your realized self to a partner with a time, touch and talk ritual and dovetailing with each other.

2. Self-disclosure helps you by reducing stress arousal, boosting the immune system, and healing the heart.

3. The most precious value of self-disclosure is the fact that it improves your altruistic pleasure in life.

25

Rest and Activity

Rest and Exercise Cycles

Life is a wave with peaks of activity and troughs of rest. When you conform to this law of nature, you conserve energy and avoid wasting it in misplaced effort. The rest and activity cycle affects both the mind end and muscle end of your mind–body.

What is Fatigue?

Fatigue is the mind–body's perception of circuit overload. This load has a "hardwire" (musculoskeletal component), a liquid media (chemical component), and a vibrational wave which interacts with the waves of nature. Just like a voltage charge in a battery depends on the chemistry inside the cell, the fatigue point in one's body has a chemical counterpart. In the human function curve, stress arousal and performance follow the pattern of an inverted U. The increase in arousal provides a linear increase of productivity until the point of fatigue. At that point, the body's biochemical reserve has reached the limit, and now increased effort gives diminishing returns on the down–slope of the curve. Now, distressful emotions are created and relationships are hampered.

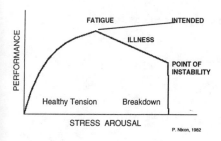

HUMAN FUNCTION CURVE

Fatigue vs. Exhaustion

Healthy fatigue is a normal feeling of tiredness after exercise. There is a recovery from this fatigue by rest and sleep. Unhealthy fatigue is exhaustion in which there is incomplete recovery and restless sleep. Exhaustion is like a battery that loses its charge gradually and gives up completely at one point. This deterioration is due to changes in the body's immune system.

CHEMISTRY OF FATIGUE

The zip or zap of your mind–body is a chemical phenomenon. How your body uses chemistry and energy depends on:

1. **Misplaced Effort**
   - Head and Heart Conflict
2. **Biological Rhythms**
   - Ultradian Healing Rhythm
   - Sleep and Wake Cycle
3. **Mindful Eating**
4. **Relationship with Self and Others**
   - Energy Quadrants of Emotions
   - Energy Exchange Vectors (Cross Checks)
5. **Reactivity Control**
   - Breathing pattern (Hyperventilation and Breath holding)
   - Heart Rate Variability (Yin–Yang Balance)
   - Restless Mind Control
6. **Physical Exercise** (Motion and Emotion)

MISPLACED EFFORT

The single most important reason we experience fatigue today is conflict in the mind. This conflict is a tug–of–war between the head and the heart. The brain tries to achieve material benefits, While the heart seeks love. This leads to unwanted muscle tensions or misplaced effort. There are two ways to solve this. One is to do your HRI and resolve the conflict. You can alternate a "report visit" - material problem solving - with a "rapport visit" of caring love by using the duck–rabbit flip flop method described elsewhere.

The other is to learn differential relaxation, which is using task specific muscles while relaxing others.

BIOLOGICAL RHYTHM

The mind–body operates in a cycle of 90 minutes of activity and 20 minutes of rest. This is our **Ultradian Rhythm.**

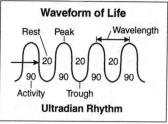

Natural cues that the body gives to take this 20 minute break are: daydreaming, the need to stretch, yawning, tension, hunger, the need to urinate, a wandering mind, or sharp drops in the level of performance.

In the graphics below you see what happens when you do

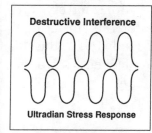

not pay attention to the rhythms of nature. The simplest way to take an ultradian healing break is to close your eyes and meditate for 5 to 10 minutes. You don't need caffeine, nicotine or drugs to stimulate you.

Meditation and Ultradian Healing Response

The meditative state is similar to the ultradian healing because in both, alpha–theta brain waves dominate. Several cultures in the world traditionally close their eyes and pray six times a day, corresponding to the ultradian healing periods. We recommend you close your eyes and drift into a brief meditative state every 90 to 120 minutes, to take advantage of this natural healing rhythm.

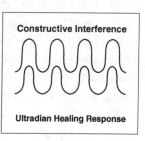

Sleep and Wake Cycle

Sleep renews energy and heals you. Insomnia can cause fatigue. The easiest way to manage insomnia is to sit up and do muscle–to–mind exercises, especially eyeball desensitization and progressive relaxation. See the section on insomnia for cybernetic management of sleep disorders.

One third of us are night people, one third are morning people. And the remaining third can go either way. Learn your own biological rhythm and organize your productive time accordingly.

Afternoon Nap

There is a clear difference between a nap and the ultradian healing response. A nap is a delta wave sleep, whereas the ultradian healing response is an alpha–theta state. You wake up slightly groggy after a nap, but you feel restful and alert after an ultradian healing response. One third of the world enjoys an afternoon siesta to recharge. And most people feel a low energy state in mid–afternoon. Unfortunately, our workaholic culture doesn't allow time for the "primordial snooze." Though it could surely raise productivity. For the elderly, heart patients, and people with chronic illness, an afternoon nap rejuvenates and replenishes energy.

MINDFUL EATING

You Are When You Eat?

You feel an urge to eat about every ninety minutes. In response, some bite their nails, nibble on the end of a pen, or light a cigarette. Caffeine, it messes up this natural rhythm. The best way to satisfy these ninety minute hunger pangs is to eat a healthy snack of fruits or vegetables. Such complex carbohydrate snacks (not candies and chocolate) in mid–morning, mid–afternoon, and at bed time, keep the insulin level even. This "grazing diet" also maintains brain serotonin and mood levels.

Eating three square meals and three round meals per day is the best solution to fatigue and mood disturbances. Fresh fruits and vegetables provide the antioxidant vitamins A, C, and E, which help to fight fatigue. Caffeine and alcohol should be minimized as mood altering foods because they create a chemical debt by undermining the body's chemical inventory.

RELATIONSHIP WITH SELF AND OTHERS

Energy Quadrants of Emotions

At any given moment, you have one emotion dominant in your mind–body. This emotion uses energy in a positive or negative way. Pay attention to your mind–body right now and figure out which energy quadrant you are in. If you are stuck with the energy drain of misplaced effort, take a healing break.

Energy Exchange Vectors (Cross Checks)

Energy Quadrants of Emotions

High + Pleasure Love Flow	*High -* Fear Anger
Low + Sleep, Rest Meditation	*Low -* Guilt, Sad Repress

You either take or give energy to each person you meet in your life. Figure out how you relate in each direction of your relationship. Vertically, you relate to your own mind–body network and your higher self. Horizontally, you relate to your spouse, partner, significant other on one side, and society at large on the other. The best way to relate to any person is through your heart by doing the HRI technique as explained elsewhere. This way, you may have an enemy in your mind, yet you can love him or her through your heart and save energy.

There are two frequent opportunities in daily life to "practice" your caring love skills. One is when you run into someone. The other is when you are on the phone. Your mind tries to be judgmental about others. All you

Higher Self

Vertical

Family Spouse, Significant Other Partner — Horizontal — Me — Horizontal — Co-workers Society

Vertical

Mind-body network

have to do is focus your awareness on your anatomical heart and experience caring love at these moments. On the phone, you may find yourself holding your breath or breathing with your chest, making you tense and stressed out. The solution is to pick up the phone during expiration and continue to breathe with a slightly prolonged expiration.

REACTIVITY CONTROL

Reactivity is an ongoing chemical reaction in your body. Your mind is a victim and witness of this chemistry. You can intervene in various ways to change and even prevent it.

Breathing Pattern

Breathing from the diaphragm helps to clear fatigue. Just think of your abdomen and let it bulge with each inspiration. This enhances the lymphatic flow, strengthens the immune system, clears free radicals, and increases blood pH level. It also conserves energy by switching from the ergotrophic, energy consuming sympathetic system to the tropotrophic, energy conserving parasympathetic system.

Heart Rate Variability

The heart rate varies depending on what emotion you have at the moment. You can deliberately focus your awareness on your heart and enter into a state of caring love to make your heart rate smooth and regular. Anger makes the heart rate erratic.

Restless Mind Control

A restless mind is the result of a restless body. It is easier to work from the muscle end to control the mind.

Body Motion: Body motion can be standing, moving the arm and body in space, structured exercises, such as yoga, aerobic, or anaerobic rituals. Whatever it is, it will change your emotions. For example, just imitate frowning with your forehead and observe your thoughts and feelings. Then, deliberately smile and observe your thoughts and feelings. Do you notice the difference?

Yoga Postures: Slow movements, as yoga postures, enhance sensory motor feedback to the brain. They send a sensation of stretch, pressure, and force of a muscle contraction into your brain's control center. You relieve unnecessary tension and decrease muscle–to–mind nerve impulse traffic.

PHYSICAL EXERCISE

Exercise clears fatigue by mobilizing energy. Do aerobic (which means "with oxygen") exercise at a rate that lets your cardiovascular system easily supply all of the oxygen your body needs to continue exercising. Walking is aerobic exercise for most people. Aerobics also helps build cardiovascular endurance, by keeping ability of the heart, lungs, and blood performing at optimum levels.

To build cardiovascular fitness, you must do aerobics within the target zone for cardiovascular fitness. This means you need to apply the proper frequency, intensity, and time. These three important factors constitute the "F.I.T. Principle." F for frequency; I is for intensity; and T for time (duration). Exercise for 20 to 30 minutes continuously, in your aerobic zone, at least 3 to 5 times per week.

Aerobic Conditioning

Start-and-stop exercise burn mostly sugar, whereas exercise sustained over 20 to 40 minutes burn mostly fat. Do stamina-building activities within 60% to 85% of your maximum heart rate.

Calculate your maximum heart rate by subtracting your age from 220. Then multiply that by 0.60 and by 0.85. Your pulse rate during exercise should be in this zone. This is like any training. You put a slight overload on your oxygen utilization system to build it up, steadily increasing frequency, intensity, or duration of exercise. Fatigue is postponed by such a training effect. The muscle activity produces lactic acid and clears the alkalosis of hyperventilation. This acid base shift increases the buffer capacity of blood. You are better able to face stress during the day and sleep at night.

Aerobic Options

Cross country skiing, swimming, cycling, jogging, running, rowing, ice and roller skating.

Recreational sports, such as tennis, basketball, soccer, and baseball, build stamina and increase both aerobic and anaerobic conditioning. However, the best physiological exercise for all ages is walking.

When not to exercise: We do NOT recommend exercise after a heavy meal. It affects your digestion. People with coronary artery disease shouldn't exercise early in the morning Incidences of heart attack increase then. Thicker blood and a morning surge of adrenaline make the heart more vulnerable.

Walking

Walking is for everyone, and therefore the most popular aerobic exercise. Serious commitment is essential to turn walking from a stop–and–go activity or casual stroll to an aerobic option. If you plan to make walking your sole aerobic exercise, the Institute of Aerobics Research suggests you walk up to three miles in 45 minutes, four to five times a week.

Walking for Health

Benefits of Walking: Walking burns calories, helping control weight and shape the body. It improves cardiovascular fitness, and posture. Walking places less stress on joints than jogging. It strengthens bones, enhances creativity, and boosts energy.

Walking is a Real Exercise: Fast walking burns enough calories and conditions the body sufficiently to maintain optimal health. Walking fast for 40 to 60 minutes burns more fat than jogging for the same length of time, because jogging burns more carbohydrates. That's why walking is a better exercise to lose fat. Abdominal obesity is the hallmark of obesity–induced health problems. If you can pinch more than an inch of love handles on your belly, you need to lose weight. Sustained walking is your best choice.

Pace Walking: Fast walking is called pace walking or race walking. This is a pleasant alternative to jogging and running. Marianne Dickerson, second place winner in the 1983 World Champion marathon, shifted to walking to recover from a running injury. She calls walking "active rest." Walking exercises the quadriceps and hamstrings better than running does. Walking uses small diameter nerves and muscles more effectively than running, which gives better feedback control to your neuromuscular system.

Motion–Emotion Cybernetics of Walking: Any movement of the body influences emotion. When you are tense and uptight, just getting up and walking around releases tension.

Walking to Relieve Panic Attacks: Research tells us that during panic attacks the major chemical change is hyperventilation, causing increased alkalinity of the blood and neuromuscular irritability. Walking around rather than sitting in one place increases lactic acid production and decreases this alkalinity in the blood. Additionally, paying attention to breathing and slowing it down cools the panic attack.

Walking to Relieve Insomnia: If you wake up at night with insomnia and a restless mind, and cannot go back to sleep, walk for a few minutes. It will help balance your body chemistry and increase its buffer system.

Walking Combat: If there is a conflict and argument with a significant other, invite that person for a walk. In five to ten minutes, each of you will take a compromising attitude because motion controls emotion. Perhaps the rhythm of bodily action unlocks the closed mind. In 1987, the Soviet Union and the United States signed the historic agreement eliminating intermediate and shorter–range missiles. During this meeting, President Reagan and Gorbachev had a heated argument and they were ready to walk out. Instead, Reagan invited Gorbachev for a walk on the beach, leading to the historical compromise.

Walkman Music: Research done at Ohio State University shows heart rate and blood lactate levels go down if you listen to soothing music during walking and strenuous exercise.

Walking Meditation: During anxious times, try to walk while effortlessly paying attention to each moment of stepping and feeling the contact of your feet with the earth. Pay attention to different parts of your body and sensations, and time your pace and muscle contractions with your breathing. Mindfulness of scenery, especially the natural trees and plants, with a beginner's mind is one of the simplest meditations you can do. The beginner's mind refers to the perspective of seeing something as if you're looking at it for the first time. An afternoon walk or bedtime stroll are ideal for walking meditation.

1. Your mind-body has biological rhythms of rest and activity every 90-120 minutes. Disturbing this natural rhythm disturbs your body chemistry.

2. Your body chemistry is affected by exercise, emotions and what you eat.

3. Human function curve (HFC) helps you to measure, monitor, and modify your fatigue and exhaustion.

4. Aerobic conditioning helps to increase the height of HFC, which affects your fatigue and exhaustion favorably.

26

Mindful Eating –

Eating to Control Stress

Mindful Eating

Eating is primordial bliss. Besides being our main source of nourishment, eating connects us to the earth, water, plants, animals, and people. A child tries to put everything in its mouth. Adults are almost as bad, biting our nails for oral gratification. On the other hand, eating creates more conflicts in our lives than any other activity, and it started with Adam's forbidden apple.

FOOD AS CHEMICALS

By now you know our brain and nervous system are connected to the rest of the body not only by the "hardwire" nerves,

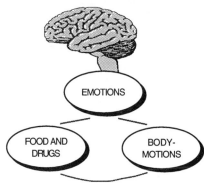

but also by the liquid media of three chemicals— hormones, neurotransmitters, and immune transmitters. Your emotions and body motions (tension or relaxation) modulate these internal chemicals. You introduce the chemicals of food and drugs into your mind-body. In this sense, **eating is either a chemical warfare - or a communion with your body chemistry.**

The chemicals of food add to the chemicals of the emotions and body motions.

CHEMISTRY OF FOOD AS FUEL

The energy your body needs to function comes from two different fuel tanks: 1) carbohydrate & protein, and 2) fat. These two types of fuel have different characteristics.

A. Thermic Effect: It takes money to make more money. Similarly, your body burns food into energy by using part of the energy from the food itself. This is called the Thermic Effect. This thermic effect of fat burning is different from carbohydrate or protein burning. Only 3% of fat is used to metabolize itself, whereas 25% of carbohydrate and protein is used to

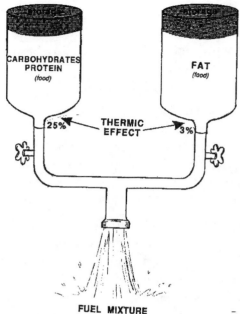

metabolize itself. In other words, the thermic effect of fuel tank #1 (carbohydrate and protein) is 25%, whereas the thermic effect of fat is 3%. The net result is, more of the fat you eat remains unused by the body and gets deposited in storage. Put another way, you need less fat than carbohydrate and protein to function well.

B. Water content: You store fat in a ratio of - 4 parts fat to 1 part water. But your body stores carbohydrate in an opposite ratio of 4 parts water to 1 part carbohydrate. Thus, you notice weight loss rapidly by carbohydrate (water) loss as compared to fat loss from storage.

C. Storage: Your body's storage capacity for carbohydrate and protein is limited. For fat, the storage capacity is unlimited! Your liver and muscles together have the total capacity of storing about 1,800 calories of carbohydrate. After this capacity is filled, food is converted into fat. A woman of normal weight can store over 100,000 calories of fat!

D. Calories per Gram: There are 9 calories contained in each gram of fat, compared to only 4 in each gram of carbohydrate or protein.

E. Exercise: The sprinting type of "stop and go" exercise burns carbohydrates and protein. Continuously sustained, rhythmic exercise over 30 to 40 minutes burns fat. Thus, to lose weight, you have to exercise at a low intensity for at least 30 to 40 minutes.

The moral of this "fuel mixture" story is that you do not get fat unless you eat fat. From the perspective of the fuel mixture, both saturated and unsaturated fat act the same way. Saturated fats have received more attention because of their atherosclerotic–producing (arteries–hardening) potential.

On an average, Americans eat more than 100 grams of fat per day. What you want to do, is switch to the other fuel tank containing carbohydrates and proteins. If you are on a regular low fat diet, an occasional excess of fat eating is metabolized rapidly along with the other type of fuel mixture. These facts are confirmed by recent Vanderbilt University research.

Our approach to cutting down fat in your diet is to check everything you eat for its fat content, and consciously switch from animal to plant food sources and from fatty foods to starches. Initially, you may want a fat-counter table. But being aware of what you eat is what really matters.

INSULIN METABOLISM AND EATING

Any food affects your insulin and glucagon secretion. These hormones affect the rest of the hormones in your body in an interdependent way. When you eat carbohydrates, your blood sugar level goes up, stimulating insulin secretion. This insulin drives an amino acid called tryptophan into the brain, which gets converted into serotonin and gives the feeling of pleasure and satisfaction. For optimum mind–body balance, insulin secretion should be even as a sawtooth instead of uneven as a roller coaster.

Excessive insulin leads to mood swings, frequent hunger, stress arousal, cholesterol and fat deposits, hardening of the arteries, and high blood pressure. Obesity, high fat foods,

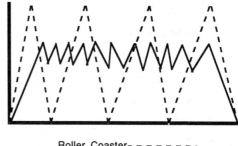

Roller Coaster- — — — — — — ·
Sawtooth ————————

simple sugars, refined and processed foods, infrequent eating, lack of physical activity, and stress increase insulin levels. The best way to balance insulin secretion is to minimize refined sugar and fat intake and eat complex carbohydrates at least six times each day. Regular table sugar is sucrose, which requires insulin for metabolism. Honey, fruits, and berries contain fructose sugar which does not require insulin for metabolism. We recommend fructose sweeteners which do not leave an aftertaste. Aspartame and saccharin leave an aftertaste. Their only value is "zero calories." Besides, these artificial sweeteners do not raise the serotonin level in your brain, required to give you a sense of pleasure. As a result, you don't feel satisfied and you want to eat more and more, which leads to "binge eating." Insulin balance is the sensitive chemical marker of your mind–body balance.

CYBERNETIC PRESCRIPTION FOR EATING

Cybernetic eating means eating controlled by the feedback and feed–forward communication from your mind–body. Our cybernetic prescription for eating is based on a holistic concept of food, digestion, absorption, and wellness. It consists of these ("**3** Wives & **2** Husbands"):

1. **Why Eat**
2. **What to Eat**
3. **When to Eat**
4. **How to Eat**
5. **How Much to Eat**

Why Eat? People eat to nourish the body, mind, and spirit: Bodily, to satisfy hunger, fulfill sensual pleasures, and repair

---

and rebuild body tissues. Mindfully, to experience love, pleasure, comfort, and reward, or to counter stress, boredom, anger, guilt, or sadness. Spiritually, to nourish the metaphoric heart and soul; to feel connected to the earth and universe from which all food comes. Traditionally, people pray before they eat, honoring this spiritual connection. In this respect, eating nourishes the entire human experience.

The pragmatic reasons to eat fall into three groups: 1) degenerative, 2) maintenance, or 3) regenerative reasons.

The typical Western diet is high in fat, protein, salt, and sugar, and low in complex carbohydrates. This is a **degenerative** diet because it increases the risk of degenerative diseases, such as atherosclerosis, coronary artery disease, osteoporosis, and cancer.

The **minimum maintenance (transitional)** diet is similar to the American Heart Association's recommendation of 30% fat, 300 milligrams of cholesterol, and three grams of sodium per day. This diet encourages complex carbohydrate intake.

The **regenerative** diet we recommend (**Stress Cybernetic Diet**) is similar to Dean Ornish's Eat More, Weigh Less Diet for Reversing Coronary Artery Disease, and McDougall's starch–based, low fat diet. This whole grain, starch–based diet consists of 75% calories from complex carbohydrates, 15% calories from protein, and 10% calories from fat. The benefits are reduction or reversal of heart disease, blood pressure, diverticulosis, hemorrhoids, diabetes, cancer, osteoporosis, and other degenerative disorders. There is concern that high carbohydrate diets may increase triglycerides in people with hereditary disorders and diabetes. Those people should consult with their physicians in planning their diets.

Do You Want to Live Healthily to be 100? According to the U.S. Census Bureau, by the year 2040, there will be more than

> DO YOU WANT TO LIVE TO BE 100?

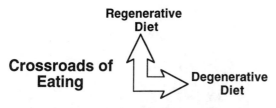

Crossroads of Eating — Regenerative Diet / Degenerative Diet

one million Americans who are over the age of 100. According to the study of Alexander Leaf, the foremost authority on aging, groups of people who currently live longer than 100 years (the Hunza in Pakistan and the Vilcabamba of Andes Mountains in Ecuador) follow this starch–based, low fat, regenerative diet.

WHAT TO EAT?

You need to decide whether to base what you eat on USDA recommendations; the degenerative diet or the regenerative Cybernetic approach to eating. In the US, dietary recommendations come from the Dietary Guidelines for Americans published by the Department of Agriculture (USDA); the Diet & Health Review published by the National Research Council (NRC); and the Surgeon General's Report on Nutrition and Health. All agree on the following recommendations:

1. Eat a nutritionally adequate diet composed of a variety of foods.
2. Eat less fat, particularly saturated fat.
3. Adjust energy intake for weight control.
4. Eat more foods containing complex carbohydrates and fiber.
5. Reduce salt intake.
6. Drink alcohol in moderation, if at all.

The baseline reference of what to eat (minimum maintenance diet) comes from the 1992 USDA food pyramid (shown on the next page). This pyramid shows that your "diet" should be distributed as follows: 40% complex carbohydrates, such as cereals and grains, another 40% fruits and vegetables, 10% dairy products, and another 10% proteins. Animal and saturated

---

The Food Pyramid

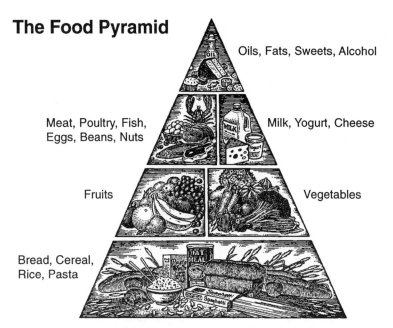

Oils, Fats, Sweets, Alcohol

Meat, Poultry, Fish, Eggs, Beans, Nuts

Milk, Yogurt, Cheese

Fruits

Vegetables

Bread, Cereal, Rice, Pasta

fat should be avoided or reduced to the minimum amount necessary to prepare the food. Refined sugars should be reduced to the absolute minimum in order to avoid the roller coaster fluctuation of insulin levels, even if you are not diabetic.

The minimum maintenance or transitional diet is a guideline that most Americans and other Westerners can follow consistently. However, a further step must be taken to promote healing and regeneration. This step involves reducing animal food sources and fat content to a minimum. The bulk of calories in the Cybernetic approach comes from complex carbohydrates in the form of whole grains, fruits, and vegetables. A small portion of the calories comes from vegetable proteins and vegetable fats.

RECOMMENDED FOOD CATEGORIES:

Cereals and Pasta: grains such as rice, wheat, corn, oats, millet, barley, and buckwheat.

Fruits and Vegetables: Humans develop a "sweet tooth" right at birth, from mother's milk. One of the basic pleasures of

Why Fruits and Vegetables?

1. Sweet Taste (Fructose) & Chewing.
2. Insulin & Mood Balance.
3. Antioxidants.
4. Folate (Anti-homocysteine)
5. Enzymes.
6. Potassium.
7. Fiber.
8. Replaces Animal Foods.

eating is sweetness. But simple sugars, such as glucose, and sucrose create insulin and mood swing disorders. So, eat fruits and vegetables which contain mostly fructose sugar. Fructose does not require a rapid surge in insulin for metabolism, unlike table sugar. Plant foods contain potassium, enzymes, and antioxidants. Research shows fruits and vegetables protect you from stroke and atherosclerosis. Homocysteine is a sulfur-containing amino acid found in a meat based diet. High levels of homocysteine increase atherosclerosis and heart disease. Plant foods contain folate, which reduces the homocysteine level in the blood.

Fiber: Fruits and vegetables provide fibers that help control constipation and intestinal disorders, diabetes, gallstones, obesity, cancer, and heart disease. There are two fiber types: insoluble and soluble. Insoluble fibers are cellulose, hemicellulose, and lignin. These create bulk in the stool, thus avoiding absorption of toxins. You get insoluble fiber in whole grains, seeds, fruits, vegetables, and legumes.

Soluble fibers include pectin and gums found in fruits, vegetables, seeds, barley, oats, and oat bran. Soluble fibers lower blood cholesterol and slow down absorption of glucose. Plant foods provide bulk and replace animal foods.

Proteins: Proteins should come mostly from vegetable sources because animal proteins invariably have a high fat content and cholesterol. The preferred sources of protein include beans and legumes (lentils, peas, red, black, kidney, navy or soybean, garbanzo, etc.). These foods provide soluble fiber and replace the meat–eater's protein sources adequately.

FATS OF LIFE

We have simplified the approach to "fats of life" into two parts: body fats, and dietary fats. Our goal is to balance body fats by regulating the intake of dietary fats.

BODY FATS

Excess of body fat leads to obesity and there are two reasons why it increases: too much dietary fat and sedentary lifestyle. Body fat is either in tissues or blood.

Blood fats include:

Lipids: Such as triglycerides, phospholipids and sterols. Ninety five percent of the lipids in food and our bodies are triglycerides.

Cholesterol: It is a sterol in blood carried by lipoproteins. Cholesterol is largely produced by the liver. Cholesterol is essential for healthy hormone production and cell function. Excess of cholesterol causes hardening of arteries, heart disease, gall bladder problems etc.

Lipoproteins: Lipoproteins (lipid and protein complex) transport lipids between liver and cells. Lipoproteins with less fat and more protein are called high density lipoprotein (HDL), and the ones with more fat and less protein are called low density lipoproteins (LDL).

Total Cholesterol: The total cholesterol includes HDL (good), LDL (bad), triglyceride (ugly), and Lp-a (deadly). The goal is to increase good cholesterol, and decrease "bad" and "ugly" cholesterols. The "deadly" cholesterol is not affected by diet or exercise.

DIETARY FATS

The fats in foods are mostly triglycerides (three fatty acids and glycerol). All fats are combinations of saturated or unsaturated fatty acids. Think of fat molecule as a sand box and hydrogen atoms as sand. The saturated molecule, or sand box, is full of sand. The mono-unsaturated box is empty in one corner. The polyunsaturated is empty in several corners. Saturated fats tend to be solid at room temperature, and unsaturated fats are liquid oils.

Saturated Fats: Mostly from animal sources - dairy products (butter, milk fat, and cheese) and fat in meats. Tropical vegetable oils- palm oil and coconut oil, and cocoa butter are also highly saturated. **Chocolate is high in saturated fats.** Saturated fat is dense in calories. It also increases your blood cholesterol levels and can clog up your arteries. Hydrogenated fats are unsaturated fats artificially hardened and saturated. Because they are less likely to turn rancid, hydrogenated oils are used mostly in deep frying in fast food restaurants. Hydrogenation and deep frying create a new form of fatty acids called *trans* fatty acids.

***Trans* Fats** increase LDL and decrease HDL. Willett's Harvard research has linked increased consumption of *trans* fats in margarine, cookies, crackers and proceed foods to heart disease. *Trans* fats come from products of ruminant animals such as beef, and from heavily hydrogenated oils commonly used in processed foods. Deep frying increases the *trans* fats in oils. Heart attack victims often have high trans fats in blood.

Polyunsaturated Fats: These are most unsaturated fats. Examples: safflower, sunflower, corn, cottonseed, sesame and soybean oils. Polyunsaturated fats may decrease both good (HDL) and bad cholesterol (LDL).

Polyunsaturated fats include omega-3 and omega-6 fatty acids. The benefits of fish oil is ascribed to the omega-3 fatty acids. At one time, the media hype focused on eating fish and fish oils to heal coronary artery disease. Fish oils thin the blood, but do not have antioxidant properties. American Heart Association and National Heart Lung and Blood Institute say that there is not enough data to recommend fish oil for prevention or treatment of coronary heart disease.

Monounsaturated Fats: These are least unsaturated fats. Examples: olive oil, canola oil, and peanut oil. Most nuts are high in mono fats. Monos reduce LDL without reducing HDL. In

---

fact, they may help to increase HDL. *There is not enough data to recommend tablespoons of olive oil as panacea for cholesterol problems.*

Essential Fatty Acids: Three fatty acids (linoleic acid, linolenic acid, and arachidonic acid) are "essential" for our body, because we cannot make them. The minimum daily requirement for these essential fats is easily met in a starch based, plant diet because most vegetables and grains have them. With a plant based diet, if your fat intake is at least 2% of total calories, you need not worry about essential fats, or about absorption of fat soluble vitamins, A, D, E and K.

Hazards of Excess of Dietary Fats:

Too much fat causes clogging of blood vessels by spasm, clot or aggregation of platelets. The platelet problem is worse with saturated fats. **Many people recall a large fatty meal preceding a heart attack.** Excess fat suppresses the immune system, which may lead to infections, autoimmune diseases, and cancer. Fat antagonizes insulin and aggravates diabetes.

Bottom Line of Fats in Life

1. Reduce all types of fat intake. Any fat is fattening, including olive oil, fish, and nuts.
2. For cooking, choose unsaturated oils over saturated and mono over poly fats.
3. If you use margarine, switch from solid to liquid type. Liquids have less of harmful *trans* fats.
4. Avoid fried foods which contain a lot of *trans* fats and free radicals. Frying in olive and canola oil produces least amount of *trans* fats. Reusing the same oil again and again for frying increases *trans* fats. *Remember a quote from one of my heart patients. " The fatty, fried food could have been my last meal !".*
5. Plant source of fats is preferred over animal sources. Starch based plant foods contain enough of essential fats for your daily requirements even if your daily fat intake is less than 2%.

Ruler for Dietary Fats

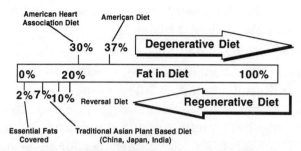

6. **Rule of Thumb for Fats** is given in the graphics. If your fat intake exceeds 20%, you are hastening your degeneration. Our typical American diet contains 37% fat. The American Heart Association recommends to stay within 30%. Reversal diet should have less than 20% fat - ideally 7-10%. A traditional diet in China, Japan, and India contain 7-10% fat, mostly from vegetable sources. *(The Americanized Asian foods contain 30-40% fat with deep fried appetizers, meats and oily main dishes competing with the traditional staples of rice, wheat, and vegetables).*

DAIRY PRODUCTS:

These should be mostly nonfat, such as egg whites, skim milk, nonfat yogurt, cheese, and sour cream.

FOODS TO AVOID:

Minimize caffeine to avoid stress arousal and insomnia. Alcohol increases fat deposits and affects your quality of sleep. High fat food and food preservatives increase free radicals in your blood. This, in turn, increases your stress arousal and decreases healing. Salts should be used in moderation, since excessive salt can promote hypertension.

MICRO– & MACRO–NUTRIENTS:

At the "micro" level, vitamins A, C, and E work on free radicals and render them harmless. At the "macro–nutrient" or gross level, these vitamins are found in fresh fruits, vegetables, and grains. Macro–biotic and vegetarian diets recommended for healing and preventing cancer and coronary artery disease, are based on these principles. Some examples are the McDougall Plan, Dr. Dean Ornish's *Eat More, Weigh Less Diet*, and Kushi's Macro–Biotic Diet.

Cooked vs. Raw Foods:

Heating food denatures (breaks down) the enzymes. In the case of fruits and vegetables, the loss of natural enzymes creates an "enzyme debt" in the food, for which your body has to compensate by secreting additional enzymes from bodily stores. This leads to an extra burden on your physiological system. If at least 50% of your food intake is in the form of fresh, uncooked fruits and vegetables, you lighten the enzyme debt on your system.

An interesting experiment compared changes in blood sugar and insulin level after eating the same calorie equivalent of fresh apples, apple sauce, and apple juice. Fresh apples caused the least fluctuation of blood sugar and insulin, apple juice the most, with apple sauce in between. This variation in metabolic changes is due to the change in fiber content and the denaturation of apples by processing. Since unprocessed foods are embedded with fiber, their absorption is gradual, and your body does not get overwhelmed by the rapid influx of sugar.

When to Eat

A baby's natural instinct is to feed whenever hungry. Many modern people try to eat three square meals each day. Jenkins' research study showed that after eating 17 meals each day for two weeks (although probably impractical for many), people reduced their cholesterol by 15%, cortisol by 17%, and insulin by 28%. In addition, these people lost weight and had balanced moods. This eating frequent, small meals is a **grazing diet**. One of its added benefits is, it corresponds to the recurring ultradian healing responses. Furthermore, this type of eating helps you regulate your mood by maintaining your brain serotonin at an even level.

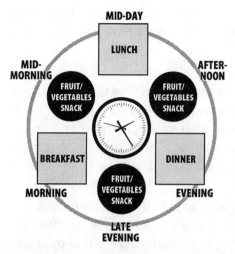

3 Square Meals and 3 Round Meals a Day

MID-DAY

LUNCH

MID-MORNING

AFTER-NOON

FRUIT/ VEGETABLES SNACK

FRUIT/ VEGETABLES SNACK

BREAKFAST

DINNER

MORNING

EVENING

FRUIT/ VEGETABLES SNACK

LATE EVENING

To make your diet more of a **"grazing"** one, add three snacks to your three square meals (mid–morning, mid–afternoon, and bedtime) for a total of six meals per day. These snacks should consist of **fresh fruits and vegetables**, rather than high–fat foods, candies, sugar, or caffeine. As noted earlier, fruits mostly have fructose sugar, which does not require an insulin surge for metabolism. So, fruit snacks help keep your insulin level and mood well–balanced. (Diabetics should consult their physicians in planning their diets.)

When you have a craving to eat, develop the habit of taking a diaphragmatic breath to become centered. Ask your mind–body *why* you want to eat and *what* you want to eat. Then, and then only, proceed to eat. After eating, observe the aftereffects on your mind–body. This simple cybernetic principle of **"foreplay, play, and replay"** provides feedback and "feed forward" information (mindfulness) to your body's intelligence system. This is called **"cybernetic eating."**

Grazing Diet Experiment:

Take two days to monitor your mood and energy levels, and how they relate to your eating patterns. On the first day, just eat your regular diet and observe your mood and energy levels.

On the second day, eat a breakfast, lunch and dinner of starch–based, low–fat, low–sugar foods. In addition, have a mid–morning, mid–afternoon, and evening snack of fruits or vegetables. (not candies, caffeine drinks, chocolate, or "chips"

---

which adversely affect your insulin level and mood). Compare your energy levels and mood variations to the first day. For the best comparison, repeat this experiment twice more at later dates.

When Not to Eat

When you feel acute stress arousal. Postpone eating to avoid the eating-as-a-pacifier conditioned reflex, as well as digestion problems. You should also avoid eating when you are angry or frustrated. Statistics show a large fatty meal at night can cause a heart attack in the morning.

How to Eat

For maximum nourishment, eat *slowly* and *mindfully*. Mindfulness means paying attention to the ambience, texture, flavor, sight, sound, and taste of food. Many civilized people normally eat in a hurry, as if the tongue were a moving conveyor belt. More food is needed to give the same amount of pleasure because contact time at each bite with the tongue and taste buds is too short to be remembered. Eating slowly also allows the flavor of the food to be aerosolized so you fully enjoy the smell of food. Chewing satisfies your biting instinct. Fast chewing sets the pace of life in general. This is why the Type A person, with hurry sickness, eats quickly. Slow eating allows enough time to get the feeling of fullness, thereby preventing overeating. Finally, reading the newspaper or talking about emotional issues interferes with the pleasure of eating and the process of digestion.

How Much to Eat

Normally, you should eat only until you feel approximately two–thirds full. If you eat mostly fruits, vegetables, and complex carbohydrates, however, you can eat until you feel mostly full because these foods are high in fiber. If you eat three additional snacks as outlined above, you will automatically avoid, or at least minimize, overeating at main meals .

Where's the Meat

In Western society, eating meat, fish, and poultry is a cultural habit and sign of prosperity. This is becoming more so in the East as well, due to "Westernization." Animal foods contain a lot of protein, saturated fat, cholesterol, and sodium, and very little carbohydrates, vitamins, or potassium. The fat in animal food has a concentrated amount of toxins from the soil, and from plants and drugs - hormones, stimulants, and antibiotics - fed to animals. Animal foods contain bacteria and parasites that can affect humans. Meat cooked over high heat can turn into carcinogens. Our cybernetic recommendation is to switch from animal foods to an entirely vegetarian diet. Reducing the quantity of meat, fish, and poultry still keeps the "addictive taste" in the tissues, which leads to a tendency for craving and over-indulgence. Total abstinence from meat products will change the tissue–embedded biochemical dependence after two to three months. Then you will not miss meat.

CYBERNETICS OF FOOD ADDICTION:

Eating is a habit. A habit becomes an addiction when you continue to do it in spite of the fact that the habit is harmful to you. The addictive agents associated with eating are: a) food components, particularly sugar, chocolate, and fat; and b) social and cultural situations.

Food Ingredients as Addictive Agents

Sugar: Americans eat an equivalent of 30 teaspoons of sugar per day. Consider the sugar content in candies, breakfast cereals, soft drinks, snacks, and cakes. When you eat these foods, the sugar in them releases endorphins from the brain, thus giving you immediate gratification. Your body absorbs sugar quickly, leading to a blood sugar rise. A large amount of insulin is secreted from the pancreas to metabolize the high amount of sugar. The next time you become hungry, you crave sugar again. You eat the same high sugar foods, and the cycle continues. Sugar is the most addictive food because it gratifies immediately. The shorter the interval between craving and satisfaction, the stronger the addiction.

Nicotine is a parallel. Smoking a cigarette gratifies in six seconds. This reinforces the habit. Nicotine gum and patch help wean from the cigarette habit because these maintain a constant blood level of nicotine, thus breaking the vicious cycle of supply and demand.

Your desire for sweetness is innate. In an experiment, sugar was gradually added to a baby's bottle while feeding. The baby's sucking frequency increased with the sugar content. Mother's milk is naturally sweet. No wonder we have expressions like "sweetheart," "sweetie pie," and "sweet dreams."

Sweetness is an Experience: Eating sugar is the easiest and quickest way to attain the sweet experience. Eating sugar moves the amino acid tryptophan from the blood to the brain. The tryptophan gets converted to serotonin, which gives you a sense of pleasure. What you actually become addicted to is the *experience* of sweetness. Eastern religions believe that the experience of heavenly bliss during meditative *samadhi* is "sweet." Sweetness is not just the sensory experience of the tongue, but also the emotional experience of the heart and soul.

Chocolate is a common addictive food. Some people say "I love chocolate." This statement is true both metaphorically and literally. Dr. Donald Klein and Michael Liebowitz, from the New York State Psychiatric Institute, published research showing that when a body is feeling love, a chemical called phenylethylamine is released. Chocolate is full of this chemical. So, when you eat chocolate, you literally feel in love. In another study, it was shown that women who crave chocolate during their premenstrual period are actually craving the magnesium contained in chocolate. Other problems include the high sugar and fat content in many chocolate products.

Social and Cultural Situations

In all cultures, "we meet to eat." We invite people out to dinner or we invite them to the house for dinner. Parties and celebrations compel us to eat. Certain food smells, such as fried chicken, pizza, barbecued meat, and coffee tempt us. TV ads reinforce addictive behavior.

Other negative impacts of social situations are untimely meals, skipped meals, overeating due to peer pressure, eating while excited or stressed, the use of alcohol, coffee or other stimulants, and so on.

Breaking the Chains of Food Addiction

1. Awareness of love hunger: inventory your relationships with your spouse, nuclear family, family of origin, friends, authority figures, food, and God, as well as with yourself (actions, thoughts, and emotions).

2. Scan the events for food hunger vs. love hunger.

3. Assess the need to gratify in the love and food hunger departments. Do not try to satisfy your emotional needs with food, as they may be unrelated to food and your body's physical needs.

4. Eat six meals of fruits and vegetables each day to prevent a roller coaster effect of craving for food and sweetness.

Hunger for Food or Hunger for Love

We have a tendency to substitute the sweet taste of food for the sweet experience of love. When you are love hungry, you have low self-esteem and you derive gratification by using addictive agents, such as sugar, alcohol, or nicotine. Then, you face the consequence of guilt and shame. This leads to a lack of intimacy and further isolation from society. The vicious cycle of love hunger starts all over again. When a baby cries, we put a pacifier in its mouth, and the baby learns eating as a source of security. This learned love of security carries into adulthood, and some eat candy or sweets when they feel insecure.

Love Hunger

Lover Hunger

Lack of Intimacy

Low Self-Esteem

Rebound of Guilt - Shame

Need for Gratification

Face Consequences

Look for Addictive Agent

Food

Feeding the "Feedback"

The axiom, **"foreplay, play, and replay,"** applies to eating cybernetics very well. Pay attention to your hunger and cravings just before you eat; observe the sensory and motor experience as you eat; and notice the immediate and delayed aftereffect on the various functions of your mind and body. Pretty soon you will be able to "read" the effects of food by simply thinking about them. This is called tapping into your body's own intelligence system to determine your need of nourishment. The other side of feedback is **"feed forward."** You start to observe the aftermath of eating a particular food and use it to decide whether to eat that food again or not. The basic principle of cybernetic feedback is "foresight and hindsight lead to insight." This is particularly true with regard to what you eat and what is eating you.

You can observe the effects of what you eat on the "pumps and pipes" of your body. Your "gut feeling" and "feeling gut" change according to what you eat. Your bowel function, urinary function, heart rate, blood pressure, sleep pattern, breathing pattern, mood, and relationship with others change according to what kind of food you put into your mind–body.

Judging the Food for Thought

When you change your food habits to the regenerative diet just explained, you will tend to judge others wrong if they are not eating what you think is the right food. This critical judgment can create conflicts in your mind and generate stress chemicals. The way to handle this conflict is to use the HRI (heartfelt resonant imaging) method and love the other person unconditionally, regardless what food they love to eat.

Why Eat? For Degeneration or ***Regeneration?***
When to Eat? Three or ***6 Meals a Day.***
What to Eat? Processed, Refined Sugar, Fat, Animal Food? or ***Natural, Starch-based, Plant Food Plus Appropriate Antioxidant Vitamins (A, C, E).***
How to Eat? Fast and Absent Minded? or ***Slow and Mindfully?***
How Much to Eat? Overeat? or ***Eat 70% of Your Capacity.***

Heart Disease and Cancer

27

Heart Resetting Tools

Part A: Orientation to Tools
Part B: Implementing the Tools

Heart Resetting Tools

PART A: ORIENTATION TO TOOLS

A *tool* is a handy instrument to modify or shape something. A tool has to be user-friendly, efficient, and take advantage of a principle such as leverage. That's what makes a wrench better than bare hands.

Our resetting tools are user-friendly, efficient, and they employ known principles to help you change behavior; control stress and anger; reverse or prevent heart disease, cancer and other degenerative diseases. And because they change the way you act or react now to a new way to act or react, we call them resetting tools.

We've developed three types:

1. **Measuring Tools:** Scales and Graphs.
2. **Monitoring Tools:** On–line and off–line data collectors.
3. **Modifying Tools:** Short and Long Rituals or Methods.

MEASURING TOOLS:

A. Human Function Curve, Vital Exhaustion Scale, and William's Anger Scale.
B. Money Function Curve and Money Style Scale.
C. Energy Exchange Vectors (Cross Checks).

MONITORING TOOLS:

Present–Moment

   On–line Monitors

A. Centering, Mindful Breathing, and Open Focus™.
B. CyberScan™ Snapshot of Behavior.
C. Heartfelt Resonant Imaging (HRI).
D. Energy Quadrants of Emotions.

   Off–line (Daily Monitors)

A. Observe Sleep and Restless mind
B. Observe Pumps and Pipes of Body

MODIFYING TOOLS

1. **HRI to Altruism.**

2. **Meditation and Imagery.**

3. **Physical Exercise.**

4. **Mindful Eating & Vitamins.**

5. **Self–Disclosure.** (Supplements of Muscle–to–Mind and Mind–to–Muscle Tools.)

The Body's Feedback System, or Cybernetics.

Consider your automatic home heating system with thermostat. It measures, modifies and controls temerpature through a constant feedback process. Similarly, you want to Measure, Monitor, and Modify your behavior; through your mind body information feedback system. This idea of control based on feedback is called **cybernetics**. Since our stress control system uses both internal awareness of feedback and machine-aided awareness of feedback (biofeedback), we use the term Stress Cybernetics.

Stress Control and Resetting the Heart involve two distinct phases using medical problem-solving models:

(1) **Self–diagnosis of life patterns.**

(2) **Self–healing by behavior modification.**

Self–diagnosis, in turn, has two components:

1. Measuring Life Patterns

You measure your life pattern with the yard sticks of the human function curve, money function curve, and energy exchange. Measurement means taking an inventory of what is there now, appraising its current value, focusing on a target, setting goals, and working on modifications of your behavior patterns.

2. Monitoring Your Behavior

Monitoring is collecting current information, just like looking in the mirror to comb your hair. You monitor yourself by taking a snapshot of your present behavior in the area of action, thoughts, and emotions. Compare your heartfelt feelings with mindfelt feelings. Assess the energy cost of your emotional state at that moment.

Self–healing occurs when you modify your behavior patterns using our cybernetic, feedback–based tools. These tools address your stress from the standpoint of your emotions, as well as the reactivity of your body. We will go into each tool and explain how to use them. First, let us go over the concepts of measuring and monitoring stress.

MEASURING LIFE PATTERNS

You measure your life patterns in three distinct areas:

1. **The Human Function Curve** assesses your life overall in areas of muscle actions, thoughts, and emotions. It also shows how stress changes your life for better or worse. You can periodically measure these against the human function curve, as well as monitor on–line with the CyberScan™ described below.

2. **The Money Function Curve** measures your relationship with money. Since you assign a symbolic monetary value to your life energy, how you relate to money has a direct impact on your stress level.

3. **The Energy Exchange Directions** tell you exactly where you spend your life energy intentionally or unintentionally.

HUMAN FUNCTION CURVE (HFC)

The HFC shows how close to wreckage and illness you are as you row your lifeboat; and indicates how to attain the "maximal self" without unnecessary wear, tear and burnout. In the HFC, the horizontal axis is stress arousal. The vertical, performance (ability to cope and adapt). You can see curve has an up–slope, a peak, and a down–slope.

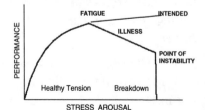

HUMAN FUNCTION CURVE

Heart Disease and Cancer

The **up–slope is healthy.** Effort earns a proportionate return, and there is healthy fatigue and recovery. **The litmus test of healthy fatigue is restful sleep.** Your muscle actions, thoughts, and emotions are balanced. The skeletal muscles feel fatigue only with exertion and recover completely with rest. Thoughts are manageable. Emotion is filled with caring love, pleasure, and a sense of humor. Any negative emotions are appropriate and short lived, as they are in childhood. Human relationships are pleasant and enjoyable.

Stress hardiness is represented by a high HFC curve. It takes a lot of stress arousal to push you off the top. A higher performance is possible at a lower level of exertion because there is no misplaced effort to waste energy. This hardiness comes from a commitment to life with a sense of challenge and control.

If the HFC curve is low, you feel exhausted from minimal exertion.Contributing factors may include: poor parenting, poverty, childhood struggles, failure, inadequate social support, uprooting, political unrest, environmental disasters, etc. These all lead to a loss of predictability of events and control in life. So, the height of the curve decides your "stress tolerance," which is the sum total of your body's "exercise tolerance" and mind's "exercising tolerance." The curve enables you to picture various factors, urges, or drives that push you on to the down–slope. Here's how to tell if you are on the down–slope. Check these major factors that affect the height of your human function curve:

1. **Exercise Tolerance** or Physical Conditioning.
2. **Caring Love** and Relationships with People.
3. **Foods** and Chemicals You Eat.

On the unhealthy down–slope. At your peak you still enjoy healthy fatigue. However, if you push beyond the peak, you hit the down–slope. Your goal is along a straight line higher and higher. But the more effort you put in, the more your returns diminish. You are beating a tired horse that pretty soon has to give up. High stress hinders the restorative power of rest and sleep. On the down–slope, your sense of challenge gives way to fear, threat, loss of control, and a feeling of being off–centered. As you continue on the down–slope, you feel a sense of **vital exhaustion,** and you reach a point of "no return."

From this **point of instability** your mind–body can fall into a complete breakdown: catastrophic illness, a heart attack or cancer.

STRESS ADDICTION

Stress addiction is covered in chapter 10. But, to review: Stress arousal makes you breathe from your chest rather than from your diaphragm, creating a chemical imbalance in the blood. When you hyperventilate, you blow out too much carbon dioxide, temporarily making your blood alkaline,and causing kidneys to excrete bicarbonate buffer. Then, when you try to sleep, you do not have enough buffer reserve to carry you through the night. You become restless. You literally experience a "sour life," due to too much acid in your blood.

This is how you develop insomnia, awaking in the early hours with a restless mind and emotional sweating. The daytime equivalent is inability to stay still, a compulsive urge to keep doing something, workaholism, and a restless mind.

The buffer loss leaves you without energy reserves for coping with extra loads. In the past, people would pay

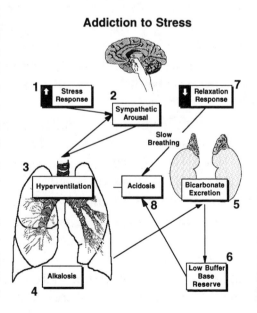

Addiction to Stress

Heart Disease and Cancer

attention to these feedback signals and take rest breaks. In today's society, you deny and suppress your mind–body signals and keep pushing despite a low energy reserve. It's like trying to drive a car on empty. Collectively, these events create an addiction to stress, as shown in the diagram. Addiction is a condition you know is harmful, but "hooked" on, and unable to escape.

The Chain of Events Creating Stress Addiction

1. An initial trigger and subsequent stress response.
2. Stress response creates sympathetic arousal in the body.
3. Sympathetic response triggers hyperventilation, or over breathing.
4. The hyperventilating creates an alkalosis condition in the blood chemistry and triggers additional sympathetic arousal in a self–feeding cycle.
5. Excessively alkaline blood chemistry triggerskidneys to excreteexcess bicarbonate.
6 This creates a low bicarbonate buffer reserve in the blood, which causes the blood chemistry to become acidic (step 8).
7. Trying to relax by slow breathing or sleep also creates an acidic blood condition due to the original slow buffer reserve.
8. The acidic blood condition triggers hyperventilation and the cycle repeats itself.

Once you are in this vicious cycle of stress leading to more stress, you unsuccessfully try various gimmicks you hear about, and once again prove that you are helpless.

In our clinic, we use a machine, called a capnometer, which measures carbon dioxide in your exhaled breath to determine your buffer level. Without such equipment, your best index of a low buffer reserve is how restless you sleep and how restless your mind is during the day.

To identify the down–slope markers of buffer failure or "sour life," identify and monitor your emotions. Then relate your emotions to your restless mind (thoughts) and restless body (muscle actions). This is easy to remember if you divide human behavior into the three parts of an iceberg: body actions (muscle contractions) at the tip, thoughts in the middle, and emotions at the base.

Reactivity of Body Actions

The most sensitive measure of reactivity to stressful circumstances is to observe your breathing patterns. When stressed, you either hold your breath or over breathe with chest breathing. You can graduate from our stress cybernetic class when you can do two things:

1. Observe your breath holding or chest breathing pattern periodically throughout the day.
2. Deliberately replace it with diaphragmatic breathing, both while discussing stressful subjects and during your own negative self–talk.

You can also note your emotional sweating, cold extremities, bowel habits and digestion. An overreactive response to minor interruptions of noise, people, or light is another indicator. Your muscles feel sore and fatigued because the lactic acid does not have enough buffer to balance it.

Stress hormones like adrenaline and cortisone change the calcium–magnesium equilibrium, leading to spasms in various tubes in the body. Here's how stress–induced spasm in these tubes can feel.

- **Spasms of the blood vessels** = cold extremities, migraine headache, or high blood pressure.
- **Coronary artery spasms** = anginal chest pain or a heart attack.
- **Gastrointestinal spasms** = heart burn, constipation, stomach pains, a spastic colon, irritable bowels, and lump in the throat feeling.

- **Bronchial spasms** = asthma.
- **Urinary spasms** = bladder problems.
- **Uterine spasms** = menstrual cramps or infertility.
- **Spasms of blood vessels in the brain** = restless mind.

Reactivity of Thoughts

Thoughts are just mental statements.When stress makes them reactive, you have a restless mind; hurry sickness; excessive competitiveness; an inability to concentrate; irrational (often self–deprecating) ideas; and, most importantly, perceptions of a loss of control and ability to manage life.

Reactivity of Emotions

Emotionally, you may first try to over control the situation with cynical mistrust, anger, rage, and aggression (Type A behavior). Stress chemicals, such as adrenaline and noradrenaline, trigger it.Your other emotional reactivity may be feelings of loss of control, defeat, despair, or a giving in–giving up feeling - the helpless, hopeless attitude in Type C behavior. This is mostly due to cortisol–like hormones. You lose the pleasure of human company because of hostility, social isolation, guilt, and sadness. You may also lose sense of humor and compassion. Emotional fatigue makes life robotic. Self–esteem is lost, and you try to do more and more to regain it, but with diminishing returns.

Peter Nixon, the originator of the human function curve, offers the mnemonic **SABRES** to help you remember key concepts and important behavior changes identified by the Human Function Curve.

S for Sleep: Awareness of quality and quantity of sleep for optimal performance.

A for Arousal: To manage struggles, hassles, and frustration without over-arousal of the sympathetic nervous system and adrenaline. Do not waste your energy with misplaced effort. Stress hardiness is accommodating loss, defeat, and despair without chronic stress.

B for Breathing: Awareness and control of thoracic breathing, breath holding, and hyperventilation symptoms: palpitation, chest pains, chest tightness, dizziness, numbness, "lump in throat," restless mind, panic, emotional sweating, muscle tension, pain between shoulders, chronic fatigue, and insomnia. Identify faulty breathing and replace it with diaphragmatic breathing.

R for Rest: To be still and at ease, like a baby or animal at rest.

E for Effort: Awareness of the personal energy cost of physical, mental, and emotional effort and the need to balance it with rest and sleep.

S for Self–esteem: Feelings of worth, confidence, control, and meaning in life.

VITAL EXHAUSTION

In healthy fatigue, you recover to the baseline. In vital exhaustion, there is no such recovery. Life is a wave — activity builds to a peak and then there is recovery. If you do not allow yourself to recover with periodic rest, daydreaming, and adequate sleep, you drain your energy reserve. This is like a battery that loses charge gradually and finally loses all power.

People who have catastrophic illness, such as a heart attack, can recall such gradual drainage of energy until the "last straw breaks the camel's back." You'll find the scale to measure vital exhaustion in the tool implementing section.

MONEY FUNCTION CURVE

In our culture today, much of our value system is based on money. We have transferred a lot of our biological energy to the symbol of money. The Money Function Curve has

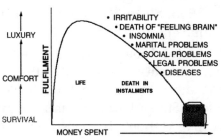

MONEY FUNCTION CURVE

- IRRITABILITY
- DEATH OF "FEELING BRAIN"
- INSOMNIA
- MARITAL PROBLEMS
- SOCIAL PROBLEMS
- LEGAL PROBLEMS
- DISEASES

LUXURY

COMFORT

SURVIVAL

FULFILMENT

LIFE

DEATH IN INSTALMENTS

MONEY SPENT

the horizontal axis of money spent and the vertical axis of fulfillment in life.

On the up–slope, money earned and spent increases along with healthy survival, comfort, and luxury.

On the down–slope, after luxury, more money spent goes to buy your death in installments. You progress through irritability, death of a "feeling brain," insomnia, marital, social, legal, and medical problems, get hit with a catastrophe and then rest in peace, having paid your last installment. Find where you are on your money function curve and decide the overall health of your position.

MONEY STYLE OF LIFE

Another aspect of your money relationship is your attitude towards it. The need and greed for money leads to other challenging issues: love, power, security, connectedness, independence, self–esteem, and control. Olivia Mellon describes the following imbalances in money styles:

Money monks, who think money is evil.

Money amassers, who constantly scheme to make more, whether they need it or not.

Money avoiders, who just do not want to think about the subject.

Money worriers, who spend every waking hour totaling up figures in their heads, imagining a financial disaster.

Hoarders, who believe the purpose of money is to save it.

Spenders, who never have a penny in the bank.

Typically, if money styles differ in a relationship, conflicts erupt. This is often the undercurrent in failures of business partnerships and marriages.

ENERGY EXCHANGE VECTORS (CROSS CHECKS)

You have a certain amount of biological energy. How you spend it is based on how you relate to yourself. Note whether you are giving or receiving energy. Caring love makes you receive energy. Hostility and resentment make you lose it.

Horizontally, map your energy flow to your spouse, significant other, and close family members on one side, and your co-workers and society at large on the other side. Vertically, see how

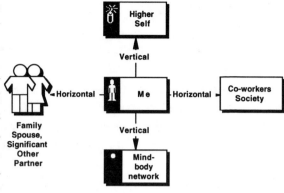

you relate to your mind–body information system and your spiritual or higher self. In all cases, caring love is the only way to fully realize your energy. Our tool, called heartfelt resonant imaging, will help you regain this energy instantly.

MONITORING STRESSFUL BEHAVIOR

Monitoring your behavior is like looking at a mirror or computer monitor. You collect immediate information about the present moment. In most cases, simply monitoring it changes your behavior. It's like the glancing eye of a teacher alerting you to behave.

You monitor in real time, regardless of what else you are doing, because the human mind is a multi–tasking, parallel processor. You can solve more than one task at the same time. Most of us rarely use our full mental capabilities. We can process 800 words per minute, yet we all speak less than 300 words per minute. Typically, we use the remaining processing power to ruminate on the past or forecast the future. Instead, you can use this processing ability to monitor your own behavior from the background all day long. You use three distinct tools to monitor yourself.

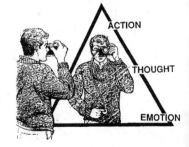

Mindfulness by CyberScan™

This is like taking a photograph.

1. You stabilize the camera (your mind) by directing your awareness to your belly button.
2. You focus on particular aspects of your behavior: action, thought, or emotion.
3. Take a snapshot. The mind will automatically develop the picture.

You can review your snapshots or make a movie by connecting several of them. This will give you a pattern of your behavior at the end of the day.

Energy Quadrants of Emotions

You spend or save energy every moment. When you have negative feelings of fear, anger, guilt, or sadness, you spend too much energy in misplaced effort, because your muscles are tense, your mind restless. When you have positive feelings of love or pleasure, your

Energy Quadrants of Emotions

High + Pleasure Love Flow	High - Fear Anger
Low + Sleep, Rest Meditation	Low - Guilt, Sadness Repression

energy is even with the "flow." When you are at rest, asleep, or meditating, you save energy. There are four energy quadrants. The two quadrants on the left side are the high positive of pleasure and flow, and the low positive of sleep, rest, and meditation. The two quadrants on the right side are the high negative of fear and anger, and the low negative of guilt and sadness.

When you take a snapshot of your behavior, focus your awareness on your energy usage. It's like watching your fuel gauge periodically.

Heartfelt Resonant Imaging (HRI)

The purpose of HRI is to use caring love as a tool to open up energy reserves. You lose energy when there is a conflict between mindfelt and heartfelt feelings. Although the human mind may judge, resent, or hate, the human heart knows only how to love. You do HRI in two simple steps. First, get oriented to the heart muscle. Second, relate the state of mind to the heart muscle. Here's how:

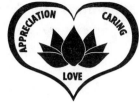

1. Focus your awareness on your anatomical heart area.
2. Ask yourself, "Can I experience heartfelt caring love towards this person, plant, animal, or object?" Your heart will always answer yes.

MODIFYING THE PATTERNS

Once you have measured and monitored your life patterns, the next task is to modify those that don't work and improve those you can improve. You do this because: 1) experiments modifying behaviors creates a before and after comparison which identifies current patterns that are not effective; and 2) modifying brings you to a new level from which you can further advance.

Summary of Modifying Human Functions

Combine four different models:

1. Dean Ornish's Life Style Changes to Reverse Heart Disease
2. Carl Simonton's Cancer Healing
3. Peter Nixon's Cardiac Rehabilitation (European model)
4. Our own experience of cybernetic research with heart rate monitoring of emotions.

    Merge them with millenniums of Eastern and Western wisdom, and you have the most effective tools for changing human functions:

Change the Mind–Body Chemistry by

1. Internal Pharmacy

    Anger Control, Reactivity Control (Restless mind control and Insomnia control), Stress control (Meditation, Self–disclosure, and Physical exercise)
2. External Pharmacy of mindful eating.

Heart Resetting Tools

PART B: IMPLEMENTING THE TOOLS

1. MEASURING TOOLS

Use each measuring tool at the beginning of the program to get a baseline. Repeat these measurements after 21 days and see the difference. Then, keep checking once a month.

2. MONITORING TOOLS

Learn the monitoring tools in the first two days by repeating them several hundred times, moment to moment. Use the monitors for the rest of your life every day.

3. MODIFYING TOOLS

Learn and repeat each tool, one per day. Add the next tool and keep practicing the previous tools until mastered. These tools should become a part of you for the rest of your life.

Right after hatching, baby chicks need light, controlled temperature, and very meticulous feeding for the next 24–48 hours. Similarly, your new born tools need close attention and nurturing by deliberate repetition over the first two days. Tennis Master Vic Braden has shown that if you repeat an act at least a thousand times, it becomes second nature. The tools

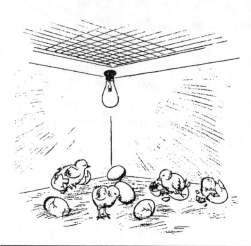

should be practiced diligently one after the other for 21 days.

The lapse of an old habit is not a relapse. Just observe your lapse and repeat the correction several times in your mind. Your mind will catch on.

Human Function Curve (HFC)

Objective

To find where you're headed, or your performance in relation to arousal.

Method

If you are on the up-slope, you sleep good, have control over your restless mind, human relationships are enjoyable, the "pipes" in your body function OK . See the pictorial "pipe" list in the monitoring section.

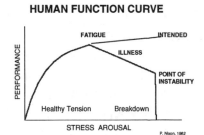

HUMAN FUNCTION CURVE

P. Nixon, 1982

If you are on the down-slope, you may wake up between 1 and 3 AM, have a restless mind during the day with a compulsive urge to do things (forced workaholism), and the "pipes" in your body do not function properly.

Result

Once you know where you are on the HFC, keep working on five major modifying tools of anger control, stress control, self-disclosure, physical exercise and food habits to stay on the up-slope most of the time.

Mastery

Repeated observation of HFC keeps you anchored to the basic purpose of human life – being connected to others in a harmonious relationship regardless of material achievements. You learn to pay attention to the affiliative motive in spite of achievement demands.

Money Function Curve (MFC)

Objective

Refocus to divert at least 50% of your energy away from money dynamics.

Method

1. Find your position on the MFC. On the up-slope, money earned and spent brings basic needs and comfort. On the down-slope, you chase money frantically, losing the human perspective of caring love and connectedness.

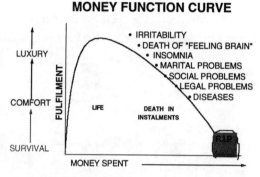

MONEY FUNCTION CURVE

- IRRITABILITY
- DEATH OF "FEELING BRAIN"
- INSOMNIA
- MARITAL PROBLEMS
- SOCIAL PROBLEMS
- LEGAL PROBLEMS
- DISEASES

LUXURY
COMFORT
SURVIVAL
FULFILMENT
LIFE
DEATH IN INSTALMENTS
R.I.P.
MONEY SPENT

2. What is your money relationship? Are you a money monk, amasser, avoider, worrier, hoarder, or spender? How does this compare to your spouse or partner? The healthy attitude to money is to divert at least 50% of energy to human relationships, regardless of money. This is done by using the flip-flop method described under Heartfelt Resonant Imaging.

Result

You accept your current level of money as abundant enough to enjoy human values.

Mastery

Ability to divide your mind-body energy system into money- based and non money-based values. Ability to have a child-like detachment from money at least half your waking time.

Energy Exchange Vectors

Objective

To realize that human relationships either give or take away energy. Caring love gains energy. Hostility loses energy.

Method

1. Vertical axis tells you about your own mind-body balance and spirituality in the form of higher self.

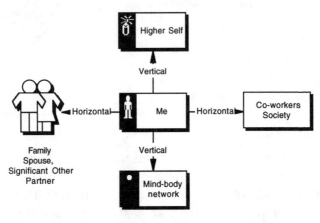

2. Horizontal axis tells you about your intimacy and rapport with your partner, spouse, and significant other as well as society at large.

Result

You are reminded that relationship problems cost you energy. You can desensitize your mind to conflicts by the heartfelt resonant imaging method. The heart will forgive, the mind may still dislike the person.

Mastery

Able to resolve major conflicts by reasoning out energy cost of resentments. Able to use caring love as a tool to energize the mind-body.

Heart Disease and Cancer

MEASURING TOOL SCALE 1

Vital Exhaustion

The following checklist will help you determine if you are on the vital exhaustion down-slope. If some statements are true, then utilizing our stress control tools will help you get back on the upslope of the Human Function Curve:

1. *I can't cope anymore.*

2. *I am not sufficiently in control.*

3. *I am not accomplishing anything.*

4. *I am spiritless.*

5. *I have come to a dead end.*

6. *I have no energy left, only sheer will power.*

7. *I cannot say "no" when I should.*

8. *I am sick of people.*

9. *I am too angry, tense, upset, irritable, indignant, or impatient.*

10. *I have too many demands made on me.*

11. *I am too pressed for time.*

12. *I am not sleeping well enough to stay healthy.*

13. *I am not keeping fit enough to stay healthy.*

14. *My work and rest periods are imbalanced.*

15. *I often have trouble falling asleep.*

16. *I wake up repeatedly throughout the night.*

17. *I often feel tired.*

18. *I feel weak all over.*

19. *I feel dejected.*

20. *I feel like crying sometimes.*

21. *I feel as if I no longer have what it takes.*

22. *I feel as if I want to give up trying.*

23. *I've been feeling hopeless lately.*

24. *I sometimes feel like I want todie.*

25. *I no longer enjoy sex.*

26. *Little things irritate me more than ever.*

27. *I frequently wake up of exhausted or fatigued.*

28. *It takes me more time to grasp a difficult problem than it did a year ago.*

29. *I have increasing difficulty concentrating on a single subject.*

30. *I am resentful and unable to forgive others.*

MEASURING TOOL SCALE 2

Protesting Heart Scale

One catastrophic illness related to vital exhaustion is a heart attack. Here are questions based on Peter Nixon's research to ask yourself about your heartbefore it falls apart in a heart attack:

- *What is it trying to say? Am I listening?*

- *Why is it protesting?*

- *What makes it protest each time? And why so often?*

- *Am I working to make it stronger, or am I too upset with myself to succeed?*

- *Am I looking for a drug or operation to keep it quiet?*

- *Is my heart experiencing caring love, both as a sender and receiver of love?*

William's Hostility Scale

TEST YOUR HOSTILITY LEVEL

Cynicism

- When in the express checkout line at the supermarket, do you often count the items in the baskets of the people ahead of you to be sure they aren't over the limit?

- When an elevator doesn't come as quickly as you think it should, do you quickly focus on the inconsiderate behavior of someone on another floor who's holding it up?

- Do you frequently check on family members or co-workers to make sure they haven't made a mistake in some task?

Anger

- When you are held up in a slow line in traffic, at the bank, or supermarket, etc., do you quickly sense your heart pounding and your breath quickening?

- When little things go wrong, do you often feel like lashing out at the world?

- When someone criticizes you, do you quickly begin to feel annoyed?

Aggression

- If an elevator stops too long on a floor above you, are you likely to pound on the door?

- If people mistreat you, do you look for an opportunity to pay them back, just on the principle of the thing?

- Do you frequently find yourself muttering at the television during a news broadcast?

If you answered "yes" to event one question in each area or to four or more overall, your hostility level is probably high.

Centering, Mindful Breathing, Open Focus

Objective

To re-focus attention from head to body; to relieve traffic congestion in your head. To enjoy the present moment mindfully, away from mind-talk.

Method

1. **Centering:** Simply focus your awareness on your belly. This centers you and balances your attitude away from mind-talk.

2. **Mindful Breathing**: Find your breath in your belly and follow your breath. Breathe with your diaphragm, making your belly bulge out during inspiration and collapse during expiration. Prolong your breathe out slightly.

3. **Open the narrow focus** of your mind by visiting different parts of your body one by one. This takes away the head centered thinking. Can you be aware of your body parts while simultaneously thinking of mundane activities? Also, open focus from "I-ness" to "You-ness" so that you do not spend all the time thinking of yourself.

4. Use these centering devices to control restless mind during meditation.

Result

Centering allows you to be present in the present. You enjoy the present moment mindfully without judgement.

Mastery

Use centering, mindful breathing, and open focus as tools to control restless automatic self-talk for the rest of your life.

CyberScan™ *Mindfulness Snapshot*

Objective

To take a snapshot of your behavior at the moment, in the areas of actions, thoughts, and emotions.

Method

1. Get centered by focusing awareness on the belly and continue to breathe. This is like stabilizing a camera to take a picture.

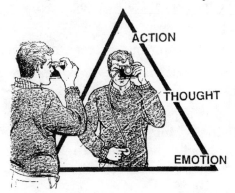

2. Now, you focus the mental camera on your behavior. Observe your muscles in different parts of the body, thought patterns, and dominant emotion. The basic emotions are: pleasure or love, fear, anger, guilt and sadness. Relate your emotion to thoughts and muscle tensions.

Result

You observe your physiology moment-to-moment as you do other things. You can connect each snapshot and observe the movie of your behavior pattern.

Mastery

Your mind is a parallel processor. You should be able to observe your action, thoughts, and emotions in the background as you talk, walk, write, etc.

Heartfelt Resonance Imaging (HRI)

Objective

To develop a conditioned response to a biological state of caring love. This will resolve the tug of war conflict between your heart and mind, and replace the biological state of anger

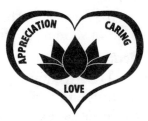

Method

1. Focus your awareness on your anatomical heart area.

2. Ask yourself: "Can I experience heartfelt caring love towards this person, animal, plant or object?"

3. Flip-Flop between mundane activities of information processing and problem solving in the left brain to intuitive caring love in the right brain.

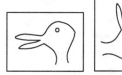

Duck-Rabbit Flip-flop

Result

Judgmental and analytical stress, frustration, and angerare covered with messenger molecules of caring love. This puts affiliation over achievement; rapport visit over report visit in life; human being over human doing.

Mastery

You should be able to do HRI with most people you meet in person and on the phone during the day.

Develop the conditioned response and HRI every time you encounter a person, animal, or plant actually, or in your mind) to heal yourself and stay connected. Use this method every time you use the phone.

Energy Quadrants of Emotions

Objective

To assess the cost of energy for positive and negative emotions.

Method

1. Get centered, take a snapshot of your muscle tension, restless mind, and positive and negative emotions in four quadrants:

High Negative: Fear, Anger

Low Negative: Guilt, Sadness, Repression.

High Positive: Pleasure, "Flow with the Moment."

Low Positive: Sleep, Rest, Meditation.

Energy Quadrants of Emotions

High + Pleasure Love Flow	High - Fear Anger
Low + Sleep, Rest Meditation	Low - Guilt, Sadness Repression

Result

Awareness of each emotion and its energy cost on your mind-body. This allows you to switch at any moment to a meditative or heartfelt feeling state to escape tension.

Mastery

Ability to switch to low positive energy conserving mode just by closing your eyes and drifting into a meditative state. Ability to recall positive imageries from the past to overlay negative emotions and negative imagery.

Off-Line Daily Physiological Monitors

Objective

To monitor your cause-and-effect physiology in the area of sleep at night; restless mind during the day; functions of various pumps and pipes in the body.

Method

1. Every morning evaluate your sleep quality, sleep interruptions in difficulty falling asleep and staying asleep. Observe your workaholic urge and restless mind during the day, and the effects of meditation on these factors.

2. Observe your body's pumps and pipes. Also your bowel habits. Relate them to your emotional conflicts and stress level.

Result

Daily feedback regulation of your physiology. Stress and its effects can be dissipated by the tools that modify the internal chemistry: HRI, Meditation-Imagery, Exercise, Mindful eating, and Self-disclosure.

Mastery

Able to change the stress-induced damage to your physiology by daily monitor.

Meditation and Imagery

Objective

To enter into an alpha-theta meditative state by momentary mindfulness, in one minute and or five minute increments. Use imagery in the meditative state for healing, personal growth, and balanced creativity.

Method

1. MINDFUL MEDITATIVE CENTERING

(One moment, Please).

Simply drift your awareness to your belly center or heart area AND CONTINUE TO BREATHE FROM YOUR BELLY.

(Belly button centering for balanced assessment at the moment, and heart area centering for accessing caring love feelings). This helps you escape your usual head-centered, intellectual state.

2. ONE MINUTE MEDITATION

Close your eyes (You can do this with eyes open as well, but closed eyes works better).

Focus your awareness on your breath as follows: Find and follow your breath in your belly, and slightly prolong your breathe-out phase.

Use a mental sound or mantra as follows: Mentally say "soo" as you breathe in and "ham" as your breathe out.

Deepen the meditation as follows: Roll your eyeballs up as if watching a sunrise and following the sun to midday over your head.

As your mind wanders, bring it back to the breath and mantra and repeat.

3. ONE MINUTE IMAGERY

Close your eyes (You can do this with eyes open as well, but closed eyes works better). Find, follow, and link your breath (as in one minute meditation) and make sure that you prolong your breathe-out three times.

Focus awareness on your heart area and ask your heart "Can I experience caring love towards me, my heart, etc.?" "Can I visualize opening up of my heart like a lotus blossoming, and my coronary arteries are opening wider and wider?"

Once experienced, you can do the imagery concurrently focusing on your heart zone and prolonging the breathe-out slightly with each breath.

Meditation Mnemonics: It is easy to remember meditation with the mnemonics,

3 P's : Place, Posture, and Passive Attitude.

3 R's : Relax Muscles, Respiration Watch, and Repeat *Mantra*.

Place: For the morning and evening meditation, sit on your favorite chair or your bed to develop a conditioned response.

Posture: Meditation is always done in the sitting position. The head, neck, and back should be straight and comfortable. Close your eyes.

Passive Attitude: You re-focus your thinking from your head to various parts of your body. The suggested body parts to be aware of are: forehead, eyes, jaw, tongue, neck, shoulders, arms, legs, and abdomen. You can do this by:

1. Contracting and relaxing muscle groups, paying attention to tension.

2. Shifting your awareness from one body part to the other.

3. Focusing on each body part and imagine it to be heavy and warm.

4. Imagining that each body part is a hollow space.

4. FIVE MINUTE MEDITATION

Sustain the one minute meditation. You will notice your mind has a tendency to wander. You solve this by visiting various body parts as outlined above. You add the bodywork and the mind work as outlined in chapter 23 on Meditation.

Additional imageries for your personal growth and to realize your greatest potential.

1. **Resolve Conflicts:** Use Heartfelt Resonant Imagery and forgive everyone causing conflict in your mind. Focus on your heart, enter into a state of caring love and forgive. Switch back and forth between the mind and heart to desensitize.

2. **Inner Guide:** Visualize your inner guide as a person, light, or idol to help you solve your problems.

3. **Abundance:** Visualize the abundance of your family relationships with father, mother, spouse, children, etc., and your house, car, work, etc.

4. **Performance:** Visualize a successful performance of an interview, public speech, etc.

5. **Healing:** Greet the afflicted organ and visualize it healed.

6. **Restful Sanctuary:** Visualize a sunny beach or a green meadow and take a mental vacation.

Result

Meditation and imagery will give you an inner road map to your thought patterns. Once you monitor your thoughts, you will be able to modify them by acting them out in the imagery theater. Mind-Body communication is direct and most effective in the restful, alert state of meditation. Your net result is stress control, healing, and a maximized you.

Mastery

You should be able to enter into a meditative state on the spur of the moment by closing your eyes and rolling the eye balls up. Take one to five minute meditative breaks every two hours and as needed. Schedule regular 5-20 minute meditative sessions for at least once and preferably twice a day.

Physical Exercise

Objective

To develop sustained, low to moderate intensity, large muscle exercise for physical and mental health.

Method

Sustained movement of the body's large muscles. The safest lifelong exercise is fast walking. Bicycling, swimming, gardening, and tennis are also effective.

F.I.T. Principle

Frequency: Exercise a minimum of 3 to 5 times a week.

Intensity: Exercise in the training zone. The training zone is figured on a maximum heart rate of 220 minus your age. Exercise hard enough to maintain your heart rate in the range of 65-80% of this maximum heart rate. Overtraining above your 80% level risks harmful free radical release and physical injury.

Time Duration: Exercise should be at least 15-20 minutes of sustained activity. For burning fat and weight loss, prolong the exercise from 45 minutes to an hour.

Latest Cooper Prescription: Kenneth Cooper, the original aerobics researcher's 1995 prescription is "Low intensity exercise, at least 30 continuous minutes 3 times a week, or for 20 continuous minutes 4 times a week."

Result

Physical exercise will control stress, insomnia, and restless mind; it will elevate mood, strengthen the immune and musculoskeletal systems; and it will prevent or heal afflictions, such as high blood pressure and heart disease.

Mastery

Develop a regular habit of physical exercise and learn the healthy habit of "exercise high." Use "motion controls emotion" logic to dissipate stress arousal.

Mindful Eating

Objective

To eat a starch-based, vegetarian, low fat, high fiber, antioxidant food 6 times a day. To switch from degenerative food habits to regenerative food practices.

Method

1. **What to eat?** Staples should be complex starch, such as rice and wheat. An easy visual formula is to make at least 50% of each meal raw fruits and vegetables, and most of the remainder starch and plant protein. Avoid fats and oils as much as possible.

2. **When to eat?** Six times a day for balancing your insulin, blood sugar, and mood. Three square meals, three round meals. Take an antioxidant vitamin mix 3 times per day.

Breakfast: Bread without butter, one banana, cereal with low fat milk or no milk. Antioxidant vitamin mix (Vitamin A - Beta carotene - 10,000 to 50,000 IU; Vitamin C - 500-2000 mg. Vitamin E -200 to 600 IU). The total amount should be divided into three parts: one at breakfast, one at lunch and one at dinner. **Mid-morning snack:** Fresh fruit or vegetable snack. Orange/Apple/Carrot/Cucumber. **Lunch:** Salad (low fat dressing), pasta, rice, bread, fruit. Antioxidant vitamin. **Mid-afternoon snack:** similar to midmorning. **Dinner:** Similar to lunch. Antioxidant vitamin. **Bedtime:** A fruit or vegetable snack.

3. **How to eat?** Mindfully slow. Observe the effects of food before, during, and after eating. Eat until you feel about 70% full.

Result

The balance of insulin, mood, enzymes, and antioxidants will keep you fit and heal your mind and body.

Mastery

Gradually wean yourself from addictive foods of fat, caffeine, sugar, salt, and animal foods.

Self-Disclosure

Objective

(1) Identify your own personal style of life by self-actualization. (2) Care and share your emotion with a partner. "Dovetail" with your partner's emotions.

Method

1. Find out who you both are in the following areas:

Perceptual types, Mind-heart conflicts, Gender differences, Physiological reactivity patterns, Money Styles, and Explanatory Styles.

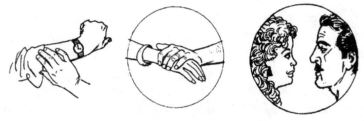

2. Share your emotions using three T's: Time, Touch, and Talk. Dedicate 5-20 minutes a day for a 3 T's session. Nonsexually and affectionately touch and talk about each other's emotions and how each positive and negative emotion affects your bodies. Then compare how emotional responses on each other's body differ. Finally, recognize common responses as "we feel, we see, we hear." This is called dovetailing.

Results

Repressed emotions get expressed; your immune system has release from pressure; and you heal by self-regulation.

Mastery

Redefine a "*difficult* person" as a "*different* person." Get feedback of immediate tension release by caring and sharing of emotions. Develop the altruistic pleasure of sharing.

28

Daily Life with Your Heart in Mind

1. Head and Heart Tug-of-War
2. Healing and Thriving with the Laws of Nature
3. New Biology of "Learned Altruism"
4. A Day in the Life of Heart Centered Living
5. 21 Days to Reset Your Heart

Daily Life with Your Heart in Mind

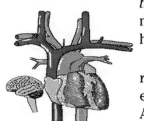

The "heart" of this book is how to reset *your* life by *resetting* your heart. That is, living as many moments in a day as possible, keeping your heart in mind.

Yes, we live in an information age rat race. We compete against time and others, and against our own achievements. As we enter the 21st century, we value our life on our economic potential, and on our problem-solving, and information-processing abilities.

Time management specialists often focus on how to maximize ourselves by economizing the dynamics of matter and motion. We are expected to do more and more in less and less time. It is a rat race, because the rat keeps running even past the finish line. A rat does not know what a clock is. Humans do. Matter and motion are only two dimensions of time. We neglect the emotional dimension. High tech gadgets will make us move faster and faster in external space. But, internally, we will remain the same. In spite of all *human doings*, we still have to live as *human beings*. To do that successfully, you will need to understand the new biology of heart-centered living.

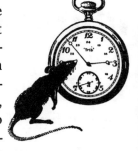

The diagram on the next page summarizes heart centered living in the hectic "information age." You have two primary driving forces in life:

(1) Affiliation, and (2) Achievement.

Affiliation for humans is the natural state just as it is for other animals. This state is helped by the internal pharmacy of endorphins. It is the "rapport visit" or rapport-producing transaction.

Daily Life with Heart in Mind

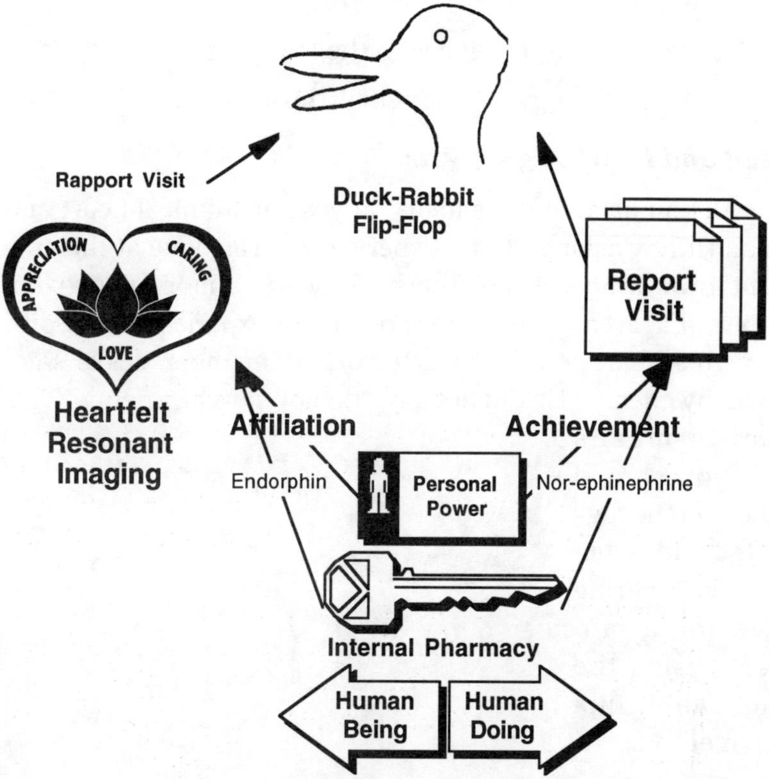

Duck-Rabbit Flip-Flop

Rapport Visit

Heartfelt Resonant Imaging

Report Visit

Affiliation

Achievement

Endorphin

Personal Power

Nor-ephinephrine

Internal Pharmacy

Human Being

Human Doing

Achievement is an unnatural state, focused on the analytical, problem-solving, money-centered life, aided by the internal pharmacy of catecholamines (Norepinephrine). It is the "report visit" or report-producing transaction.

You need both affiliation and achievement in life. You can focus your awareness on your heart and experience caring love with every human interaction, yet stay connected with normal daily activities. The duck–rabbit picture horizontally looks like a duck, and vertically like a rabbit. You can flip-flop them instantly, just as you can the report–rapport transaction. It's an innovative way for you to heal and thrive.

Heart centered living produces these results:

- Removal of the tug–of–war between your head and heart.
- Healing and thriving with the laws of nature.
- A new biology of "learned altruism."

Head and Heart Tug–of–War

All you have to do is focus on your anatomical heart and do an HRI by asking, "Can I experience caring love at this moment towards myself and others?" Stay in that moment of truth, with your heart as your vantage point, and experience the world from this heart-centered framework. Remember, Jesus said, "love thy enemy." He did not say, "do not have an enemy." This simply means that you should get out of the tug–of–war and be human with caring love for a moment, using the duck-rabbit flip-flop method.

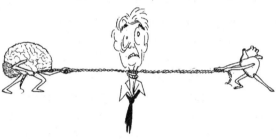

Heal and Thrive with the Laws of Nature

The *meaning* of life is being interdependent - connected to each other and the universe. There is a wave form of life involving rest and activity, production and consumption, love and let love, give and take, and so on. If you let your mind–body settle in the man–made frenzy, your mind–body's internal intelligence system will take over and manage itself. HRI and meditative moments allow you to maximize the power of this intelligence system, and thus thrive naturally.

NEW BIOLOGY OF "LEARNED ALTRUISM"

If you want to learn the art of altruism based on the science of human behavior, here are some practical tips:

Paradoxes of Altruism: Paradox means "amazing but true." Consider the following paradoxes.

1. Does Exhibitionistic Altruism Work?

A "rich and famous" celebrity tries to gain name, fame, and news media attention by the "act" of altruistically feeding homeless people, or donating to charitable causes with an *acknowledged* receipt. The celebrity will of course create "news." But the true value of altruism is in the heart-centered *experience,* with the release of endorphins, and the harmony of the heart's rhythms (heart rate variability). This experience is possible for you only by developing **biological sensitivity.**

2. Does the Alcoholics Anonymous model work?

The self–help models, such as alcoholics anonymous, help people heal by developing interactive sensitivity to each other. **Being involved and active in measuring, monitoring, and modifying each other's problems in life takes you out of helplessness.**

3. Beggar in Front of Rockefeller Center.

Imagine famous stars hosting a charity ball in the grand auditorium of New York's Rockefeller center. The dignitaries who attend are annoyed by panhandlers outside. Yet, they spend $100 per person as an acknowledged charitable contribution. Where is the biological value here? The only *condition* to enjoying altruism is to be *unconditional.*

The beggar in front of Rockefeller center does not envy the riches of the rich and famous that walk by. He envies the more successful beggar next to him. Human emotion, like water, finds its own level.

4. Tandem Bike Model (Choice and Control)

Volunteer hospital workers enjoy a "helper's high," while the nurses and doctors in the ward suffer from the burn out of

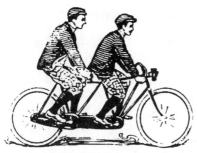

over-care and compassion fatigue. When you are forced to help someone, you become helpless and burn out. Caretakers of Alzheimer's patients suffer from immune suppression, while someone who watches Mother Teresa's movie of caretaking, empowers his/her immune system. An orthodox Hindu performs a ritual of donating money with the spiritual quest of altruism, but hesitates to contribute to a community event *he* did not start. The common thread through all this is *choice* and *control*. If you are riding a bicycle built for two, no matter how good a cyclist you are, you cannot control the balance if your partner is in the front seat.

5. Celebration of Life

The *meaning* of life is an altruistism. When you share your pleasure in life with others, it is a celebration. In Sanskrit, *seva* refers to altruism, *utsava* refers to festivity and celebrating the joy. When you are enjoying a scene, you naturally look at the person next to you and say, *look at that!* Your innate urge is to celebrate your life with someone.

Which kind of altruism will not help you biologically?

If you help others for the sake of compulsion, guilt, or because you read that it is good for you, you will not alter your biology. Two factors make altruism biologically viable: **control** and **choice**. When *you* are the giver or sender of altruistic love, *you* maintain the control and choice. When you hug someone or shake hands with someone, *you* maintain the control and choice. The bottom line is, it is *you* who must initiate and send caring love to get the biological benefit. You can do it, if not every moment, at least every other moment (duck–rabbit flip–flop) as and when you remember it. You can *remember to remember* by following this daily life with heart–in–mind routine:

A DAY IN THE LIFE OF HEART CENTERED LIVING

1. WHEN YOU WAKE UP:

A. Meditate for a moment: Stretch your body with a "baby stretch." Sit up in bed, meditate for a minute or two. Do your heartfelt resonant imaging to start your day with your heart in mind. Do meditation and HRI all day long.

B. Healing Imageries: Breathe out three times, and enter into healing imagery to observe the affliction or disorder in any body part to be healed. Do this every time your mind gets trapped in negative imageries of the illness or problem.

C. Cybernetic Evaluation of Sleep: Evaluate the quality and quantity of sleep and observe how your heart–mind conflicts affect your quality of sleep. Close your eyes and visualize solving the head–heart tug–of–war in favor of the heart.

D. Smiling Feedback: As you brush your teeth, smile and do your HRI towards each part of your body. Send healing imageries to any afflicted body parts. Feel the difference in your body as you experience the smile.

E. Observe the pumps and pipes of the body: Relate your bowel function, muscle tension, and heart symptoms to your stress and notice the changes as you modify stress levels.

2. MORNING MEDITATION AND YOGA STRETCHING

Do simple stretching or yoga for at least five minutes and meditation for at least five minutes. Ideally, 20 minutes of yoga and meditation will give you optimal yin–yang balance.

3. EAT SIX MEALS A DAY.

Eat three square meals (breakfast, lunch, dinner) and three round meals (fruit and vegetable snacks mid morning, mid afternoon, and at bedtime). Eat starch-based, low fat, mostly vegetarian food. Eat slowly and mindfully.

4. PHYSICAL EXERCISE

If you have confirmed coronary artery disease, it is better to exercise in the afternoon. The heart is vulnerable due to thicker blood and the adrenaline surge in the morning. Otherwise, many people prefer morning exercise. Walking is by far the best exercise. Remember, we are not made to be sedentary. Keep moving your body by taking a "walk break" periodically.

5. EMOTIONAL EXERCISE

We recommend you daily do deliberate crying to release pent up "cry chemicals," and deliberate smiling and laughing to keep your humor tuned up. You'll find these rituals in the appendix.

6. USE THE RESETTING TOOLS

Measure your life pattern at least once a month, ideally once a week, with the following measuring tools:

A. Human Function Curve, Vital Exhaustion, Protesting Heart Scale, and William's Anger Scale.

B. Money Function Curve and Money Style.

C. Energy Exchange Vectors (Cross Checks).

Monitor your day at least once every hour by centering, mindful breathing, and open focus™.

Check your behavior iceberg in the area of action, thoughts, and emotions.

Examine your energy exchange quadrants of emotions, and modify them by changing each state and observing the results.

Do your HRI with every person you meet, and during every phone call.

7. ULTRADIAN HEALING BREAKS

Observe the 90–20 minute rhythm of the ultradian healing response to synchronize yourself with nature. Take a few minutes meditative break every 90 minutes. Eat a fruit or vegetable at this time to keep your insulin and mood level even. You may want to do an

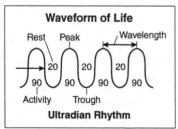

extended 20 minute meditation in the evening before or after dinner. Do your healing imageries at least 6 times a day during the ultradian healing breaks.

8. SELF–DISCLOSURE

Every day do a time, touch, and talk ritual to disclose your pent up emotions and discover how these emotions affect *your* body.

9. BEDTIME RITUAL

Recall the results of your daytime behavior, monitoring and visualizing how you could have done it differently to solve *your* head–heart conflicts. Meditate and do your healing imageries for a few minutes just before your sleep.

21 DAYS TO RESET YOUR HEART

Research tells us that if you repeat the new behavior consistently for 21 days, the new behavior becomes second nature. We have found the following guidelines in practicing our heart resetting tools. You must practice each tool several hundred times (almost a thousand times) on the first day. New behavior is mastered by the number of repetitions rather than the duration of each session. Most of the tools given in this book can be "practiced" in a one minute session. This allows you to use the tools while while meeting your daily obligations of home and work.

On the second day, you briefly repeat the previous day's tool and move on to the next. On the third day, continue with the previous learning. This is a cumulative system and on the 8th day you will have learned most of the tools. In the second and third week, you repeat the process.

21 Days to Reset Your Heart

Practice to Mastery — Week 3

Drill to Skill — Week 2

7 Self-Actualization Self-Disclosure

6 Rest and Activity: Aerobic Training, Ultradian Healing Breaks

5 Mindful Eating: Starch based low fat food 6 times a day (3 Square meals, 3 Round meals)

4 Meditation and Imagery: Five Minute, One Minute and One Moment Tools

3 Modifying Tools: Heartfelt Resonance Imaging (HRI) and Anger Control

2 Monitoring Tools: Centering, Mindful Breathing, Open Focus; CyberScan Snapshot; Energy Quadrants; and Biological Monitoring

1 Measuring Tools: Human Function Curve, Money Function Curve, Energy Exchange Vectors, Exhaustion, Protesting Heart, and Anger Scales

Week 1

WEEK ONE

A. Measuring Tools

Day 1. Human Function Curve, Money Function Curve, Energy Exchange Vectors, Vital Exhaustion questions, and Anger scale.

B. Monitoring Tools:

Day 2. Centering, Mindful Breathing, Open Focus™: CyberScan Snapshot; Energy Quadrants; and Biological Monitors: Muscle Tension, Gut Function, Restless Mind, & Insomnia.

C. Modifying Tools:

Day 3. Heartfelt Resonant Imaging for anger control.

Day 4. Meditation and Imagery.

Day 5. Mindful eating.

Day 6. Rest and activity.

Day 7. Self-actualization and Self-disclosure.

WEEK TWO

Repeat cycle of Measuring, Monitoring, and Modifying behavior patterns to learn more and make effective changes; drill the Modifying tools to build skill.

WEEK THREE:

Continue practicing the Modifying Tools to develop subtle awareness of behavior; Tools will become second nature, and you will have a sense of mastery.

Now your heart is reset for stress control, healing and maximal self. Live the rest of your life with your heart in mind.

How to Handle Lapse and Relapse:

Your mind has a "default setting" of lapsing into judgmental head-centered vigilance of "what is in it for me." Simply ask yourself the question, "where am I, in the head or heart?" If in the head, drop down to the heart level.

Appendix

Pill Power for Heart Disease

Medications are a serious matter. Modern medical science has several drugs to strengthen the heart and even reverse coronary artery disease. But often, those taking such drugs don't take as prescribed because they don't like to be reminded they are in less than optimal health, or they are concerned about side effects.

So, prevention is still the best treatment for any disease. But heart disease is like a fire. If your fire retardants don't work, wouldn't you call the fire department once you knew your house was on fire?

Prevention of heart disease has two levels: primary (before you know that you have heart disease) and secondary (to stop or regress the diagnosed disease). High risk groups should act as if their needs were for secondary prevention. The chemical goal of secondary prevention is to bring the LDL cholesterol level below 90-100 mg/dl.

An easy-to-understand analogy for heart and blood vessels is that of pump, pipes and fluid. Especially when it comes to drug therapy. Pump drugs act on mechanical or electrical properties of the heart. Pipe drugs act on pipe clogging (sticky cholesterol, or blocking clots), pipe kinking (anginal drugs), or pipe narrowing (high blood pressure drugs). Drugs acting on the blood either thin it or prevent the clumping of platelet particles.

PUMP DRUGS

Digitalis is the major drug acting on the **pumping action of the heart**. It increases heart muscle contractions and slows down the heart's electrical activity. Digitalis is used for congestive heart failure in which fluid accumulates due to an ineffective heart pump.

Electrical disturbance in the heart affects rate and rhythms of the heart. **Cardiac arrhythmia** can be harmless or dangerous depending on which part of the heart they originate in and how they progress. Some drugs change heart rhythms: beta-blockers, calcium blockers, digoxin, quinidine, procainamide (Pronestyl), Disopyramide (Norpace), Phenytoin (Dilantin), mexiletine (Mexitil), tocainaide (Tonocard), flecainide (tambocor), propafenone (Rythmol), moricixone (Ethgmozine), and amiodarone (Cordaraone). Some drug side effects can actually aggravate arrhythmia.

PIPE DRUGS

Drugs for angina: Nitrates are drugs acting on coronary arteries to relax the kink or spasm. Short acting nitrates treat the pain of angina, or prevent a kink from physical or mental stress. Long acting nitrates give all day protection from kinks. We administer nitrates under the tongue (nitroglycerin tablets), by spray (Nitrolingual spray), skin ointment, skin patch, or intravenous injections for heart attack or severe angina in the hospital.

Drugs for Angina and Hypertension: Beta-blockers block the action of adrenaline on the heart and blood pipes. They slow the heart rate and relax the spasm and narrowing of pipes. Beta-blockers include atenolol (Tenorin), betaxolol (Kerlone), metoprolol (Lopressor), nadolol (Corgard), propranolol (Inderal), timolol (Blocardren), acebutolol (sectral), carteolol (Cartrol), penbutolol (Levotol), pindolol (Visken), and labetalol (Normodyne).

Calcium blockers prevent entry of calcium into muscle cells, thereby relaxing the pipes. Calcium blockers are: diltiazem (Cardizem, Dilacor), Verpamil (Calan, Verelan), nifedepine (Procardia), nicardepene (Cardene), isradipine (Dynacirc), feldipine (Plendil), and amiodipine (Norvasc).

Ace inhibitors reduce the hormone (Angiotensin Converting Enzyme) that constricts the pipes and retains salts. Ace inhibitors include captopril (Capoten), enalapril (Vasotec), lisinopril (Prinivi, Zestril), benazepril (Lotensin), fosinopril (Monopril), quinapril (Accupril), and ramipril (Altace).

Older blood pressure medicines act directly and relax the pipes. Among them: hydralazine (Apresoline), alpha blockers such as prazosin (Minipress), terazosin (Hytrin), doxazosin (Cardura), and drugs that block sympathetic activity, such as clonidine (Catapres) and guanabenz (Wytensin).

Diuretics or fluid pills decrease salt content and volume of blood in the pipes, relaxing them and the heart. Examples: hydrochorothiazine (Diuril), furosamide (Lasix), spirinolactone (Aldactone), and triamterene (Dyrenium).

Declogging the Pipes ("Degreasers"): These are the drugs that lower bad cholesterol and triglycerides and increase good cholesterol.

Bile acid binders prevent absorption of bile acid from the intestines, so the liver won't over-produce cholesterol. Examples: cholestyramine (Questran).

Nicotonic acid or niacin reduces the production of VLDL and LDL in the liver. It also increases the HDL.

Gemfibrozil or Lopid reduces cholesterol synthesis and also decreases triglycerides.

"Statins" inhibit the enzyme HMG-CoA reductase, reducing cholesterol synthesis. Examples: lovastatin (Mevacor), pravastatin (Pravachol), simivastatin (Zocor), and fluvastatin (Lescol).

Probucol or Lorelco reduces cholesterol and has some antioxidant properties.

What these drugs do:

Drugs acting on blood clots are clot busters, clot dissolvers, and clot preventors.

Clot busters rapidly clear the clots during the first six hours of a heart attack. Examples are: streptokinase, urokinase, and tissue plasminogen activator.

Clot dissolvers are heparin, given by injection.

Clot preventors are simple aspirin and Coumadin drugs.

We list these drugs to show the action on different aspects of heart and blood vessel disease. You should consult your own physician for specific dosage and indications. In general, know these eight facts about any drug you take: 1. Generic and trade name. 2. Dosage. 3. How it works. 4. Interactions with other drugs and food, and activity. 5. Whether taken with meals, before, or in between. 6. Side effects. 7. What are the restrictions and changes in activities. 8. How long to take the drugs.

"De-greasing" Power of Drugs

Drug	↓ LDL	HDL ↑	↓Triglyceride
Bile Acid Binders	15-30%	◄─►	◄─►
Nicotinic Acid	10-25%	15-31%	25-30%
Gemfibrozil	10-15%	15-25%	35-50%
Statins (HMG CoA Inhibitors)	20-40%	5-10%	10-20%
Probucol	10-15%	↓ 20-25%	◄─►

Sense of Humor Revisited

Humor has both psychological and physiological benefits. Laughter convulses the entire body and shakes up your messenger molecules, such as endorphins. In fact, Norman Cousins healed his incurable neurological disease by watching funny movies.

The word humor is from the Latin root meaning flexible or fluid. Humor is not just telling jokes, but also "being available" to experience joy. A sense of humor is the ability to perceive, enjoy, and express what is comical or funny. Humor is a state of mind-body in which the dominant emotions are pleasure, peace, love, and joy. Humor, like any other emotion, has two purposes: subjective experience and visible expression. There are hidden and visible expressions of humor. The hidden are in your mind-body — where only you can see them. The visible expressions are what others see, and they get the message filtered through their own "state" at the moment.

What is the Problem?

"What you see is what you get." But, the eyes do not see what the mind does not know. We point this out to remind you that humor requires a shift in perspective to experience some surprise, absurdity, or paradox in or around you. Humor requires some level of manipulation or "play" with your perceptions to get into experiencing something funny.

Basically, a lack of humor goes with an inflexible, narrow focus. Exercises in this section will help you to shift your focus from narrow seriousness to an open focus of joy.

What Went Wrong? (Why We Lose Our Sense of Humor)

We started smiling when we were six or eight weeks old. It was not a response to a joke, but a pristine expression of love and security. A smile is an exchange of energy. Babies smile and kiss at the same time. As we grew, we narrowed our focus on school and work, with many of us becoming workaholic.

Play for a workaholic is "working" at play. Work is an imposition. But play is a deliberate celebration of life. To learn to play again, you have to find the child within who has the perspective to play. Children smile and laugh 400 times a day, whereas for adults, it's 15 times or less. Adults think negative thoughts three fourths of the time. In our workaholic culture, adults weaken their smile muscles due to disuse. The kinetics of the smile muscle system gets overlaid with the kinetics of negative emotions such as fear, anger, guilt, and sadness.

What is the Solution? (Revive the Smile Apparatus)

Humor, like a coin, has two sides: a muscle side and a mind side. There are two direct approaches to stimulate a sense of humor: tickling the mind (mind-to-muscle) or tickling the body (muscle-to-mind).

Tickling the Mind:

1. **Learn to observe the fun within your own automatic self-talk** as if you were a spectator watching a movie. After all, your thoughts happen on their own. If you do not try to rationalize them, you may find them absurd, full of surprises and

paradoxes. If you learn to laugh at yourself, your feelings about others become empathetic and sympathetic, not cynical and sarcastic. This applies the "beginner's mind" to a sense of humor.

2. **Acknowledge that you are not the center of the universe.** The center is the ultimate power, God, or whatever your belief system calls it; but not you. This spiritual perspective takes away your desire to control everything and end up getting angry (Type A) or depressed (Type C) when you lose control.

3. **Do not confuse your mission in life what you do for a living.** Your career is a way of earning your livelihood, but your true mission in life is to connect with others with love and compassion. This is the perspective of altruistic self-transcendence. Always think, "How can I help someone?"

4. **Learn the art of forgiveness.** Changing your judgment of self and others leads to forgiveness. Separate the person from the event, using the argument that an offending event or events are minuscule part of the whole person. Look for the good parts. Learn to live with heart in mind.

5. **Develop the beginner's mind of a child to see more fun in life.** Observe fun in your actions, thoughts, and emotions. Find beginner's mindfulness in eating, exercise, relationships, and spirituality.

6. **Catalogue your list of positive past experiences**, especially those from childhood. Keep this list in the top of your mind and replay it all day to replace the negative emotions of blahs (mood swings) and blues (prolonged depression).

7. **Get centered for momentary pleasure.** Healing pleasure is a moment-by-moment experience. On a graph, it resembles a saw tooth design of a small ups and downs, rather a roller coaster pattern. Many people think that pleasure in life is an expensive vacation, a lavish birthday party, or taking refuge in a drink or drug. Research tells us that healing pleasure happens with the small release of pleasure chemicals throughout the day. Pennies, after all, build up to a dollar.

Tickling the Body (Kinetics of a Smile)

Every emotion has a counterpart in a body motion. You can retrain your smile and laugh muscles to experience a sense of humor. Practice the following eight stages of smiling:

1. Mona Lisa Lip Smile: This is the minimal smile. There is reluctant intention. Practice by saying "ooo" and "eee." It is similar to a kissing movement, while pulling the lips back sideways.

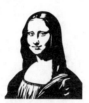

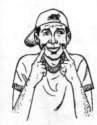

2. Zygomaticus Pumping: Put two fingers on your cheek and feel the major smile muscle, the zygomaticus, pulling the corners of your mouth toward your ears.

3. Twinkle the Eyes (Wrinkle the Eye Muscles): The hearty smile causes your eyes to squint, creating "crows feet" at their edge. You contract the orbicularis oculi muscle around the eyes.

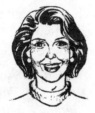

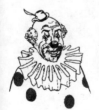

4. Clown Face: The forehead wrinkles (frontalis muscle contraction) and the lower jaw pulls down, exposing the lower teeth (platysma muscle contraction).

5. Giggle: When you add sound to the smile, it is like the teen age giggle. The vocal cord and upper chest muscles vibrate. The females are more adept at, or perhaps are more comfortable with giggling.

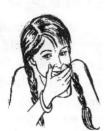

6. Belly Laugh: Put a hand on your stomach and say "aa ha ha" or "ho ho" or "he he." Usually the head is thrown back slightly. Men are better with belly laughter, while women tend to cover their mouths, due perhaps to our culture thinking women should not laugh boisterously.

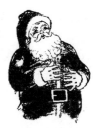

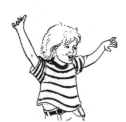

7. Dancing Laugh: Laugh until you dance like a happy child.

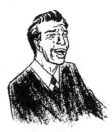

8. Tears of Joy: This is laughter until you cry. The neurotransmitter "delivered to the wrong address," creating happy rather than sad tears. They contain more of the d-lysozyme enzyme than tears of crying. This "humor molecule" is supposed to enhance the immune system.

Note: In all stages of smiling, the anal sphincter also participates, contracting during active laughter and relaxating in between. Incidentally, when you are tense and stressed out, the internal anal sphincter gets very tight as a sign of sympathetic arousal and misplaced effort. That is why constipation gets worse during protracted stress arousal. Smiling not only reflects the gut feeling, but also is felt in the gut.

ACTION PLAN FOR DEVELOPING A SENSE OF HUMOR

1. **Make a Joy List** of all humorous things you experienced since your childhood. Your own past humor experience is your best resource. You have lived through it. You can easily recall and replay this state again and again. As you ruminate on this list, it stays at the top of your mind. In our stress clinic, one of our executives, familiar with writing a "to do" list, calls the joy list a "ta dah!" list.

       Heart Disease and Cancer

2. **Use the beginner's mind** to look for something funny. Get centered by thinking of your belly button, and notice the fun things in your surroundings, in others, and in your own body movements, thoughts, and emotions.

3. **Use meditative drills to explore**, enhance, and sharpen the sensation of joy and humor in your mind-body. Live with heart in mind.

4. **Morning smile drill**: Every morning do your "ooo" and "eee" smile in front of the mirror and loosen up your smile muscles for smiling the rest of the day. Do the eight stages of smiling in front of the mirror and record the experience of the "state" in your memory.

5. **Get tickled**: At least once a week, ask your partner to tickle you and you tickle your partner so that your humor muscles perk up for the week.

6. **Laughing Place**: During your meditation, create a familiar place, including surroundings and people you have fun with, and make this a laughing place. Retreat into this laughing place every morning when you meditate. It keeps your laughing place at the surface of your memory.

7. **Howl for Joy and Peace**: During your morning meditation, ask your inner guide to provide you with the most peaceful, blissful, and joyful mind-set without judgmental intrusions.

8. **Amplify Your Humor Response**: When you feel the slightest experience of a "sense of humor", expand on it by recruiting more muscle-to-mind resources. Example: add a chuckle, giggle, belly laugh or dance to make it a *multimedia* experience.

The Power of Crying

Is crying good for you? If so, how do you cry well? Only humans cry for purely emotional reasons. Two thousand years ago, Aristotle said, "crying cleans the mind," and modern scientific experiments prove it. There is a hierarchy to crying and laughing.

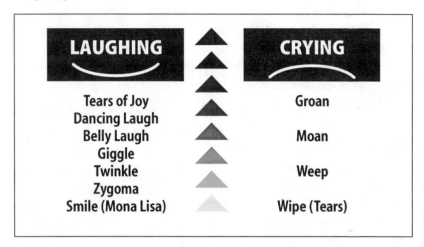

LAUGHING		CRYING
Tears of Joy		Groan
Dancing Laugh		
Belly Laugh		Moan
Giggle		
Twinkle		Weep
Zygoma		
Smile (Mona Lisa)		Wipe (Tears)

Relearning Your Expression of Sorrow and Pain

As children, we all knew how to cry, moan, and groan. "Big boys do not cry. Big girls should suppress their sorrow in public." This social constraint has become a habit. UCLA psychologist, Margaret Keemeny, featured on Bill Moyer's Healing and The Mind TV series, studied the effect of expressing negative emotions. She found that even short term expression of negative feelings, such as sadness, would enhance the function of natural killer cells, thereby making the immune system stronger. More interestingly, their group, led by Ann Futterman, studied the "method trained" actors as they acted sad feelings, and found the immune system of each actor was stimulated. Pennebaker of Southern Methodist University found that the immune system of medical students who expressed their negative emotions became stronger.

What is in Tears?

William Fry, a psychiatric biochemist, found tears wept in sorrow have a different chemical composition than "onion cutting tears." Emotional tears have an abundance of endorphins, hormones, and catecholamines. Letting your tears flow freely leads to a cathartic effect, dissipating pent up chemicals. Crying releases enkephalin, a stress chemical that relieves pain. Crying restores balance and communicates your feelings. Suppressing tears denies this important mode of emotional experience. Paradoxically, the depressed person is unable to cry as much as his or her physiology wants. Crying releases tension and gets rid of the toxic chemicals of the stress reaction.

Why Do Women Cry More Than Men?

Women cry four times more often than men do. At the other end of the pendulum, women laugh about four times more often than men do. In one study, 85% of the women and 73% of the men reported that they felt better after crying. One of the hormones released in tears is prolactin, which is higher in women. In fact, after menopause, the prolactin level falls and more women have dry eyes after menopause.

Relearning Crying

You can relearn to cry by placing your hands on your upper chest near your collar bones and breathe in and out like a dog panting. Deliberately bring the feelings of sadness and build up your emotional tears until they flow out freely. If you get pains in your neck and head muscles, stop for a few moments and cry again. This crying catharsis can be done in front of your significant other - it works even better. Another way is to monitor your crying drills in a mirror, tape recorder, or video camera. This gives you cybernetic feedback.

Relearning Moaning and Groaning

Human beings have the instinct to groan away emotional and physical pain. Groaning promotes deep diaphragmatic breathing and makes the whole body go into rhythmic convulsions just like a good laugh.

You can feel the vibrations of groaning all over your body. In fact, the sounds of groaning have the primordial sound of "Om" in them. A groan is much stronger, louder, and more forceful than a sigh. The difference between a groan and a sigh of relief is that a sigh marks the end of tension and groaning means that tension is still bottled up.

Patients coming out of surgery groan with pain because the pain is still there. The groan acts as an opening of the release valve for the pressure and pain built up inside. Moaning is a gentler type of groaning after the big pressure is let out. Moaning is a response to continuous low intense pain such as the pain of college examinations.

You can lie down or sit up and groan and moan for one to ten minutes and feel the difference. It is your natural instinct and nobody has to teach you that. One good place to groan without wasting your "groaning time" is while driving in your car. You can feel relieved immediately.

Learned Smiling and Laughing

Depressed people have forgotten how to laugh. Just looking at the mirror and continuously smiling is shown to change the level of endorphins and adrenaline levels in the blood for the rest of the day. Learn to smile, laugh, and dance again as if you were training for a smiling and laughing competition.

Conundrum and Paradox of Eating

by Kusum and Jyoti Bhat

A **conundrum** is a riddle with no right answer. For example, "Forty cups on the table, two broke, how many remain? Two or thirty eight?" This is a conundrum.

A **paradox** is something that is "amazing but true." Eating can be a communion with your heart, or a heartbreak with chemical warfare.

1. Indian Paradox

People of Indian origin are mostly vegetarians, yet they have a relatively high rate of coronary artery disease (CAD). Why? Besides the inherited destiny of Lipoprotein [Lp-(a)] and diabetes, westernization and mechanization have given Indians apple type obesity, insulin resistance, and free radical supply by stress, toxins, and excess of fat and refined sugar in the diet.

2. Japanese Paradox

Japanese people have the lowest incidence of CAD. Is this because of Japanese tea with flavonoids (natural plant color with antioxidant power) or Japanese tea parties where people meet each other with a trusting heart (*amae*)? The new problem in Japan is workaholic people dropping dead at work with heart attacks, called karoshi.

3. French Paradox

French people have the second lowest incidence of CAD despite their smoking and fat eating habits. Is it due to wine? If so, is it red wine with its antioxidants? The French are the number one wine drinkers in the world. But they also have the highest death rate due to alcoholic liver disease (of all industrialized countries).

---

4. Italian Paradox

Italians have a low incidence of CAD. Can it be the olive oil benefit? Italians are second to the French in wine drinking and liver disease as well.

5. Mediterranean Pyramid

Mediterranean countries, like Italy, Greece, Spain, and the island of Crete, have ten times less CAD compared to Americans. Scientists focused on the Mediterranean pyramid of eating. The base of this pyramid is made of complex carbohydrates (bread, pasta, rice, couscous, polenta, bulgar, grains, and potato). The next level of the pyramid is made of fresh fruits and vegetables, followed by olive oil. As you go to the top of the pyramid, you add dairy products and fish. Finally, the apex is made of sweets and red meat.

6. Trans-Fatty Acid, the Margarine Paradox

Harvard researchers Willet and Ascherio attribute 30,000 annual deaths from CAD in America to the fat in margarine; and cookies, crackers, chips, and processed foods which contain similar fats. The more solid the margarine is, the more it has trans-fatty acid. Your body does not like the trans-fatty acid. The Willet study published in *Lancet* looked at 90,000 women and found that there was a 50% increase in CAD due to margarine use. Liquid vegetable oils, as opposed to solid in room temperature oils, have the least amount of harmful trans-fatty acids.

7. Frying Pan to Fire

When you deep-fry foods, they oxidize, and fatty acid changes from *cis* to *trans* form. The longer duration of frying, high heat, and the repeated use of the same oil creates a lot of toxic trans-fatty acids, which, in turn, create free radicals in the blood. Free radicals attack normal cells and destroy them, causing aging, hardening of arteries, or cancer. The modern culture eats fried foods such as french fries, tempura, egg rolls, samosas, and pakodas. The taste of fried foods puts you into the fire of free radicals.

8. Live On Olive Oil?

The glory of olive oil is partly a commercial hype. Canola oil (rape seed) is almost as good as monounsaturated fats. Olive oil creates less trans-fatty acid in frying. Any fat is fattening, including oil from olives.

9. Your Cup of Tea

Second to water, humans worldwide drink tea. Tea contains fluoride for teeth and polyphenols as antioxidants. Green tea (direct drying) is common in China. Black tea (fermented before drying) is common in western countries. Both kinds of tea have antioxidants. Although it has less caffeine than coffee, too much tea will caffeinate you.

10. Carotenoids (Carrot's Cousins)

Beta-carotene is a precursor of vitamin A, and is a powerful antioxidant. There are over 600 carotenoids which give fruits and vegetables yellow, orange, and red colors. Ten carotenoids are identified in broccoli, six in apricots, five in tomatoes, and over 20 in the blood of vegetarians. Eat all colors of fruits and vegetables and you will get an assortment of carotenoids.

11. Alcoholic Ominous

Alcohol increases the good cholesterol, HDL, and t-PA factor to dissolve blood clots. Should you follow the French and start drinking? The French drink red wine and have less CAD. The Kaiser study in California looked at 81,000 people who preferred white wine and found the same salutary result of wine. One or two drinks can be medicinal, but two too many will make you "alcoholic ominous." Can you count after two drinks?

12. "Recap" Your Sugar and Fat Tooth

The craving for refined sugar and fat can be retrained over a month or two by replacing them with the right sugar and low fat foods. If you switch from whole milk to low fat milk, the first few days your brain will crave the gliadin chemicals in the fat. After a month, you will dislike whole milk because your teeth will be recapped and your taste buds will be resensitized. The same is true with a high protein diet. Scientists say that 12% protein in your food is enough. Animal foods are rich in fat and protein, and they put a load on your kidneys and increase calcium excretion. You can recap your sweet tooth with fructose sugar, which does not require insulin for metabolism. Besides having "fructose capped" teeth, you'll appreciate the sweetness of fruits and vegetables more. Artificial sweeteners, such as saccharin and aspartame, give you the taste of sweetness in your mouth, but they still deprive your brain of serotonin-based pleasure. This is the bittersweet aftertaste of a sugarless sweetener.

13. Where's the Meat?

Animal food is high in fat, protein, and toxic chemicals. Fats clog the pipes, proteins overload kidneys, and toxins release ferocious free radicals. *Killed animals' meat kills you in slow installments.*

14. Fish Smells the Same

Fish contains a lot of omega-3 fatty acid, which thins the blood and reduces plaques in the arteries. If you walk on thin ice, you may end up having a hemorrhagic stroke. Fish oils demand more vitamin E in your system. Recent research has shown that large doses of fish oil suppress your immune system. Eat fish rather than fish oil. Too much fish is fattening.

15. Nut–But Don't Bolt It!

Research has shown that eating almonds and walnuts decreases the risk of heart disease. Like olive oil, they contain mono fats. But what about other nuts, like cashews and peanuts? Scientists still have not cracked this yet. Nuts are good for you, but don't bolt on them, because they will grease you with too much fat.

16. Eat When You're Not Hungry!

Eat three square meals of breakfast, lunch, and dinner and three round meals of fruit and vegetable snacks in between. This in-between eating, even if you are not hungry, keeps your insulin level and mood even, and you don't *gulp* your main meals later.

---

17. Fat Is Fatal, If Ignited

Research has shown that if you eat a large, fatty meal when you are angry, the fat is ignited by your angry atoms. This fire goes directly to your coronary arteries or arteries in the brain and clogs the pipes with sticky grease.

18. Chew When You're Angry

If you are angry and frustrated, bite a carrot. Watch your biting instinct when you are upset. It is better to chew the carrot rather than "chew" somebody else out, including yourself.

19. Nutrients or Nourishment

Science focuses on micro or macro nutrients. But nourishment is the *process* where food becomes a part of you. You get connected to everything else in the universe by eating. You return to nature by eating. Your nature has to align with Mother Nature first. That is nourishment.

20. The Final Word

The final word on conundrums and paradoxes is to ask GURU what you can eat. If you break GURU into G-U-R-U, it is "Gee, you are you." You are what you eat. Who are you? Observe yourself before, during, and after you eat something. This is called foreplay, play, and replay. Foresight and hindsight gives you insight.

The ABC's of Yoga Postures

The scientific guidelines for reversing heart disease include yoga and meditation as major tools. In our clinic we prescribe the ten postures and shavasana below.

What is Yoga?

Yoga means to unite, or "yoke." Union by yoga has eight parts: lifestyle (*yama*–restraints, *niyama*–observances), yoga postures (*asanas*), mindful breathing (*pranayama*), open focus (*pratyahara* -sensory withdrawal, *dharayna*–passive attention), meditation (*dhyana*), and union (*samadhi*).

Yoga postures unite your mind and body—here and now in the present moment. During yoga postures, your head-centered restless mind focuses on your body parts, and there is a nonverbal symbolic communication between your mind and body. This is a right brain based, intuitive state, which literally "yokes" your mind-body. Yoga improves the strength and flexibility of your muscles. The bottom line benefit of yoga stretching is the lengthening of muscle fibres, which thereby reduces the muscle-to-mind traffic. This clearing of traffic congestion reduces the negative effects of time pressure and restless mind by replacing the adrenaline-dominant chemistry with the endorphin-dominant chemistry of love and connectedness.

The essential features are summarized as the ABC's of yoga postures: Awareness, Breathing, and Control Signals.

Awareness:

Become aware of 4 different states of the muscles:

Normal tension at rest, stressful tension of misplaced effort, tension during voluntary contraction, and feeling of voluntary stretching. The "muscle sense" is awareness of the muscle during contraction and stretching.

Become aware of the following points in breathing during yoga postures:

1. Forward bending (postures in which the abdomen is

collapsed) is done during exhalation. Backward bending (postures in which the abdomen expands) is done during inhalation.

2. Each posture has three parts: move to position, hold the stretch, and let go. You move to position during inhalation or exhalation as indicated above. You stay in the position of stretching for at least three breaths. Remember to prolong your exhalation to twice the length of inhalation.

Breathing Exercise

Alternate nostril breathing. Do the following exercises to balance your energy flow and shift to an intuitive right brain connection at the beginning of your yoga work out. Opening your left nostril activates your right brain.

1. Inhale and exhale naturally with both nostrils, prolonging the exhalation.

2. Inhale through both nostrils, close your right nostril, and exhale through your left nostril.

3. Alternately inhale through your left nostril and exhale through your right nostril, and vice versa. Do this exercise for a minute or two rhythmically.

Note: Prolong your breathe out (exhalation) to twice the length of your breathe in (inhalation) phase by slightly tensing your glottis.

Control Signals

With each posture, feel the stretch sensation, or control signal, and feel your comfortable "stretch zone."

Ten Minute Yoga Stretching

The ten postures and corpse posture (*shavasana*) (shown on the next page) are simple and most people can perform them. These postures combine a sequence of forward bending, backward bending in the lying down position, standing and sitting positions. Each posture takes about a minute, and overall the sequence takes 10 minutes. If you have more time, you can stay in the "stretch position" longer than a three breath duration. If you have less time, do not rush through postures; instead, skip a few postures.

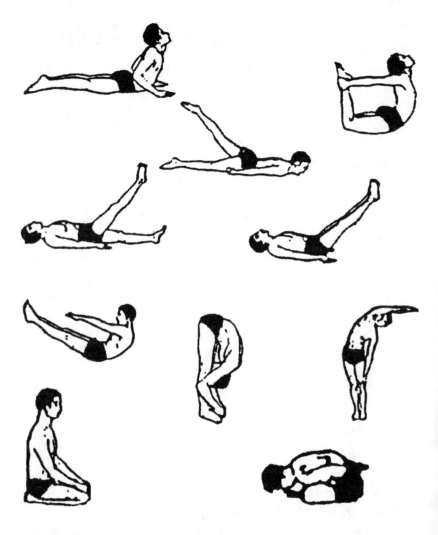

In **shavasana**, or corpse posture, close your eyes and visit different parts of the body. This is also known as body scanning. One variation of shavasana is to stay with each body part for a one breath duration and proceed to the next. Another variation is to gently contract each body part with awareness and move on to the next.

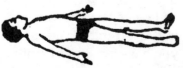

Experiental Meditation Exercises

These exercises interface between your conscious and sub-conscious mind. Use them to compare the different factors that affect your meditative state. Doing each exercise verifies your personal *"before and after"* changes that occur in each variation.

Do these exercises one at a time, both with eyes open and closed. Take a short break of a minute or two between each one, center yourself in the belly button area and do your abdominal or pyramidal breathing. Each exercise takes only a minute or two; so many, if not all, can be explored at a single sitting.

Exploring each exercise leads you to experiencing the components of the total meditation experience. It's as if you are gradually sampling your way through the selections on a buffet table, tasting each item to see what you might want to eat the next time.

1. **Place:**
Experiment with different locations: your bed, favorite chair, office chair, parked car. Sit with your eyes closed, observing your thoughts. Notice if there are any differences in your thoughts relative to your location.

2. **Posture:**
Observe your thoughts, with eyes closed and open, in these positions: sitting, standing and lying down; with and without a headrest; with and without a backrest.

3. **Body Scanning:**
Do a baseline check-in, then mentally visit different parts of your body and check-in. Do this with your eyes open and then closed; compare the difference.

4. **"I-ness" Exercise:**
Narrow focus on the sense of "I-ness" in your head and and the "I-ness" in your abdomen. Narrow focusing is when you

purposely focus on one area with one of your senses, such as sight or hearing, and ignore all other sensations or information. Next, center on your belly button or abdomen. Compare the difference.

5. **Open Focus:**

Narrow focus on a single tree or a star, noticing the tension and sensation you're experiencing. Then spread your focus to experience the background of the tree or night sky. Add in your other senses (sounds, smells, objects you're touching.) Check-in to see if you feel more relaxed.

6. **Relax Muscles:**

Observe the thoughts and tensions in your body before and after contracting different groups of muscles to experience the changes. Observe the control signal of tension in each muscle as you contract it.

7. **Respiration Watch:**

Observe your thoughts and level of attention, ignoring your breathing. Then do the same thing while taking a rhythmic ride with your breath.

8. **Repeat Mantra:**

Repeat the sound mentally ("so" as you breathe in and "hum" as you breathe out) and observe your thoughts while making the sound. Compare the differences between linking the sound to breath and not linking. As your mind wanders, return to the sound, or the breathing, and observe how your wandering mind refocuses.

9. **Tick-Tock Eyeball Movement (horizontal):**

Observe your thoughts before, during and after the tick-tock movements. Move eyes to the left ("tick") and to the right ("tock"). Continue for two minutes. Synchronize with your breath and notice your thoughts.

10. **Sunrise-to-Sunset Eyeball Movements (vertical):**

Observe your thoughts in relation to where your eyes are as you roll them up. Behind closed eyes, imagine you are looking to the east and watching the sun rise. Follow the sun until it is directly above your head at noon. Then, follow the sun as it sets behind your head.

11. **Voice Exercises:**

Observe the tension and relaxation sensations and mind-talk before and after the "ooo-eee" lip movements, the tongue roll, and "turning down the volume" of the vocal cords. Say "ooo" and "eee" repeatedly. Then curl your tongue up, down and stick it out. Picture a control knob going down as you mentally lower your voice from ten to one.

12. **Thought-Labeling Baby Sitter:**

Try being each type of baby sitter with your thoughts—over-controlling, neglectful, and then observant, but not controlling. Observe the effects on your thoughts.

13. **Mind-Set Change/Retreat Sanctuary:**

Check into your mood and level of tension. Imagine a beach scene or green vista, with great sensory detail. Observe your experience before and after.

14. **Heartfelt Resonant Imaging (HRI):**

Check into your mood and level of tension. Do the HRI while picturing someone you resent. Center yourself, then focus on your anatomical heart area. Ask your heart, "Can I experience caring love towards this person?" Compare what your heart says, versus what your mind says.

Do another HRI towards someone you love. Check-in again. Do the HRI towards a body part that has, or is, troubling you. Check-in again. Do the HRI, imagining yourself as a baby. Check-in again.

15. **Inner Guide:**

Check-in. Imagine your inner guide giving you some valuable or inspirational messages. Check-in again.

16. **Healing Imagery:**

Check-in. Imagine a body part that is in need of healing.

Network Resources for
Heart Disease Reversal and Cancer Healing

We are thankful to Lawrence Spann, PA-C, MHS, Program Director of Heart Disease Reversal Clinic & Rice Diet Program at the Duke University Medical Center for providing us with the addresses for the Heart Reversal Program. They are reproduced here for reference only and does not constitute an endorsement by the author or the publisher.

HEART DISEASE REVERSAL NETWORK

CALIFORNIA

Cardiology Associates of Marin & San Francisco

Total Atherosclerosis Management
2 Bon Air Road
Larkspur, CA 94939
(415) 927-6173 (Voice)
(415) 927-6168 (Fax)
Vicki Chase, RN, Program Director
Mark Wexman, MD, Medical Director

Heart First
Heart Disease Reversal Program

1860 Mowry Ave., Suite 202
Fremont, CA 94538
(510) 713-1030 (Voice)
(510) 792-9686 (Fax)
Bonnie Batty, RN, Program Director
Jeffrey Carlson, MD, Medical Director

McDougall Program at St. Helena Health Center

Deer Park, CA 94576
800-358-9195 (Voice)
(707) 963-6248 (Voice)
(707) 963-6461 (Fax)
DorAnne Doneski, NP, MS,
   Program Director
John McDougall, MD, Medical Director

Preventive Medicine Research Institute

900 Bridgeway, Suite 2
Sausalito, CA 94965
(415) 332-2525 ext. 237 (Voice)
(415) 332-5730 (Fax)
Terri Merritt, MS, Program Director
Lee Lipsenthal, MD, Medical Director

Sequoia Hospital District– Cardiology Education

170 Alameda de Las Pulgas
Redwood City, CA 94062-2799
(415) 367-5734 (Voice)
(415) 366-7644 (Fax)
Liz Robinson-Carlson, RN, MS, CCRN,
   Patient Educator
Tom Hinohara, MD, Medical Director

Stress Cybernetix Institute

2182 East Street
Concord, CA 94520
(510) 685-4224 (Voice)
(510) 685-6997 (Fax)
Thomas Browne, PhD, Program
   Director
Naras Bhat, MD, Medical Director

COLORADO

Lutheran Medical Center– Cardiac Rehabilitation

8300 W. 38th Avenue
Wheatridge, CO 80033
(303) 425-2327 (Voice)
(303) 467-8971 (Fax)
Colleen Hatton, PT, Program Director
Gary Han, MD, Medical Director

COLORADO (CONT.)

Preventive Cardiology Services

2750 Broadway
Boulder, CO 80304
(303) 440-3057 (Voice)
(303) 449-9380 (Fax)
Lisa Scatera, MS, Program Director
Ronald Jenkins, MD, Medical Director

CONNECTICUT

Griffin Hospital–
Cardiac Rehabilitation

130 Division St.
Derby, CT 06418
(203) 732-7458 (Voice)
(203) 732-7449 (Fax)
Marge Deegan, RN, Program Director
Kenneth V. Schwartz, MD, Medical
    Director

ILLINOIS

Swedish Covenant Hospital–
Cardiac Rehabilitation

5145 N. California
Chicago, IL 60625
(312) 989-3804 (Voice)
(312) 728-3584 (Fax)
Corinne Murphy-Hines, MS,
    Program Director
Noel D. Nequin, MD, Medical Director

MICHIGAN

Blodgett Memorial Medical
Center – Preventive Cardiology
and Rehabilitation

1840 Wealthy SE
Grand Rapids, MI 49506-2968
(616) 774-7936 (Voice)
(616) 774-5030 (Fax)
Pam Kushmaul, RN, Program Director
Ronald Vander Laan, MD, Medical
    Director

MINNESOTA

Minneapolis Heart Institute–
Cardiac Rehabilitation

920 East 28th St., Suite 180
Minneapolis, MN 55407
(612) 863-3970 (Voice)
(612) 863-3801 (Fax)
Amy Amberg, Senior Coordinator
Barry Welge, MD, Medical Director

NEW JERSEY

Cardiac Rehabilitation–
Northwest Covenant Medical
Center

Dover Campus
Jardino St.
Dover, NJ 07801
(201) 989-3388 (Voice)
(201) 989-3532 (Fax)
Linda Aldrich, RN, Coordinator
Barry Howell, MD, Medical Director

Hackensack Medical Center–
Cardiac Preventive and
Rehabilitation Center

30 Prospect Ave.
Hackensack, NJ 07601
(201) 996-3792 (Voice)
(201) 996-3555 (Fax)
Christine Krieger, RN, Program Director
Joel Landzberg, MD, Medical Director

Monmouth Medical Center–
Cardiac Rehabilitation

300 Second Ave.
Longbranch, NJ 07740
(908) 870-5067 (Voice)
(908) 870-5253 (Fax)
Mary E. Cary, RN, Program Director
Jeff Daniels, MD, Medical Director

NEW JERSEY (CONT.)

Newton Memorial Hospital–
Cardiac Rehabilitation

175 High Street
Newton, NJ 07860
(201) 579-8349 (Voice)
(201) 383-9869 (Fax)
Dee Bale, RN, BSN, Program Director
Richard Redline, MD, Medical Director

Overlook Hospital–
Cardiac Rehabilitation

99 Beauvoir Ave.
Summit, NJ 07902
(908) 522-2945 (Voice)
(908) 522-3584 (Fax)
Cathy Pinch, RN, Program Director
John Gregory, MD, Medical Director

Pascack Valley Hospital–
Cardiac Rehabilitation

250 Old Hook Road
Westwood, NJ 07675
(201) 358-3609 (Voice)
(201) 358-3625 (Fax)
Mary Lyon, RN, Program Director
Theodore Goldberg, MD, Medical
    Director

NORTH CAROLINA

Duke University Medical Center–
Heart Disease Reversal Clinic
and Rice Diet Program

Box 3099 - DUMC
Durham, NC 27710
(919) 286-2243 (Voice)
(919) 286-0720 (Fax)
Lawrence Spann, PA-C, MHS, Program
    Director
Robert A. Rosati, MD, Medical Director

PENNSYLVANIA

Lower Bucks Hospital–
Cardiac Rehabilitation

501 Bath Rd.
Bristol, PA 19067
(215) 785-9855 (Voice)
(215) 785-9769 (Fax)
Kevin Ryan, RRT, Program Director
Srinivas Atri, MD, Medical Director

St. Lukes Hospital–
Lifestyle Management

801 Ostrum St.
Bethlehem, PA 18015
(610) 954-3175 (Voice)
(610) 954-4651 (Fax)
Michael Conway, Program Director
Tom Dale, MD, Medical Director

OHIO

Community Hospital–
Coronary Prevention and
Rehabilitation Center

3135 Imperial Blvd.
Springfield, OH 45505
(513) 325-1155 (Voice)
(513) 232-6611 (Fax)
Pat Cooper, MS, Program Director
Narinder Saini, MD, Medical Director

OREGON

Oregon Research Institute

1715 Franklin Blvd.
Eugene, OR 97403-1983
(503) 484-2123 (Voice)
(503) 484-1108 (Fax)
Deborah Toobert, PhD, Research
    Project Director

SOUTH CAROLINA

GHS Heart Institute–
Heart Life

875 West Faris Rd.
Greenville, SC 29605
(803) 455-7726 (Voice)
(803) 455-8447 (Fax)
William Webster, IV, PhD, Program
   Director
Edward Lominach, MD, Medical
   Director

TEXAS

Mother Frances Hospital–
Healing Your Heart Program –
Regional Wellness Center

800 E. Dawson
Tyler, TX 75701
(903) 531-4379 (Voice)
(903) 531-5095 (Fax)
Patrick Dunn, MS, MBA, Program
   Director
Noah Israel, MD, Medical Director

WISCONSIN

University of Wisconsin–
Choice to Renew
(Cardiac Retreats)

131 Quadt, Stevens Pt., WI 54481
(715) 346-4420 (Voice)
(715) 346-4655 (Fax)
Anne Abbott, PhD, Program Director

AUSTRALIA

Sydney Adventist Hospital–
The Beat Goes On
Cardiac Rehabilitation Program

185 Fox Valley Road
Wahroonga, NSW 2074, Australia
61 2 487 9880 (Voice)
61 2 489 3148 (Fax)
Jenel Ruthven, RN, Program Director
Russell Butler, MD, Medical Director

John Hunter Hospital–
Cardiac Rehabilitation Program

Locked Baq No. 1
New Castle, NSW 2310
Australia
61 4 921 3000 (Voice)
61 4 921 4210 (Fax)
Kerry Inder, CNS, Program Director
Peter Fletcher, MD, Medical Director

393 Medical Centre

393 Military Rd.
Mossman 2088
Australia
61 2 969 1633 (Voice)
61 2 969 1454 (Fax)
Russell Lee, RN, Program Director
Malcolm Parmenter, MD, Medical
   Director

CANADA

ADOPT (Adhere to Dean
Ornish's Program Today)

136 Collier Street
Toronto, Ontario M4W 1M3, Canada
(416) 962-5863 (Voice)
(416) 962-9187 (Fax)
Support group for heart patients
   coordinated by
Toronto Rehabilitation Centre Board

INDIA

Universal Healing
Charitable Trust

36, Jain Society, Ellisbridge
Ahmedabad - 380 006
Gujarat, India
079 441 942 (Voice)
079 456 733 (Fax)
Jayant V. Zalavadia, Program Director
Ramesh Kapadia, MD, Medical Director

RESOURCES FOR CANCER HEALING:

CONNECTICUT

Exceptional Cancer Patients

1302 Chapel Street
New Haven, CT 06511
(203) 865-8392 (Voice)
(203) 497-9393 (Fax)

Exceptional Cancer Patients (ECaP) was founded in 1978 by Bernie Siegel, MD, author of Love, Medicine, and Miracles and other books. Siegel is one of the most famous advocates of mind-body approaches to cancer which "help people find the strength to grow and change in the face of serious health problems."

CALIFORNIA

Simonton Cancer Center– New Patient Program

P.O. Box 890
Pacific Palisades, CA 90272
(310) 459-4434

Carl Simonton and his former wife, Stephanie have coauthored the widely read book, Getting Well Again, addressing mind-body healing methods of cancer. The Simonton center has residential programs for cancer patients.

CALIFORNIA

Residential Programs for People with Cancer–Commonweal Cancer Help Program

P.O. Box 316
Bolinas, CA 94924
(415) 868-0970 (Voice)

Founded in 1985, Commonweal is a nonmedical education program on complementary therapy of cancer. The president of the institute, Michael Lerner has a comprehensive book, Choices in Healing, Integrating the Best of Conventional and Complementary Approaches to Cancer. This book has addresses and phone numbers of several self-help support groups and residential care facilities for complementary therapy of cancer.

Epilogue

Eclectic Medicine for the 21st Century

One of my patients (Mr X) happened to read this book on the day of his heart attack. He was perplexed by the systems of medicine. He felt guilt and fear of having omitted or committed to systems of treatment. Here is how he resolved it.

1. "What is my problem?" Use physical and chemical diagnosis by modern high tech medicine.

2. "What is the solution (treatment)?" Mr X reasoned, the *logic* of modern medicine overlapped the *bio-logic* of Nature's healing. He used an eclectic blend of the Three Eras of Medicine (as prompted by Larry Dossey in his book, *Healing Words*).

Three Eras of Medicine

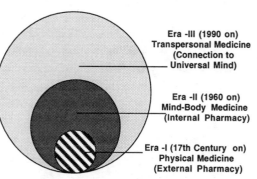

Era -III (1990 on)
Transpersonal Medicine
(Connection to Universal Mind)

Era -II (1960 on)
Mind-Body Medicine
(Internal Pharmacy)

Era -I (17th Century on)
Physical Medicine
(External Pharmacy)

Era-1 started with the Cartesian dualism of mind-body split which has been the foundation of modern medicine since the 17th century. Its focus is on physical diagnosis, organ specialists, chemical tests, external pharmacy, and therapies such as surgery and radiation. Mr X underwent the treatment including clot busters, angiogram, angioplasty, and even bypass surgery. Now, his fear was how to prevent re-clogging of coronary arteries. In addition to the doctor-prescribed drugs, diet and exercise, he started looking at other eras of medicine.

Era-II began with the concept of Psycho-neuro-immunology in the 1960s. Invoking internal pharmacy by meditation and imagery, and psychophysiological self-regulation by biofeedback are major features of this era. Ornish's reversing heart disease, Simonton's cancer healing, and Peniston's addiction healing are examples.

Era-III began in the 1990s with transpersonal healing focused on *meaning of life* and connectedness. Boosting the immune system by self-disclosure, experience of altruism, and spirituality (including prayer) are markers of this era. Heart centered living and joining the cyberpace of Universal mind has become the meaning of life as a biological experience and electronic web.

Because Mr. X is used to the concept of diagnosis and treatment of modern medicine, using this book, he tabulated the three eras of medicine into the following table. He divided the diagnosis into measuring (comparing to a standard) and monitoring (moment by moment watching).

Diagnosis and Treatment
(Confusion in Choice Delays Healing)

Era	Measure	Monitor	Modify
I **Physical Diagnosis** (External Pharmacy)	Physical Exam Blood Test X-ray EKG MRI etc.	Symptoms Vital Signs Blood Tests Other Tests	Medications Surgery Radiation Physical Therapy Mindful Eating
II **Mind-Body Medicine** (Internal Pharmacy)	Human Function Curve Money Function Curve	Mindfulness by CyberScan Energy Quadrants	Meditation- Imagery Exercise Biofeedback
III **Transpersonal Healing** (Connectedness)	Energy Exchange Vectors	Heartfelt Resonant Imaging (HRI) (Heart Centered Living)	Biological Altruism Self-Disclosure Spirituality

He made a mind-body diagonal to keep a visual impression of his progress. The functions of the mind-body change either by body chemistry (food, motion, and emotion) or by behavior (action, throught, and emotion.) The emotion is a common denominator.

Mind-Body Diagonals

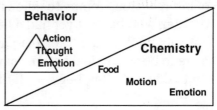

In the chemical area: Watch my abdominal obesity, blood pressure, heart rate, respiration, blood sugar, and lipid pattern: good (HDL), bad (LDL), ugly (triglyceride), and deadly (Lp-a).

In the behavioral area: "Watch my anger level, sleep, restless mind, gut function, and relationship. This is where different measuring, and monitoring tools came in handy."

When it came to modifying actions, he made a list of five items: Anger control, meditation and imagery, mindful eating, self-disclosure, and exercise. He started the heart centered living right away by moment by moment control of anger (Heartfelt Resonant Imaging). He became a total vegetarian, with starch based, low fat (minimum use of oil, *no fried food*) natural food (*fresh fruits and vegetable snacks to replace cookies and crackers*), and started on antioxidant supplements. He started one minute, and five minute meditation and imagery several hundred times a day, in addition to a 20 minute session every day. He started a time, touch, and talk session with his partner every day. On exercise and prescription drugs, he followed his doctor's advice.

One scientist friend asked Mr. X, what is the validity of mind-body medicine and transpersonal healing in the 21st century? Mr X quoted the literature of Ornish-Simonton reversal of heart disease and cancer; Harvard-HeartMath research of biological value of altruism and caring love; Spiegel study of group support and Byrd's double blind study of power of prayer to heal the heart.

Now, Mr X is home after his hospitalization. The eclectic choice this book offers gave him solace. He prayed every day, petitioning God for speedy recovery. He felt better with a prayer of intercession, hoping to guide his high stressed out business partner, who has not yet had a heart attack, to prevent it. Mr X got this book as a gift for his partner, with a note, "you don't have to be sick to feel better. I saw light after a crack. All is well that ends well. But, begin with this book."

End Notes

End Notes

The end is the beginning. We began our Heart Resetting Program (Sav–a–Heart Program) based on the following scientific and traditional sources and resources. Much of it came as feedback from thousands of people who attended our worldwide seminars and weekly Sav–a–Heart Group sessions.

INTRODUCTION, WHY READ THIS BOOK, PICTURE TOUR, BASIC QUESTIONS OF REVERSAL.

Two major scientific breakthroughs make our program unique, user–friendly, and quickly implementable *even on the day of heart attack or cancer diagnosis*. These two factors are: **heart rate variability and emotions**, and **new advancements in biofeedback.** The anger control tools were developed based on HeartMath Research (of Boulder Creek, California, Phone: 408–338–9861) on how heart rate changes with emotions and McClelland's Harvard research on how the immune system changes with emotions.

We use standard clinical biofeedback equipment (J & J, I–330) to measure, monitor, and modify heart rate on–line and teach people how to replace anger with caring love. The new biofeedback modality of alpha–theta brain wave feedback helped us to perfect our method of teaching meditation (CyberZen™). With this method, we are able to train a person to meditate in one office visit. We have trained hundreds of doctors and clinicians in this method so that they can teach meditation to their clients in less than an hour.

LIFESTYLE CHANGES VS REACTIVITY CHANGES

The main component of Ornish–Simonton programs is lifestyle changes, such as diet, exercise, meditation–imagery, and self–disclosure. The extra dimension we have added is moment by moment replacement of anger with caring love at the mind end, and moment by moment change of body reactivity at the muscle end. This is analogous to fixing the roof leak, and mopping the wet floor simultaneously. The clinical biofeedback instruments have helped us to prove to the client that this model works at every step.

As I write this end note, I can recall the following major authorities that influenced my thought process.

MEDICAL MODELS

1. **Peter Nixon's Human Function Curve (HFC):** Nixon is from Charing Cross Hospital, London. HFC and hyperventilation model are used to measure and monitor the stress response and workaholism of modern life.

2. **Dean Ornish's Reversing Coronary Artery Disease**: Ornish, published his landmark research in the prestigious medical journal, *Lancet,* July 1990. For our patients, we recommend two bestseller books by Ornish: *Reversing Coronary Artery Disease* and *Eat More Weigh Less.* Ramesh Kapadia, a cardiologist at Ahmedabad, India, has used a variation of the Ornish model successfully and has published it in his book, *Primer of Universal Healing,* Navajeevan Publishing House, Ahmedabad, India.

3. **Kenneth Cooper from Cooper Institute, Dallas:** Cooper is the originator of aerobics in 1968. Cooper guidelines are used in prescribing exercise for cardiac prevention and rehabilitation. Cooper's two books, *Aerobic Program for Total Well Being* and the new book, *Antioxidant Revolution* are recommended.

4. **Covert Bailey:** We recommend his new book, *Smart Exercise* to read about the aerobic exercise principles and their relationship to body fat and cardiovascular fitness.

5. **HeartMath Research, Boulder Creek, California:** The connection between brain and heart in relation to positive and negative emotions and heart rate variability is a new concept. The effect of caring love on immune system and DNA is also a new concept.

6. **David McClelland from Harvard:** He is a researcher on motivation. We have used his well respected theories of motivation, achievement, affiliation, and power in designing our program. The bifurcation of human motives into achievement or affiliation has been used as a model to create our duck–rabbit icon by our staff artist, Jay Mazhar. Additionally, we use his model of the Mother Teresa Effect in which caring love changes the immunoglobulin levels in the saliva.

7. **Robert Eliot:** We have used the "hot reactor" model of Eliot in which the heart disease prone people react with high blood pressure and rapid heart rate when challenged with mental and

physical stress.

8. **Redford Williams:** His model of hostility and its harmful effects on the heart. We have used his two books *Trusting Heart* and *Anger Kills* to design our anger control models.

9. **Carl Simonton and Bernie Siegel:** In the area of cancer healing we have used Simonton's *Getting Well Again*, and Siegel's *Love, Peace and Joy.* These are good models for meditation, imagery, social support, and mind–body healing.

10. **David Spiegel's Group Support Model:** Group support and self–disclosure doubled the longevity of breast cancer patients in Stanford. We have used this model of supportive expressive therapy. The James Spira modification of the Stanford model is used at Duke Uni. for coronary artery patients. We used this model in choreographing our self–disclosure system.

CYBERNETIC MODELS

1. **Biofeedback:** The modern biofeedback computers are built on the principle of real time on–line feedback with your own body physiology. The control by feedback communication is used at every step of designing our program. Eric Peper from Berkeley, California, and Robert Fried from New York have inspired me in formulating the breath connection to life using biofeedback monitoring. Elmer Green from Kansas has inspired my concepts of "scientific spirituality." Eugene Peniston's model of alpha–theta training or "electronic meditation" in modifying human behavior.

2. **Neurolinguistic Programming (NLP):** I was impressed by Anthony Robbin's NLP based seminars, tapes, and books. The process of using submodalities to keep the imagery from fading is taken from NLP.

3. **Kyzen:** The cybernetic principle of focusing on the process rather than outcome has created the new Japanese work culture of total quality management. The moment of truth is the point of contact that makes the impact. We have used the Kyzen principle in our moment by moment heart resetting by replacing anger with caring love.

ANCIENT AND TRADITIONAL MODELS

The largest laboratory in the world is behind our own closed eyes. The ancients worked in this perennial laboratory and gave us a lot of wisdom we are now trying to prove by scientific methods. Mark Twain once said, "the ancients have stolen our best ideas."

1. **Bhagavadgita, Upanishads, and Yogasutra:** I am fortunate that my parents taught me Sanskrit so that I could reach the original Vedic science texts. I have used the wisdom of Bhagavadgita in anger control (2nd chapter, called *sankya yoga*, or yoga of knowledge) and meditation (6th chapter, called *dhyana yoga*, or yoga of meditation). *Mandukya* Upanishad was helpful in formulating the levels of consciousness and relating to Universal Mind. Patanjali's Yogasutra has been my constant companion in designing experiments on self–regulation. The chakra system parallels our belly button centering (*Manipura* chakra) and heart centering (*Hridaya* chakra).

2. **Bible:** We have used the message from Jesus "love thy enemy." This is a strong message to differentiate heartfelt and mindfelt feelings. Bible's message of self study, "go to the kingdom of heaven within" matches with Patanjali's *"tapaha swadhyaya ishwara pranidhanamiti kriya yogaha"* (meditation, self–study, and surrender to God). This tallies with the success of biofeedback therapy.

3. **Buddhism:** The breath centered meditation is inspired by Buddhism and Zen. Buddha was known as *ajatashatru*, which means, one who is incapable of getting angry. Every human heart is built with this model. We use this to explain the unconditional love that springs from every heart but masked by the judgemental brain.

4. **Islam:** We use the model of five or six times a day praying in the Moslem system as a parallel to our six times a day meditation and imagery.

5. **Qui Gong:** We have used the concept of energy meridians in formulating the mind–body dialogue.

General References

1. Ornish, Dean et al. (1990). Can lifestyle changes reverse coronary heart disease? *The Lancet,* 336 (8708), 129–33. Ornish, Dean et al. (1983). Effects of stress management training and dietary changes in treating ischemic heart disease. *JAMA,* 249 (1), 54–59. Ornish, Dean. *Dean Ornish's Program for Reversing Coronary Artery Disease: The Only System Scientifically Proven to Reverse Heart Disease Without Drugs or Surgery.* New York: Random House, 1990.

2. Eliot, R. (1984). *Is it Worth Dying For?* New York: Bantam Books.

3. Lerner, M. (1994). *Choices in Healing.* Cambridge, Mass: The MIT Press.

4. Simonton, C., Mathew–Simonton, S., and Creighton, J.L. (1978). *Getting Well Again.* New York: Bantam Books.

5. Siegel, Bernie. (1990). *Peace, Love and Healing.* New York: Harper Perennial.

6. Siegel, Bernie. (1986). *Love, Medicine and Miracle.* New York: Harper Perennial.

7. LeShan, L. (1977). *You can Fight For Your Life: Emotional factors in the Treatment of Cancer.* New York: M. Evans and Co.

8. Gordon, N., and Gibbons, L.W. (1990). *The Cooper Clinic Cardiac rehabilitation Program.* New York: Simon and Schuster.

9. Robbins, A. (1991). *Awaken the Giant Within.* New York: Summit Books.

10. Kabat–Zinn, J. (1990). *Full Catastrophe Living.* New York: Delacorte Press.

11. Simon, H.B. (1994). *Conquering Heart Disease.* New York: Little Brown and Co.

12. Dacher, E.S. (1991). *PNI, Mind–Body Healing Program.* New York: Paragon House.

1. CROSSROADS: VICTIM OR VICTOR?

• Selye, H. (1974). *Stress Without Distress.* New York: Signet Book.

• Childre, D.L., (1994). *Freeze Frame, Fast Action Stress Relief.* Boulder Creek, CA: Planetary Publications.

• Ornish, D., Brown, S., Sherwitz, L., et al. (1990). Can Life Style Changes Reverse Coronary Artery Disease? *Lancet,* 336, 129–33.

- Frasure Smith, N., Lesperance, F., Talajic, M. (1993). Depression following Myocardial Infarction: Impact on 6–month Survival. *JAMA*, 270, 15, 1819–1825 and 1860–1861.

2. LEARNED HELPLESSNESS

- Seligman, M. (1990). *Learned Optimism*. New York: Pocket Books.
- Visintainer, M., Volpicelli, J., Seligman, M. (1982). Tumor Rejection in Rats After Inescapable Shock, *Science*, 216,437–9.
- Langer, E.J., Rodin, J. (1976). Effect of Choice and Enhanced Personal Responsibility for the Aged: A Field Experiment in an Institutional Setting. *Journal of Personal and Social Psychology*, 34, 191–9.

3. LEARNED OPTIMISM – SELF–EFFICACY

- The office of Prevention, California Department of Mental Health, organized a research study involving the Stanford psychologist, Kenneth Pelletier, and Steven Locke of Harvard University to find out what enables human beings to make a state of personal efficacy leading to self–mastery and sense of control in life. The research reviewed more than one thousand top scientific publications in the field of mind–body illnesses, aging, lifestyle changes, and social support. The findings were published under the title, *Personal Efficacy: A Research Database.* According to the findings, the self–efficacy concept of Bandura is the antidote to learned helplessness.

  The model of learned helplessness and learned optimism is true in animals and man. Seligman from the University of Pennsylvania has studied this phenomenon for the last 25 years. This model is working to turn around people with life long problems of depression, anger, test anxiety, athletic choking, posttraumatic stress disorder, and most importantly, depression and defeat that follows catastrophic illnesses, such as heart attack and cancer.

- Bandura, A. (1977). Self–efficacy, Towards a unifying Theory of Behavior change. *Psychological Review*, 84, 191–215.
- Bandura, A. (1977). *A Social Learning Theory*. Englewood Cliffs, New Jersey: Prentice Hall.
- Pelletier, K. (1994). *Sound Mind, Sound Body, A New Model for Lifelong Health*. New York: Simon and Schuster.

- Seligman, M. (1990). *Learned Optimism.* New York: Pocket Books.
- Seligman, M. (1994). *What You Can Change and What You Can't. The Complete Guide to Successful Self-Improvement.* New York: Alfred A. Knopff. This book is a good reference on the cognitive psychology of how to change your thinking patterns. The contemporary leaders in cognitive restructuring are: Albert Ellis, Donald Meichenbaum, and Martin Seligman. The essential principle is to study the antecedents of each behavior, question the behavior, and reframe. It is like hiring a defense attorney in your favor and restating or reframing the negative thoughts into a positive frame.

4. COMMON WAR FRONT: RADICAL ATTACK

- Cooper, Kenneth H. (1994). *Antioxidant Revolution.* Nashville, TN: Thomas Nelson Publishers.

  A very good reference on the latest research on antioxidants with particular focus on coronary artery disease and cancer. The antioxidant way of living is summarized in four points: triple antioxidant supplement, low intensity exercise, cooking and eating the antioxidant way, and lifestyle changes. Kenneth Cooper is the physician from Cooper Center, Dallas, who coined the word "aerobics." His new research shows that strenuous exercise increases free radicals.

- Sinatra, S.T. (1992). *Lose to Win, A Cardiologist's Guide to Weight Loss and Nutritional Healing.* New York: Lincoln Bradley Publishing. This book covers preventive cardiology and antioxidant supplements in great detail.

Beta Carotene

- Gaziano, J.M., Manson, J., Ridker, P.M., Buring, J.E., Hennekens, C.H., (1990). Beta Carotene Therapy for Chronic Stable Angina. *Supplement to Circulation*, 81(4), Abst. 0796.

  A study of physicians aged 45 to 80 years showed 50% reduction in coronary events in five years by using beta carotene.

Vitamin C

- Johnson, C., Meyer, C., Srilakshmi, J. (1993). Vitamin C Elevates Red Blood Cell Glutathione in Healthy Adults. *American Journal of Clinical Nutrition,* 58, 103–105. A vitamin C dose of 500 mg increased the level of another antioxidant, glutathione.

Coenzyme Q10

- Greenberg, S.M., Frisheman, W.H. (1990). Co–enzyme Q10: A new Drug for Cardiovascular Disease. *Journal of Clinical Pharmacology*, 30, 590–608.

- Langsjoen H,. et al. (1990). *American Journal of Cardiology*, 65, 512–523. Q10 helps patients with heart failure and low cardiac output.

- Kamikawa T., et al. (1985). Effects of Coenzyme Q10 in Exercise Tolerance in Chronic Stable Angina Pectoris. *American Journal of Cardiology*, 56, 247.

  Q10 acts on energy factories — the mitochondria of cells. After age 35–40, the liver produces less q10 in the body, and supplements are needed. If Q10 drops 25% or more, the energy level drops significantly.

Flavonoids

- Hertog, M.G.L. et al. (1995). Flavonoid Intake and Long–term Risk of Coronary Artery Disease and Cancer in the Seven Countries Study. *Arch Intern Med*, 155, 381–386.

  A cross cultural correlation study showed that the intake of antioxidant flavonoids is associated with lower mortality from coronary artery disease in different countries. The main source of flavonoids intake was vegetables, fruits, tea, and wine.

5. MEMBRANE WAR: HEART DISEASE

- Simon, H.B. (1994). *Conquering Heart Disease*. New York: Little Brown and Co.

- The sudden cardiac death research is adapted from Eliot, R.S., From *Stress to Strength*, (1994). New York, London, Bantam Books.

6. NUCLEAR WAR: CANCER

- Quilllin, P. (1994). *Beating Cancer with Nutrition*. Tulsa, OK: The Nutrition Times Press.

- Fischer, W. (1992). *How to Fight Cancer and Win*. Canfield, OH: Fisher Publishing Co.

7. RISK AND DISEASE

- Lawn, R.M. (1992). Lipoprotein (a) in Heart Disease. *Scientific American*, June issue, pp 54–60.

- Brown, M.S., Goldstein, J.L. (1984). How LDL Receptors Influence

Cholesterol and Atherosclerosis. *Scientific American*, November issue. (1995). Homocysteine and atherosclerosis. *The McDougall Newsletter (March–April)*, 9,2.

- Godsland I. F., Stevenson, J. C. (1995). Insulin Resistance: Syndrome or tendency?. *Lancet*, 346:100-03.

Coronary Artery Disease in Indians Study (CADI)

Coronary artery disease among Indians has emerged as a prototype of a high risk population. A cardiologist from Chicago, Enas Enas, has emerged as a world authority on this subject. He studied over 2000 Indian physicians and their families, and confirmed that CHD is 5 to 10 times higher in the Indian population than in the American population, and 20 times higher than in the Japanese. The exact reason for this high risk is still under investigation. Inheritance of Lp (a), insulin resistance, apple type obesity, low HDL, and high triglycerides are more prevalent in Indians. I have selected the following scientific articles for serious readers on this subject.

- Enas, E.A., Mehta J.M., (1995). Malignant Coronary Artery Disease in Young Asian Indians: Thoughts on Pathogenesis, Prevention and Therapy. *Clinical Cardiology*, 18, 131, pp 131–135. Enas, E.A., Yusuf S., Mehta, J.L. (1992). Prevalence of Coronary Artery Disease in Asian Indians, *American Journal of Cardiology*, Editorial. 70, 945–949. Prabha, J., Enas, E.A., Yusuf, S. (1993). Coronary Artery Disease in Asian Indians: Prevalence and Risk Factors. *Asian and Pacific Islander Journal of Health*, 1, 2.
- Editorial. (1986). Coronary Artery Disease in Indians Overseas. *Lancet*, i: 1307–08.
- Balarajan, R. (1991). Ethnic Differences in Mortality from Ischemic Heart Disease and Cerebrovascular Disease in England and Wales. *BMJ*, 302, 56–64.
- McKeigue P.M., Miller G.J., Marmot M.G. (1989). Coronary Artery Disease in South Asian Overseas: a Review. *Journal of Clinical Epidemiology*, 42, 597–609. McKeigue P.M., Shah, B., Marmot, M.G. (1991). Relation of Centra Obesity and Insulin Resistance with High Diabetes Prevalence and Cardiovascular risk in South Asians. *Lancet*, 337, 382–86.
- Shaukat, N., Douglas J.T., Bennet J.L., DeBono D.P. (1995). Can Physical Activity Explain the Difference in Insulin Levels and

Fibrinolytic Activity Between Young Indo–origin and European Relatives of Patients with Coronary Artery Disease? *Fibrinolysis*, 9,1–9.

- Editorial. (1995). Westernized Asians and Cardiovascular Disease: Nature or Nurture? *Lancet*, 345, 401–402.
- Bhatnagar, D., Anand, I.S., Durrington, P.N. (1995). Coronary Risk Factors in People from Indian Subcontinent Living in West London and Their Siblings in India. *Lancet*, 345, 405–409.
- Sharma, S.N., Kaul, U., Wasir, H.S., et al. (1990). Coronary Arteriographic Profile in Young and Old Indian Patients with Ischemic Heart Disease: A Comparative Study. *Indian Heart Journal*, 42, 365–369.
- Krishnaswamy, S., Prasad, N.K., Jose, V.J. (1989). A study of Lipid Levels with Coronary Artery Disease. *International Journal of Cardiology*, 24, 337–345.
- Sait, Shehnaz. Asian Indians Genetically Prone to Heart Disease: Chicago Cardiologist Discovers the "Deadly" Cholesterol Link. AAPI Journal, Spring 1995, a thesis submitted for Masters in Journalism, Columbia College, Chicago, March, 1994. Reprints of this review can be obtained from CADI Research, 3510 Hobson Road, #301, Woodridge, IL, 60517.

8. CYBERNETIC MODEL OF STRESS

This model is based on Everly and Benson's model. Everly, G. Jr. (1989). *A Clinical Guide to the Treatment of the Human Stress Response*. New York: Plenum Press.

9. YIN AND YANG OF MIND BODY

The yin–yang concept is based on standard human physiology of the nervous system and Chinese energy based mind–body systems.

- Algra, A. (1994). Using Heart Rate Variability Data to Assess Sudden Death Risk. *Noninvasive and Invasive Methods of Cardiac Diagnosis*. 11,7,11–21. Algra, A., Tijssen, J.G.P., Roelandt J.R.T.C., et al. (1993). Heart Rate Variability from 24 hour electrocardiography and the 2 year risk for sudden death. *Circulation*, 88, 18.
- Kleiger, R.E., Miller, J.P., Bigger, J.T., et al. (1987). Multicenter Postinfarction Research Group, Decreased Heart Rate Variability and Its Association with Increased Mortality After Acute Myocardial Infarction. *American Journal of Cardiology*, 59, 256.

10. ADDICTION TO STRESS

Based on Peter Nixon's work on hyperventilation. Reactivity is based on Robert Eliot's work on "hot reactors" as published in his book, *Is It Worth Dying For?*

11. WHAT IS RELAXATION?

1. Stroebel, C.F. (1982). *QR: The Quieting Reflex.* New York: Putnam and Sons.
2. Benson, H. p.254–255 in The relaxation response by Benson (Ch. 14 Mind–Body Medicine by Golman), Benson has shown that sleep reduces the metabolic rate by 8%, as compared to the meditative state, which reduces the metabolic rate up to 12%.
3. Gelhorn, E. (1958). Physiological basis of neuromuscular relaxation. *Archives of Internal Medicine*, 102, 392–399.
4. Gelhorn, E. (1957). Autonomic imbalance and hypothalamus. Minneapolis, MN: University of Minnesota Press.
5. Where does this go – Kindling? Weil, J.A. (1974). *Neurophysiological model of emotional and intentional behavior.* Springfield, Illinois, Charles C. Thomas, 1974.
6. Television and stress: Johnston, W.M., Graham, C.L., Davey, C.L. The Psychological Impact of Negative TV News Bulletins. *Psychological Society of London Conference.* December, 1994, as quoted in *Mental Medicine Update Newsletter* by Sobel, D.S. and Ornstein, R.O., IV:1, 1995.

12. MIND–BODY DIALOGUE

1. Ader, R. (Ed.). (1981). *Psychoneuroimmunology.* New York: Academic Press.
2. Siegel, B. (1989). *Peace, Love and Healing.* New York: Harper Perennial. Achterberg, J. (1985). *Imagery in Healing.* Boston: Shambala.
3. Benson, H., Klipper, M. (1976). *The Relaxation Response.* New York: Avon books.
4. Silva, J., and Stone, R. (1989). *The Silva Mind Control Method for Getting Help from the Other Side.* New York: Pocket Books, Simon and Schuster.

13. EMOTIONS OF HEART EVENT

This chapter is based on my discussions with several cardiologists and my patients.

- Kawachi, I., Sparrow, D., Vokonas, P.S., Weiss, S.T. (1994). Symptoms of Anxiety and Risk of Coronary Artery Disease: The Normative Aging Study. *Circulation*, 90, 2225–9.

14. NEW BIOLOGY OF EMOTIONS

- Thompson, J.G. (1988). *The Psychobiology of Emotions*. New York: Plenum Press.

- Tomkins, S.S. (1984). *Affect Theory*, in Scherer, K.R., Ekman, P. (Eds.) *Approaches to Emotion*. Hilsdale, NJ: Lawrence Earlbaum Associates.

15. HOW ANGER KILLS YOU

- Redford Williams from Duke University is the authority on anger and heart disease. He followed the footsteps of Friedman and Rosenman, the orginators of the type A behavior concept. In our Sav–a–Heart clinic, we recommend two books by Williams:

  Williams, R. (1993). *Anger Kills*. New York: Harper Collins Publishing. and

  Williams, R. (1989). *The Trusting Heart*. New York: Random House Publishing.

- Two references for Type A Behavior are: Friedman, M. and Ulmer, D.U. (1984). *Treating Type A Behavior and Your Heart*. New York: Faucett Crest. and Friedman, M. and Rosenman, R.H. (1974). *Type A Behavior and Your Heart*. New York: Faucett Crest. These two books cover the basic discovery of type A behavior and how to alter it by behavioral changes.

- Lonely heart—Berkman, L.F., Breslow, L. (1983). *Health and Ways of Living: The Alameda County Study*. New York: Oxford University Press.

- Swedish Study— Orth–Gomer, K., Unden, A.L., Edwards, M.E. (1988). Social Isolation and Mortality in Ischemic Heart Disease. A ten Year Follow up Study of 150 Middle–aged Men. *Acta Medica Scandinavica*, 224, 205–15.

- Reed study of Honolulu—Reed, D.W., McGee, D., Yano, K., Feinlab, M. (1983). Social Networks and Coronary Heart Disease Among Japanese Men in Hawaii. *American Journal of Epidemiology*, 117, 38–96.

- Tecomsheh, hating your own spouse—Julius, M., Harburg, E.,

Cottingham E.M., et al. (1986). Anger Coping types, blood pressure and all cause mortality: A follow up at Tecomsheh, Michigan (1971–83). *American Journal of Epidemiology*, 124, 220.

- Anginal reduction by supporting wife—Medalie, H., and Godbourt, U. (1976). Angina Pectoris Among 10,000 Men II: Psychosocial and Other Risk Factors as Evidenced by Multivariate Analysis of Five Year Incidence Study. *American Journal of Medicine*, 60, 910–21.—Three mile island story—Fleming, R; Baum, M.M., Giarrel, R., Gatchel, R.J. (1982). Mediating Influences of Social Support on Stress at Three Mile Island. *Journal of Human Stress*, 8, 14–22.

- Ohio Medical students and NK cells– Research as quoted by Padus, E., in Emotion and your Health, by Prevention Magazine, Rodale Press, Emmaus, Pennsylvania, 1992., p103.

- Japanese *amae* — as quoted by Williams, R. (1989). *Trusting Heart*. New York: Times Book.

Japanese People and Heart Attacks

- Doba, N., Hinohara, S., Williams, R.B. (1983). Studies on Type A Behavior Pattern and Hostility in Japanese Male Subjects with Special Reference to CHD. *Japanese Journal of Psychosomatic Medicine*, 23, 321–28.

Anger and Adrenaline, Noradrenalines

- Maranon, G. (1924). Contribution a l'etude de l'action emotive de l'adrenaline. *Revue Francaise d'Endocrinologie*, 2, 301–325.

- Thompson, J.G. (1982). *Psychobiology of Emotions*. New York: Plenum Press.

16. THE MOTHER TERESA EFFECT–LOVE AS A TOOL

- McClelland, D.C., and Kirshnit C. (1988). The Effects of Motivational Arousal Through Films on Salivary Immunoglobulin A. *Psychol Health*, 2, 31052.

- McClelland, D.C., and Jemmott J.B. (1980). Power Motivation, Stress and Physical Illness. *Journal of Human Stress*, 6, 6–15.

- McClelland, D.C., Ross, G., Patel, V. (1985). The Effect of an Academic Examination on Salivary Norepinephrine and Immunoglobin Levels. *Journal of Human Stress*, 11,52059.

- Rein, G., Atkinson, M., McCraty, R. (1994). The Physiological and Psychological Effects of Compassion and Anger. *Psychosomatic Medicine*, 56,171–172.

- Spiegel, D., Bloom, J.R., Kraemer, H.V., Gottheil, E. (1989). Effect of Psychological Treatment on Survival of Patients with Metastatic Breast Cancer. *Lancet*, 2, 888–891. Spiegel, David. (1994). *Living Beyond Limits*. New York: Times Book. The studies from the University of San Francisco and pet owner studies from UCLA are quoted by Spiegel in chapter, Social Support: How Friends, family and groups can help? in Mind–Body Medicine by Goleman, D. and Gurin, J., Consumer Reports Book, New York, 1993.
- Carnegie, D. (1944). *How to Stop Worrying and Start Living*. New York: Simon and Schuster. The Rockefeller story is quoted from this source.
- Pelletier, K. (1994). *Sound Mind, Sound Body: A Model for Lifelong Health*. New York: Simon and Schuster.

17. REACTIVITY LEVELS OF THE HEART

The references for this chapter overlap the chapters: Breathing and the Heart, Heart Rate Variability, Restless Mind Control, and Insomnia Control.

18. BREATHING AND THE HEART

- Peter Nixon from Charing Cross Hospital in London is recognized as the foremost expert on hyperventilation and the heart. I have discussed several issues of hyperventilation and the heart with Peter Nixon in formulating our heart resetting program. A lot of the information on hyperventilation and its effects presented in this book is based on Peter Nixon's research. Nixon, PGF. (1993). The Broken Heart—Counteraction by SABRES. *Journal of the Royal Society of Medicine*, 86, 4680471.
- Robert Fried from New York and Eric Peper from Berkeley, California have guided me in the area of hyperventilation and biofeedback monitoring. Robert Fried is a pioneer in the capnometric study of hyperventilation. Eric Peper is known for the effortless breathing model.
- Fried, R. (1987). *The Hyperventilation Syndrome*. Baltimore, MD: The John Hopkins University Press. Fried, R. (1993). *The Psychology and Physiology of Breathing*. New York: Plenum Press.
- Peper, E. (1990). *Breathing for Health with Biofeedback*. Montreal: Thought Technology. Peper, E., and Crane–Gockley, V. (1990). Towards Effortless Breathing. *Medical Psychotherapy*, 3, 135–140.

- Yasue,H., Nagao, M., Omote, S., et al. Coronary Arterial Spasm and Prinzmetal's Variant Form of Angina Induced by Hyperventilation and Tris–buffer Infusion. *Circulation*, 58,1, 78, pp56–62.

19. HEART RATE VARIABILITY AND EMOTIONS

1. Childre, D.L. (1994). *Freeze Frame, Fast Action Stress Relief.* Boulder Creek, California: Planetary Publications.
2. Levey, M., and Martin, P. (1989). Autonomic Control of Cardiac Function, in *Physiology and Pathophysiology of the Heart.*
3. McCraty, R., Atkinson, M., and Tiller, W. (1994). New Electrophysiological Correlates of Mental and Emotional States via Heart Rate Variability Studies, Proc Isseem Conference, Boulder, CO.
4. Lynch, J. (1990). *The Language of the Heart.* New York: Basic Books.

20. RESTLESS MIND CONTROL

1. McGuigan, F.J. (1981, 1992). *Calm Down, A Guide to Stress and Tension Control.* Dubuque, Iowa: Kendal Hunt Publishing Co.
2. Shapiro, F. (1989). Eye Movement Desensitization. A New Treatment for Post–traumatic Stress Disorder. *Journal of Behavioral Therapeutics and Experimental Therapeutics,* 20, 211.
3. Jacobsen, E. (1938). *Progressive Relaxation* (2nd ed.). Chicago: University of Chicago Press.
4. Wolpe, J. (1990). *The Practice of Behavior Therapy.* New York: Pergamon Press.
5. This is the model of yoga taught by Dean Ornish in his coronary artery reversal program and Jon Kabat Zinn in his University of Massachusetts Medical Center stress clinic. Feuerstein, G., Bodian, S. (1993). *Living Yoga, A Comprehensive Guide for Daily Living.* New York: Perigee Books. Lysebeth, A.V. (1968). *Yoga Self–taught.* New Delhi: IndiaVikas Publishing.
6. Bailey, Covert. (1994). *Smart Exercise, Burning Fat, Getting Fit.* New York: Houghton Mifflin Company.
7. Cooper, K. (1994). *Antioxidant Revolution.* Nashville, TN: Thomas Nelson Publishers. Cooper, K. (1982). *The Aerobics Program for Total Well Being.* New York: Bantam Books.
8. Benson, H. (1975). *The Relaxation Response.* New York: William Morrow and Company.

9. The inspiration for the open focus based tools comes from material presented by Les Fehmi and George Fritiz in annual AAPB Biofeedback workshops. Readers interested in attending these workshops, contact the Association for Applied Psychophysiology & Biofeedback, 10200 West 44th Avenue, Ste #304, Wheat Ridge, CO 80033.

10. Orwin. (1971). Respiratory Relief: A New and Rapid Method for the Treatment of Phobic States, *British J of Psychiatry*, 119–635.

21. INSOMNIA CONTROL

1. Morin, C. (1993). *Insomnia, Psychological Assessment and Management.* New York: Guilford Press.

2. Bootzin, R.R. (1972). Stimulus Control Treatment of Insomnia. *Proceedings of the American Psychological Assn.,* 7, 395–396.

3. Benson, H.B., and Stuart, E.M. (1992). *The Wellness Book.* New York: Birch Lane Press.

4. Wolpe, J. and Wolpe, D. (1988). *Life Without Fear.* Oakland, CA: New Harbinger Publications. Wolpe is the authority on systematic desensitization of emotions. Emotions cannot be changed by logic, but have to replaced by another emotion. This is a stimulus based change of behavior. The Bootzin method of insomnia control is a stimulus based therapy.

5. Suin, R.M. Anxiety Management and Training, A Behavior Therapy. Suin has the anxiety management model which directly works on the reactivity of the mind and body. This is a response based change of behavior. Progressive relaxation and eyeball desensitization are response based therapies.

22. BIOFEEDBACK–REACTIVITY MONITOR

• Schwartz, M.S. (1987). *Biofeedback, A Practitioner's Guide.* New York: The Guilford Press.

• Basmajian, J. (1989). *Biofeedback Principles and Practice for Cllinicians.* Baltimore, MD: Williams and Wilkins.

23. MEDITATION AND IMAGERY

• The concept of meditation given in this book is based on ancient traditions and new computer based alpha–theta training. Meditation started as early as 2,500 years ago with Buddhism, and is recorded in *Vedas* and *Upanishads* in the 2nd century B.C.

Bhagavadgita, the Hindu sacred book, has its sixth chapter dedicated to meditation. Patanjali's *Yogasutra* goes into details of eight parts of yoga and meditation. In the 6th century, Buddhism was carried to China and 600 years later to Japan. Meditation is known as *dhyan* in the Hindu system, which changed to *Chan* in China and *Zen* in Japan. Zen was introduced to America in the early 1950's. Transcendental Meditation (TM) was introduced in America by Maharishi Mahayogi in 1959. Herbert Benson made the TM meditation secular under the name *Relaxation Response*. Simonton showed the value of meditation in cancer healing and Ornish proved the value of meditation in reversing heart disease. Peniston used the alpha–theta brain wave training to heal addictions in late 1980's.

- Physiological proof of inducing altered states quickly by prolonging the expiration. Cappo, M. and Holmes, S. (1984). The Utility of Prolonged Respiratory Exhalation for Reducing Physiological and Psychological Arousal in Non–Threatening and Threatening Situations. *Journal of Psychosomatic Research*, 28(4), 265–273. Gerlad Epstein, an expert in imagery therapy, uses this method, and I had the privilege of learning it from him.

1. Benson, Herbert. (1975). *The Relaxation Response*. New York: William Morrow.

2. LeShan, Larry. (1975). *How to Meditate*. New York: Bantam Books.

3. Roshi, Suzuki. (1970). *Zen Mind, Beginner's Mind*. New York: Weatherhill.

4. Smith, J.C. (1986). *Meditation*. Champaign, IL: Research Press.

5. Goleman, D. (1988). *The Meditative Mind*. New York: Jeremy D Tarcher Perigee Books.

6. Csikszentmihali, Mihaly. (1990). *Flow, The Psychology of Optimal Experience*. New York: Harper Perennial.

7. Ornish, Dean. (1990). Can Lifestyle Changes Reverse Coronary Artery Disease? *Lancet*, 336,129–134.

8. Simonton, Carl, et al. (1978). *Getting Well Again*. New York: Bantum Books.

24. SELF–DISCLOSURE

- Pilsuk, M., and Parks, Susan. (1986). *The Healing Web, Social Networks and Human Survival*. Hanover, N.H.: University Press of New England. This book gives the role of social connections and group support for human health and well being.

- Berkman, L.F., and Syme S.L. (1979). Social Network, Host Resistance, and Mortality: A Nine Year Follow up Study of Alameda County Residents. *American Journal of Epidemiology*, 109, 186–204.
- House, J.S., Landis, K.R., Umberson, D. (1988). Social Relationships and Health. *Science*, 241, 540–545.
- Spiegel, D., Bloom, J.R., Kraemer, H.C., Gottheil, E. (1989). Effect of Psychosocial Treatment on Survival of Patients with Metastatic Breast Cancer. *Lancet*, 2, 888–891.
- Spiegel, D., Social Support: How Friends, Family and Groups Can Help, in Mind Body Medicine, ed. Goleman, D. (1993). New York: Consumer Report Book, 331–350.

25. REST AND ACTIVITY

1. Erickson, M. (1980). *The Collected Papers of Milton H Erickson on Hypnosis* (4 vols), R. Rossi, (Ed.) New York, Irvington. Rossi, E. (1991). *The 20 Minute Break, Using the New Science of Ultradian Rhythms.* Los Angeles: Jeremy P Tarcher, Inc. Rossi, E. (1993). *The Psychobiology of Mind–Body Healing, New Concepts of Therapeutic Hypnosis.* New York: W.W.Norton & Company.
2. Perry, S., and Dawson, J. (1988). *The Secrets Our Body Clocks Reveal.* New York: Ballantine Books.
3. Reingberg, A. and Smolensky, M.H. (1983). *Biological Rhythms and Medicine.* New York: Springer–Verlag.

26. MINDFUL EATING–EATING TO CONTROL STRESS

The cybernetic approach for stress-free eating is based on the eclectic synthesis of information from the following sources:

1. Ornish, D. (1993). *Eat More, Weigh Less.* New York: Harper Collins.
2. McDougall, John A. and Mary A. (1983). *The McDougall Plan.* Piscataway, NJ: New Century Publishers, Inc.
3. Katahan, M. (1989). *The T Factor Diet.* New York: Bantam Books.
4. David, Marc. (1991). *Nourishing Wisdom.* New York: Bell Tower.
5. Heller, R.F. (1991). *Carbohydrate Addict's Diet.* New York: Penguin Books.

6. Humbart, Santillo. (1993). *Intuitive Eating.* Prescott, AZ: Hohm Press.

7. Quillin, P. and N. (1994). *Beating Cancer with Nutrition.* Tulsa, OK: Nutrition Times Press.

8. Brodie, J. (1982). *Jean Brodie's Nutrition Book, A Lifetime Guide to Good Eating for Better Health and Weight Control.* New York: Bantam Books.

9. Wurtman, J. (1988). Carbohydrate Cravings: A Disorder of Food Intake and Mood. *Clinical Neuropharmacology,* 1, S139–145. Wurtman, J. & Danbrot, M. (1986). *Managing your mind and mood through foods.* New York: Rawson Publishing. Brzezinski, A., Wutman, J., Wurtman, R., Gleason, R. & Greenfield, D. (1990). d–Fenfluramine suppresses the increased calories and carbohydrate intake and improves the mood of women with premenstrual depression. *Obstetrics and Gynecology,* 76, 296–301. Moline, M. (1993). Pharmocologic strategies for managing premenstrual syndrome. *Clinical Pharmacology,* 12, 181–196.

10. Pritikin, R. (1990). *The New Pritikin Program.* New York: Simon and Schuster.

11. Physician's Committee for Responsible Medicine, Washington, D.C.

12. Kushi M. with Jack, A. (1983). *The Cancer Prevention Diet .* New York: St. Martin's Press.

13. Shils, M.E., Olson, J.A., Shike, M. (Eds.). (1994). *Modern Nutrition in Health and Disease, 8th ed., Vol. 2.* Philadelphia, PA: Lea & Febiger.

14. If you want to live to be 100: Leaf, A. (1973). "Every day is a gift when you are over 100," *National Geographic,* Jan. issue, p. 96.

15. Jenkins's research study of the grazing diet: Jenkins–David, J.A., Wolever, T., Vuksan, V., et al. (1989). Nibbling Vs Gorging: Metabolic advantages of Increased Meal Frequency. *New England Journal of Medicine,* 321:14, 929–34.

16. Butchko, H.H. & Kotsonis, F.N. (1991). Acceptable daily intake vs. actual intake: The Aspartame example. *Journal of the American College of Nutrition,* 10 (3), 258–266. Rolls, B.J. (1992). Effects of intense sweeteners on hunger, food intake, and body weight: A review. *American Jrnl of Clinical Nutrition,* 53, 872–878.

17. Apple, applesauce, and apple juice: G. Haber. (1977). Depletion and Disruption of Dietary Fiber, Effects on Satiety, plasma Glucose, and serum Insulin. *Lancet*, 2, 679.

18. Sheldon, M., Lashof, J.C., and Buffler, P.A. (1995). *Nutrition 1995, University of California, Berkeley Wellness Reports*. New York: Health Letter Associates Inc. This book covers the controversies of eating as they stand in 1995.

19. Fats of Life: The hazards of excess of dietary fats is an alarming yet a scientifically validated fact. The reader can find more details in the book, *McDougall Plan*, pages 76-90. Additional references are: Cullen, C. (1954), *Intravascular Aggregation and Adhisiveness of Blood Elements Associated with Alimentary Lipemia and Injection of Large Molecular Substances*. Circulation, 9:335. Friedman, M. (1964), *Serum Lipids and Conjunctival Circulation After Fat Injestion in Men exhibiting Type-A Behavior Pattern*. Circulation, 29:874. O'Brien, J. (1976), *Acute Platelet Changes after Large Meals of Saturated and Unsaturated Fats*. Lancet, 1:878. Olivia, P. (1981), *Pathophysiology of Acute Myocardial Infarction*. Ann Int Med. 94:236.

   Trans Fats: Willet, W.C. & Ascherio, A. (1994), *Trans Fatty Acids, Are the Effects Only Marginal?* Am J of Public Health 84:722-24.

27. HEART RESETTING TOOLS

The principles of self–directed change in behavior are largely based on Albert Bandura's behavior modification principles and Richard Lazarus's approach to coping with stress.

- Watson, D.L., Tharp, R.G. (1989). *Self–Directed Behavior*. Pacific Grove, CA: Brooks–Cole Publishing Company.

- Lazarus, R.S., Folkman, S. (1984). *Stress, Appraisal and Coping*. New York: Springer Publishing Company.

- The Human Function Curve is based on Peter Nixon's cardiac rehabilitation program. Nixon, P.G., Human Functions and the Heart, in *Changing Ideas in Health Care*, Ed. Seedhouse, D., & Cribb, A. (1989). New York: John Wiley and Sons, pp. 31–65. Nixon, P.G.F. (1986). Exhaustion: Cardiac Rehabilitation's Starting Point. *Physiology*, 72, 5.

- The vital exhaustion scale is based on the Myocardial Infarction Rotterdam Study as quoted by Appels, A., in the chapter "Loss of Control, Vital Exhaustion and Coronary Artery Disease" in the book by ed. Steptol, A. (1989). *Stress, Personal Control and Health*. New York: John Wiley and Sons.

- The Money Function Curve is based on Dominguez, J. and Robin, V. (1992). *Your Money or Your Life*. New York: Viking Penguin Books. The Money Style is based on Mellon, O., as quoted by Barret, K. (1994). I Love you, but Hate the Way You Spend Money. *Redbook*, Nov. issue, p. 56–60.

- The Energy Exchange Vectors are based on the life space planning concept taught by Barbara Peavy in Stress Management Education classes conducted by the American Association of Physiology and Biofeedback.

- The CyberZen™ concept of taking pictures of your own behavior is based on the parallel processing mode of the human mind.

- The Heartfelt Resonant Imaging (HRI) concept is based on the principle of Magnetic Resonant Imaging (MRI). In MRI, you send a radio wave question to the proton of the cell and the answer is a MRI image. In HRI, you send a thought wave question to your heart and get an answer in the form of love, appreciation, and caring. My radiologist friend, Ram Rao, helped to formulate this model.

- The energy quadrants of emotions are based on sports psychologist, James Loehr's Mental Toughness Training, Nightingale Conant Audio series, 7300 N. Lehigh Ave., Niles, Illinois, 60714.

28. DAILY LIFE WITH YOUR HEART IN MIND

- Cousins, Norman. (1979). *Anatomy of an Illness*. New York: Bantam Books.
- Ornstein, R., Sobel, D. (1989). *Healthy Pleasures*. New York: Addison Wesley Publishing, Inc.
- Hageseth, C. (1988). *A Laughing Place*. Fort Collins, CO: Berwick Publishing Co.
- Klein, A. (1989). *Healing Power of Humor*. Los Angeles: Jerermy P. Tarcher, Inc.

EPILOGUE
Eclectic Medicine for the 21st Century
- Dossey, L. (1993). *Healing Word*. New York: Harper-Collins.
- Byrd, R. C. (1988). *Positive Therapeutic Effects of Intercessory Prayer in a Coronary Care Unit Population*. Southern Medical Journal, 81:7,826-29.

APPENDIX
Pill Power for Heart Disease Reversal

- Enas Enas, cardiologist from Chicago,Illinois contributed for this chapter. General reference on this topic came from Rosenman, R.S., Frauenheim, W.A., Tangney, C.S. Dislipidemias and Secondary Prevention of Coronary Heart Disease, (1994). Disease a Month, Vol XL, 8:369–464.

Sense of Humor Revisited

- Cousins, Norman. (1979). *Anatomy of an Illness*. New York: W.W.Norton and Co.
- Hageseth, C., III, (1988). *A Laughing place, Art and Psychology of Positive Humor in Love and Adversity*. Fort Collins, CO: Berwick Publishing Company.
- Killinger, B. (1991). *Workaholics, The Respectable addicts*. New York: Simon and Schuster, p.130–131.
- Klien, A. (1989). *Healing Power of Humor*. Los Angeles: Jeremy P Tarcher Inc.
- Fry, William, F. Jr. (1986). Waleed A. Salameh, eds. *Handbook of Humor and Psychotherapy*. Sarasota, FL: Professional Resource Exchange.

Power of Crying

- Frey, W.H. (1980). Not so Idle Tears. *Psychology Today*, Jan. issue, 91–92.
- Fairfield, K.A. (1984). Good Cry, Tears, Scientists Find, Hold Clues to Everything from Eye Disorders to General Health. *Forbes*, 134, Nov. 5 issue, 232–34.
- Frey, W.H. (1985). *Crying: The Mystery of Tears*. New York: Harper Row.
- Ornstein and Sobel, The Healing Brain, 43–44.
- Poole, W. (1993). Institute of Noetic Sciences publication, The Heart of Healing. Atlanta, GA: Turner Publishing.

Conundrum and Paradox of Eating

- More information on this subject can be found in the U.C. Berkeley Wellness Letters, and Nutrition–1995 published by the University of California School of Public Health, Health Letter Associates, Inc., New York, 1995.
- The ABC's of Yoga. M.N. Rao, PhD, our staff yoga teacher, contributed to this chapter.

Additional Reading

KEY REFERENCES TO BROADEN YOUR HORIZONS

1. Ornish, D. (1990). **Dean Ornish's Program for Reversing Coronary Artery Disease.** New York: Random House.

2. Ornish, D. (1993). **Eat More Weigh Less.** New York: Harper Collins Publishers.

3. Eliot, R., and Breo, D.L. (1984). **Is it Worth Dying For?** How to Make Stress Work for You–Not Against You. NY: Bantam Books.

4. Eliot, R. (1994). **From Stress to Strength.** NY: Bantam Books.

5. Simonton, C.A., Mathew–Simonton, S., and Creighton, J.L. (1978). **Getting Well Again,** The bestselling classic about Simonton's revolutionary lifesaving self–awareness techniques. New York: Bantum Books.

6. Siegel, Bernie S. (1990). **Peace, Love and Healing,** Body–Mind Communication and The Path to Self–Healing. New York: Harper Perennial.

7. Cooper, Kenneth H. (1994). **Antioxidant Revolution.** Nashville, TN: Thomas Nelson Publishers.

8. Williams, Redford and Williams, Virginia. (1993). **Anger Kills,** Seventeen Strategies for Controlling the Hostility that can Harm Your Health. New York: Harper Perennial.

9. Benson, Herbert with Klipper, M.Z. (1976). **The Relaxation Response.** New York: Avon Books.

10. McDougall, John E. and Mary A. (1983). **The McDougall Plan.**, New Century Publishing, Piscataway, NJ.

11. Childre, Doc Lew. (1994). **Freeze Frame,** Fast Action Stress Relief, A Scientific Proven Technique. Boulder Creek, CA: Planetary Press.

12. Rossi, Ernest L. (1991). **The 20 Minute Break.** Reduce Stress, Maximize Performance, Improve Health and Emotional Well Being Using the New Science of Ultradian Rhythms. Los Angeles: Jeremy P. Tarcher, Inc.

13. Jon Kabat–Zinn. (1990). **Full Catastrophe Living,** Using the Wisdom of Your Body and Mind to Face Stress, Pain, and Illness. New York: Delacorte Press.

Index

Index

A

Actions, in iceberg model 151
Activity/rest cycle 303
Addiction cycle **336**, 336–339
Addictions
    food 329
    stress **336**
Ader, Robert 130
Age, as a risk factor 82–83
Aggression 138, 167
Alkaline blood 213–214
Alpha brain waves 257
Altruism, biology of 192
Altruistic egotism 41–45, 193
Anger
    biological cost of 175
    as cause for heart attacks 95–96, 138, **182**, 182–183
    chemical effects of 169
    costs of 419–420
    expression of 168, 170–171
    in health professionals 179–181
    in iceberg model 167
    intrapersonal cost 176
    learning 174
    in legal professionals 181
    origins of 172–174
    replacing with caring love 179
    social cost of 179
    solutions for 183–185
    as yang 114
Angina 22, 75, 376
Antioxidants
    cancer and 93
    food sources of 67, 70–71
    recommended daily intake 72
    references 414
    theory of 62, 66
Arrhythmia. *See* Cardiac arrhythmia

Arteriosclerosis 86
Ascorbic acid. *See* Vitamin C
Atherosclerosis 23, 88
Athletic choking 53

B

Beta brain waves 257
Beta carotene. *See* Vitamin A
Biofeedback
    described 219, 249
    explained 252–254
    modalities 249–254
    references 423
Body-mind medicine 33
Bohr effect 213–214
Bootzin technique 245
Brain
    brain waves **257**
    breathing and 215
    dominance, left or right 290
    evolution of 162–163
    heart and 205–207
    yin and yang functions 112
Brain wave feedback (EEG) 251
Breathing.
    See also Hyperventilation
    anxiety and 213
    bad habits 217
    clearing fatigue 306
    described 212
    diaphramatic 216–217
    heart and 213, 421–422
    mindful 352
    stress and 212–213
    as stress indicator 338
    sudden cardiac death and 215–216
Brown, Michael 86

C

D

E

Internal toxins 65
Intimacy 291
Irritable gut 44
Isolation 137, 141, 178

J

James-Lange theory 156
Job strain 141

K

Kaplan, cancer research 194
Kindling 126–127

L

LDL cholestorol 85–87
Learned altruism 367–368
Learned helplessness
    biology of 53–54
    described 50–51, **56**
    examples of 52–54, 291
    in heart attacks **145**
    references 413
    research in 51–52
Learned optimism
    basic requirements 58–60
    described **58**, 144
    examples of 291
    in heart attacks **145**
    references 413–414
Learned pessimism 291
Life patterns
    forces that sink the ship 39
    measuring 334, 342
    references 408
    sedentary lifestyle 88, 137
Limbic system 106
Lipoprotein (a), as a risk factor 86
Liquid media
    heart rate variability and 224
    imagery and 275
    messenger chemicals 131, 151

restless mind and 229
    in stress response 107
    variances in 189, 206
Locus ceruleus 106
Love.
    See also Caring love
    expression of 168–169
    as yin 114

M

Magnesium 209, 214
Materialistic centering 157
McClelland, David 190
Measuring tools 17–18, 146, 345
Meat 326
Medications
    pipes of your body 376–378
    pumps of your body 375–376
Meditation 357
    21 day routine 271–277
    defined 238, 256, 257
    exercises 395–397
    five minute 267–270, 358–359
    how to meditate 259–261
    imagery and 45
    instructions for 262–264, **265**
    models 411
    one minute 266, 357
    purpose for 257–258
    references 423–424
    time for 270–271
    ultradian healing and 303
    validations for 256
Meditative state 257
Membrane wars 63–64
Messenger chemicals 130–131
Metabolic changes 214
Mind-body 418
    in cancer 33
    caring touch, chemistry 281–282
    communications 131–135
    healing 33, 135
    imagery 132–133
    medicine 34
    network, elements of 131

T

Temperature feedback 250
Temporomandibular disorders 45
Test anxiety 53
Theta brain waves 257
Thoracic breathing 217
Thoughts
    caring love and 195
    defined 280
    gender differences 290
    in iceberg model 151
TMJ. *See* Temporomandibular
    disorders
Tomkin's model of nerve traffic 161
Toxins, as a cancer risk factor 93
Type A personality 170
Type C personality 170, 172

U

Ultradian healing response 303
Ultradian rhythm 236, 303

V

Validation 294–295
Vegetables 318
Vertical intimacy 281
Vibrational waves 205, 206–207, 229
Vibrational whisper 107, 131, 275
Vital exhaustion 349–350
Vitamin A 67, 70, 414
Vitamin C 67, 70, 414
Vitamin E 67, 70

W

Walking 308–310
Whirlpool effect 254
Williams, Redford 83

Y

Yin and yang
    described 110, **111**
    functions 113
    heart rate variability and 225
    heartfelt feelings and 159
    imbalance 84
    mindfelt feelings and 159
    references 417
Yoga 233–235, 392–393, **394**

General Information

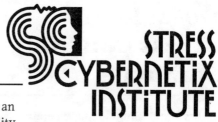

STRESS CYBERNETIX INSTITUTE

The *Stress Cybernetix Institute* is an educational and treatment facility located at Concord, in the San Francisco Bay Area.

MISSION:

Do-able Stress Control for the 21st Century. The word *do-able* means it is affordable in time and money. The methods take advantage of the concurrent parallel processing of the human brain. This allows you to implement the tools despite the time pressure of the 21st century information age.

OBJECTIVE:

Training people to defocus from the judgmental, head centered, achievement mode of living to non-judgmental, heart centered, affiliative mode of living at least 50% of waking hours.

METHODS:

Anger control by biologically learned altruism, control of learned helplessness by changing physiological reactivity. Biofeedback is used to demonstrate the efficacy of methods. Life-style modification by do-able tools of meditation and imagery, mindful eating of starch based, low fat food, self-disclosure to boost immune system, and rest and activity to match the biological rhythms.

MEDIA:

Two major books, *"Do-able Stress Control for the 21st Century"* and *"How to Reverse and Prevent Heart Disease and Cancer"* and two videos, *"Uprooting Anger"* and *"Meditation Prescription"*, have been published. Audios, CD-ROM, and interactive learning media are at various levels of preparation. Dr. Bhat has appeared on Radio and Television shows as an invited guest. Dr. Bhat has given hundreds of seminars, and workshops worldwide. He is also a popular speaker for - doctor's lunch presentations in the hospitals - and for rotary clubs and large corporations.

PEOPLE:

Naras Bhat, MD, FACP is the founder and medical director of the Stress Cybernetix Institute. Dr. Bhat is an Internal Medicine and Immunology specialist who has done research on psycho-neuro-immunology methods for mind-body healing. He is assisted by **Thomas Browne Jr., PhD(C)**, a certified neurotherapy specialist. Dr. Browne has extensive training on changing physiological reactivity using biofeedback and brain wave monitoring.

Stress Cybernetix Institute
2182 East Street, Concord, California, 94520. Phone: 510/685-4224.

Do-able Stress Control Seminars

Dr. Naras Bhat conducts seminars worldwide to train the audience on "Do-able Stress Control for the 21st Century." The seminar teaches you how to take advantage of the parallel processing mode of the human mind and to control stress arousal in spite of the time pressure.

SEMINAR OUTLINE:

1. *Cybernetics Model of Stress:* How the Eastern disciplines of Yoga, Qui Gong, Zen, Kaizen, and Suzuki system integrate with the Western science of biochemistry, behavioral science, neurolinguistic programming (NLP) and the cybernetics of control theory and mind–body self-regulation.

2. *Cyber-Physiology:* How to tap into your body's own intelligence system. How to differentiate between normal and abnormal stress arousal. The chemical basis of stress and workaholism and why stress is an addiction.

3. *Restless Mind Control:* How to take a picture of your own mind. How to use muscle-to-mind and mind-to-muscle tools to control the restless mind.

4. *Insomnia Control:* How to intercept insomnia and drift into sleep as a seamless continuum of proactive chemical change in mind–body.

5. *Meditation and Imagery:* How to meditate anytime, anywhere, in five minutes, in one minute and even in one moment.

6. *Mindful Eating* to balance insulin and mood swings.

7. *Healing and Balance:* How to heal afflictions such as coronary artery disease, cancer, irritable bowels, headaches, fatigue, anxiety and stress disorders, anger control, reactivity control, self-disclosure, rest and activity,

8. *Maximal Self:* How to achieve your maximal self by biologically integrating the achievements and affiliations in life.

Please contact: *Stress Cybernetix Institute,* 2182 East Street, Concord, California, 94520. Phone: 510/685–4224.

Uprooting Anger Video

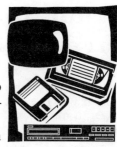

Anger is the #1 killer in the world. This video will train you to uproot the deadly anger permanently.

Naras Bhat, MD, a world renowned expert on "Do–able Stress Control for the 21st Century" brings you the breakthrough research of new biology of anger and caring love as a practical tool in daily life.

CONTENTS:

1. **What is Anger?** What is the chemistry of anger? Type A and Type C behavior. Where anger comes from? Nurture of anger as a conditioned reflex and how to undo it. How anger kills you at the atomic, cellular, body organ and social level.

2. **New Biology of Altruism and Caring Love** (Mother Teresa Effect). How the immune system and rhythms of heart beat change with endorphins of caring love.

3. **The Tool (Heartfelt Resonant Imaging, HRI):** New scientific discovery to replace the anger chemistry with endorphins instantly and use this skill rest of your life.

INNOVATIVE APPROACH:

The tool given in this video is based on the most crucial discovery of 20th century – the skyrocketing anger in our life is a biological reflex, and it can be unlearned within a week. This learning can be measured as a change in blood chemicals, and a change of heart rate pattern.

WHAT YOU WILL LEARN:

- How to biologically replace anger with caring love and altruism and do it with control and choice all day long.
- How to reactivate the suppressed sense of humor.
- How to live with the heart in mind.
- How to heal and thrive in the stressful information age.

Meditation Prescription Video

Meditation is not a mystic ritual, but a doctor prescribed tool. *The skill of meditation can be learned like learning to ride a bicycle.*

Naras Bhat, MD, a world renowned expert on "Do–able Stress Control for the 21st Century" brings you the breakthrough research of meditation as a therapeutic tool in the doctor's office.

CONTENTS:

1. *What is meditation?* Meditation, an alpha–theta state, is an interface between the conscious mind and the subconscious mind. Anybody can learn to enter and exit this state by choice.

2. *Why meditate?* For stress control, healing afflictions and maximal self by personal growth and creativity.

3. *Why people fail to meditate?* The problems of a lack of time, inability to concentrate, and a restless mind are solved by proven methods given in this video.

3. *How to meditate?* The easy steps to meditate are: 3 P's (Place, Posture and Passive Attitude), and 3 Rs of Relax muscles, Respiration watch and Repeat mantra.

INNOVATIVE APPROACH:

The tool given in this video is based on the scientific discovery that meditation is a biological state rather than a ritual. The crucial task in meditation is how to tap into the newly described mind–body network called Psycho–neuro–immunology.

WHAT YOU WILL LEARN:

- **How to meditate** anywhere and anytime, in five minutes, in one minute or even in a moment.
- **How to overcome restless mind** and distractions during meditation.
- **How to** use meditative state to **rewrite the blueprint of your mind** and heal.
- **How to forgive, control anger,** retreat into mind–set sanctuary, use inner guide for problem solving, and creative visualization for peak performance.
- How to incorporate **meditation as a way of life** despite time pressure of modern life.

Doctor's Doctor Program

Naras Bhat, MD has trained thousands of physicians, psychologists, nurses and health professionals on how to implement *"physician heal thyself"* principle and reverse the burn-out process called compassion fatigue. The doctor's doctor program is available in three formats:

WEEKEND RETREATS:

The participants come to our Stress Cybernetix Institute in Concord, California for two days of intensive training. Each person will have hands on experience in our cybernetics laboratory with computer feedback. The heart rate variability monitoring confirms that the anger control is learned at a biological level.

Special emphasis is given to train health care professionals on how to use the clinical contact with the client to enter into an endorphin based affiliative state and switch from catecholamine based frustrations and anger by our unique "duck-rabbit flip-flop method".

WORKSHOPS:

One day and half a day workshops which covers our "Do-able Stress Control for the 21st Century" topics. Additionally the seminar focuses on the high incidence of coronary artery disease, addictions, insomnia, relationship problems, professional burn out, and stress disorders in health care professionals.

Health professionals are trained in handling their own stress and this in turn trains them to train their clients.

APPRENTICESHIPS:

We are developing new programs to train health care practitioners to implement our cybernetic methods in their office using our learning resources and multimedia teaching aids.

Do-able Stress Control Newsletter

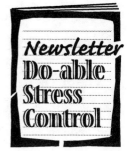

We live in an era of paradigm shift. The way we learn depends on what media is dominant in contemporary life. The world of virtual reality is real now with interactive television, CD–ROM, e–mail, Internet/World Wide Web and so on.

Thousands of our audience are using the cyberspace media to spread the message of our cybernetics research. You can keep in touch with us by receiving our regular newsletter on *"Do–able Stress Control."*

The newsletter covers the schedules of our seminars, workshops, new publications and learning resources. New advancements and research findings in stress control, healing various afflictions and achieving creativity and maximal self are covered in each issue.

Our research department is getting feedback from our worldwide audience to measure, monitor and modify do–able stress control for the 21st century.

FREE NEWSLETTERS:

You can be a part of this network and receive **FREE INTRODUCTORY NEWSLETTERS** by sending us the following information:

Your name, address, city, zip code,
phone & fax numbers and e–mail address
to the following address:

Stress Cybernetix Institute
Att: Newsletter Department
2182 East Street
Concord, California, 94520
Phone: 510–685–4224
Fax: 510–685–6997
E–mail: SAVAHEART@AOL.COM
24 Hour Orderline: 1–800–887–HART

SAV-A-HEART Program

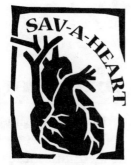

SAV-A-HEART is an educational and training program conducted at Concord, California. Sav-a-Heart by *Seva* or biologically retrained altruism. *Seva in Sanskrit means "you are also included in my agenda."*

OBJECTIVE:

Anger control by learned altruism using the innovative tool called Heartfelt Resonant Imaging. This resets the heart from judgmental head centered living to non-judgmental heart centered living. Escape from learned helplessness by controlling physiological reactivity of stress arousal. This resets the immune system from a whirlpool effect of give up – given up state.

METHOD:

There are two pathways by which Sav-a-Heart is achieved.

1. *Supportive Expressive Group Therapy:* Each week, **Dr. Naras Bhat** and **Dr. Thomas Browne**, conduct a two hour session at Mt. Diablo Medical Center, Concord, in the San Francisco Bay area. *The admission is free for these classes.* The group session involves a review of mind-body physiology, and interactive learning to control anger and stress. Tools to measure, monitor, and modify anger and stress arousal are learned in a group setting. The major tools include: anger control, meditation and imagery, self-disclosure, mindful eating, restless mind control and rest and activity.

2. *Individual Sessions:* Each person is trained on a one to one basis using computer feedback of heart rate variability and other physiological monitors such as hand temperature, emotional sweating, respiration, muscle tension and brain wave feedback. These individual sessions awaken the suppressed immune system by removing the person from the whirlpool effect of learned helplessness.

HOW TO PARTICIPATE:

We welcome the general public to attend our weekly night group sessions as our guest. Please call or write to the Stress Cybernetix Institute for further information. We are in the process of making video recordings of major sessions so that people who cannot personally attend these classes can benefit. Please contact: *Stress Cybernetix Institute,* 2182 East Street, Concord, California, 94520. Phone: 510/685-4224.

Order Form

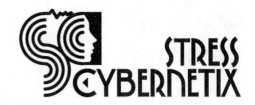

STRESS CYBERNETIX

1. **Uprooting Anger**
   Video $ 29.95 x ___ =

2. **Meditation Prescription**
   Video $29.95 x ___ =

3. **How to Reverse and Prevent**
   Heart Disease & Cancer Book $19.95 x ___ =

4. **Do-able Stress Control**
   Newsletter   FREE   = $ 0.00

                                Sub-total : _____

         California State Sales Tax (8.25%) : _____

              Shipping/Handling per Order : $ 5.00

                              TOTAL : _____

Name: _____

Street Address: _____

City: _____

State: _____ *Zip* _____

Phone: _____

Please make out check   ***Stress Cybernetix Institute***
in the name of   Att: Order Department
STRESS CYBERNETIX   2182 East Street
and mail it to: Concord, California, 94520
                                     Phone: 510–685–4224

24 HOUR ORDERLINE: 1-800-887-HART

Order Form   **Stress Cybernetix Institute**